The Athlete's Guide to
Sports
Supplements

Kimberly Mueller
Josh Hingst

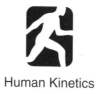

Human Kinetics

Library of Congress Cataloging-in-Publication Data

Mueller, Kimberly, 1976-
  The athlete's guide to sports supplements / Kimberly Mueller, Josh Hingst.
    pages cm
  Includes bibliographical references.
  1. Athletes--Nutrition. 2. Athletes--Health and hygiene. 3. Dietary supplements. I. Title.
  TX361.A8M83 2013
  613.2'024796--dc23

                                              2012049778

  ISBN-10: 0-7360-9369-9 (print)
  ISBN-13: 978-0-7360-9369-9 (print)

This publication is written and published to provide accurate and authoritative information relevant to the subject matter presented. It is published and sold with the understanding that the author and publisher are not engaged in rendering legal, medical, or other professional services by reason of their authorship or publication of this work. If medical or other expert assistance is required, the services of a competent professional person should be sought.

The web addresses cited in this text were current as of March 2013, unless otherwise noted.

Acquisitions Editor: Tom Heine; **Developmental Editor:** Anne Cole; **Assistant Editors:** Claire Marty and Tyler Wolpert; **Copyeditor:** Ann Prisland; **Permissions Manager:** Martha Gullo; **Graphic Designer:** Nancy Rasmus; **Graphic Artist:** Kim McFarland; **Cover Designer:** Keith Blomberg; **Photograph (cover):** Jason Allen; **Photo Production Manager:** Jason Allen; **Printer:** Versa Press

Human Kinetics books are available at special discounts for bulk purchase. Special editions or book excerpts can also be created to specification. For details, contact the Special Sales Manager at Human Kinetics.

Printed in the United States of America   10 9 8 7 6 5 4 3 2 1

The paper in this book is certified under a sustainable forestry program.

Human Kinetics
Website: www.HumanKinetics.com

United States: Human Kinetics
P.O. Box 5076
Champaign, IL 61825-5076
800-747-4457
e-mail: humank@hkusa.com

Canada: Human Kinetics
475 Devonshire Road Unit 100
Windsor, ON N8Y 2L5
800-465-7301 (in Canada only)
e-mail: info@hkcanada.com

Europe: Human Kinetics
107 Bradford Road
Stanningley
Leeds LS28 6AT, United Kingdom
+44 (0) 113 255 5665
e-mail: hk@hkeurope.com

Australia: Human Kinetics
57A Price Avenue
Lower Mitcham, South Australia 5062
08 8372 0999
e-mail: info@hkaustralia.com

New Zealand: Human Kinetics
P.O. Box 80
Torrens Park, South Australia 5062
0800 222 062
e-mail: info@hknewzealand.com

E5146

The Athlete's Guide to
Sports
Supplements

CONTENTS

SUPPLEMENT FINDER

■ Beneficial
□ Possibly beneficial

Supplement	Fuel usage	Aerobic capacity	Anaerobic endurance	Strength, power, and hypertrophy	Strength and power endurance	Psychological	Hydration	Recovery	Joint support	Immunity	Antioxidant	Body composition	Notes
Acetylcysteine		□			□			□					
Arginine			□	□	□								
Astragalus										□			
Avocado soybean unsaponifiables									□				
Beetroot		■	■										
Beta-alanine			■		□								
Beta glucan								■		■			
Boron								■	■				More research needed; appears beneficial only in deficient states
Boswellia serrata								□	□				
Branched-chain amino acids (BCAAs)				■				■					
Caffeine	■			■	■	■		■				□	
Calcium												□	
Capsicum								■	■		■		
Carbohydrate	■			■	■	■		■					
Casein				■				■					
Cat's claw									□				
Chitosan												□	

The supplements listed here include only those that have demonstrated health- and performance-oriented benefits through well-controlled and replicated scientific research. Chapter 3 includes additional supplements that either require further research or don't have demonstrated benefits.

>continued

Supplement	Fuel usage	Aerobic capacity	Anaerobic endurance	Strength, power, and hypertrophy	Strength and power endurance	Psychological	Hydration	Recovery	Joint support	Immunity	Antioxidant	Body composition	Notes
Choline		☐			☐								Only beneficial for longer duration endurance exercise or short-burst, high-intensity efforts lasting longer than 2 hours
Chondroitin									☐				
Cinnamon								☐			■	☐	
Citrulline malate	☐				☐			☐					
Cocoa		☐								☐	■		
Coconut								☐		☐		☐	
Coenzyme Q10								☐			■		
Colostrum				☐				☐		☐			
Cordyceps sinensis		☐											
Creatine				■	■			■					
Curcumin								☐		☐	■		
Devil's claw									☐				
Ecdysteroids				■				☐					
Egg protein				■				■					
Elderberry										☐			
Fenugreek	☐							☐		☐			
Fiber												■	
5-HTP								☐					
Folic acid		☐											
Garlic								☐		■	■		
Ginger								☐	☐	■	■		
Ginseng		☐				☐		☐					
Glucosamine									☐				
Glutamine	☐							☐		☐			
Grape seed								☐	☐	☐			

Supplement	Fuel usage	Aerobic capacity	Anaerobic endurance	Strength, power, and hypertrophy	Strength and power endurance	Psychological	Hydration	Recovery	Joint support	Immunity	Antioxidant	Body composition	Notes
HMB								□					
Hydroxycitric acid												□	
Iron		■						■		■			
Isomaltulose	■							■					
Leucine				■				■					Beneficial only when complete protein intake is inadequate
Magnesium	■	■	■		■				■				Beneficial for deficient populations only
Medium-chain triglycerides (MCTs)												■	
Melatonin								□					Possibly beneficial but only for jet lag
MSM									□				
Omega-3 fatty acids	□	□				□		□	□	□		□	
Phosphate salts	■	■	■		■			■					Beneficial for high-intensity endurance activity (e.g., time trials)
Phosphatidyl-serine		□		□					□				
Piperine												□	
Potassium	■						■		■				Replacement via sport drink beneficial for prolonged activity
Probiotics										■			
Pycnogenol		□						□	□				
Quercetin		□						□		□	■		
Resveratrol	□	□						□		□	■	□	
Rhodiola rosea	□					□		□		□			

>*continued*

Supplement Finder >continued

Supplement	Fuel usage	Aerobic capacity	Anaerobic endurance	Strength, power, and hypertrophy	Strength and power endurance	Psychological	Hydration	Recovery	Joint support	Immunity	Antioxidant	Body composition	Notes
S-adenosyl methionine (SAMe)								□	□				
Salt							■						
Sea buckthorn		□						□					
Selenium					□			□		□			
Sodium bicarbonate and sodium citrate	■		■		■								Beneficial primarily for female athletes engaged in short, high-intensity activities
Soy protein				■				■			■		
Superoxide dismutase								□			■		
Synephrine												□	
Tart cherry								■			■		
Thiamine	□				□	□							
Tyrosine		□			□								Only beneficial in warm environments
Undenatured type II collagen									□				
Vitamin C					□			□	□	□	■		Possibly beneficial for ultra-athletes
Vitamin D				■				■				■	
Vitamin E								□			■		Possibly beneficial for ultra-athletes
Whey protein				■				■					
Willow bark									□				
Withania somnifera								□		□			
Zinc		■						■		■			Beneficial for deficient athletes; possibly beneficial in nondeficient population

PREFACE

> Doctors and scientists said that breaking the four-minute mile was impossible, that one would die in the attempt. Thus, when I got up from the track after collapsing at the finish line, I figured I was dead.
>
> Roger Bannister (after becoming the first person to break the 4-minute mile in 1952)

Each year, there are a handful of athletes who defy odds and break performance barriers once believed to be impossible. In 2010 professional baseball player Ichiro Suzuki became the first major league baseball player to string together 10 consecutive seasons of 200+ hits. In the same year, Tony Gonzalez of the Atlanta Falcons became the first tight end in National Football League history to record 1,000 career receptions and 12,000 career receiving yards. In 2011 Patrick Makau of Kenya set the world record for the marathon by running a blazing 2:03:38 in Berlin, leaving many to wonder if a sub-2-hour marathon is indeed realistic. In 2012 several athletes performed at record-breaking levels during the Summer Olympics in London.

The science of training athletes has come a long way in the last 100 years. Top-level sport scientists are developing new methods of training, strategies for nutrition and supplement use, recovery protocols, and psychological tools to assist athletes in optimizing their abilities. This is in large part why performance milestones continue to be broken. This book is designed to shed light on the truths behind the most popular performance-focused nutritional supplements.

Chapter 1 focuses on what you, the athlete, coach, or health professional should know about supplements. We address the history of the sports supplement industry and provide you with insight into the manufacturing practices and regulation of sports supplements. We give you the tools to assess, evaluate, and purchase supplements to fit your needs and the needs of your athletes. Common questions are addressed, especially concerning the efficacy of supplement use in sports.

Chapter 2 explores the performance keys that are often targeted by supplement industry marketing, including claims that these key performance indicators can be enhanced through supplementation with various ingredients. This chapter will give you a better understanding of how supplements might be beneficial, and which areas of performance they will affect. In general, the cardiovascular, muscle, and psychological systems may all be influenced through specific nutritional supplements. To specifically address how a particular supplement may be ergogenic (i.e., enhance physical performance), each system is examined closely. For example, the section on the cardiovascular system addresses aerobic capacity, anaerobic endurance, and fuel usage. The section on muscle performance looks at muscle size and composition, neurological function, strength and power production, and resistance to fatigue. The section on psychological aspects notes several nutrients that may affect cognitive performance. There are also several outside variables that have a profound impact on performance in sport, including hydration status, overall recovery of body systems, and an athlete's body composition. Most athletes will tailor their training to focus on one or several of these performance factors. For example, a football player who is unable to hold his position will work on building muscle size and composition during the off-season while a marathon runner will increase weekly distance run as a means of boosting aerobic capacity. In addition to training, athletes will often seek nutritional guidance from a sports dietitian to learn about whole foods and ergogenic supplements that may help give them a legal performance edge on their competition.

Chapter 3 provides an alphabetical guide to the most popular performance-focused supplements marketed today. For each supplement, you'll find a description of the ingredient along with common supplement names and food sources, a discussion of the latest scientific research practical applications for dosing, recommended performance daily intake (if applicable), deficiency and toxicity symptoms (if applicable), and drug or supplement interactions (if applicable). Some supplement descriptions include information about additional performance benefits as a separate section; these other uses are not detailed in the research discussion. As you flip through the supplement guide, you'll see that each performance variable is assigned a symbol that will serve as a quick reference tool. If a supplement has been proven to be beneficial for a particular performance variable, the supplement entry will be marked with the corresponding black symbol; if the research shows that a supplement is possibly beneficial, the entry will be marked with a gray version of the corresponding symbol. You can use the supplement finder (located at the beginning of the book) to quickly identify supplements that have demonstrated benefits based on these performance variables.

Our final chapter explores the unique nutritional challenges athletic populations have to overcome in order to perform at peak and details the supplements that may help them excel. This chapter also includes nutritional recommendations for the following categories of athletes:

- Master's-level athletes
- Child and adolescent athletes
- Female athletes
- Injured athletes
- Athletes with diabetes
- Athletes with food allergies or intolerance
- Vegetarian athletes
- Athletes competing in heat or cold
- Athletes competing at altitude

Finally, a complete list of references and resources can be found at www.humankinetics.com/products/all-products/Athletes-Guide-to-Sports-Supplements-The.

ACKNOWLEDGMENTS

When esteemed publisher Human Kinetics first approached me about taking on this project a few years ago, my athlete mentality of "go after it" immediately came to the fore, and I enthusiastically took on the monumental challenge, one that had been a prominent part of my career bucket list since becoming a registered dietitian over 10 years ago. I will forever be grateful for this wonderful opportunity to help dispel the myths and discuss the truths that exist in the nutrition field and dietary supplement industry and ultimately create an important reference tool for all involved in the training and development of athletes.

Much like in a sport where a team of people, including coaches, teammates, parents, trainers, doctors, dietitians, and others all aid in the success of an athlete, the completion of this project could have not been accomplished without the invaluable support of several key players over the years. My undergraduate and graduate studies and athletic career at both Illinois State University and Florida State University certainly laid the groundwork for my career passion as a sports dietitian. In particular, research collaboration with professors Dr. Robert Cullen and Dr. Dale Brown as well as work on the nutrition and dietary supplement front with former team physician Dr. Bryan Barootes of Illinois State University really opened my eyes to the nutritional issues in sports and fostered my determination to help fellow athletes successfully and safely achieve peak performance. I am thankful for these career-paving experiences and the breakthrough research revelations and work fellow sport science colleagues continue to do. Their efforts no doubt have contributed to some of the mind-blowing performances that have made history in recent years. Most importantly, though, I'd like to extend a huge amount of gratitude to my brilliant colleague and coauthor, Josh Hingst, for the thousands of hours he has put into our project and to the team of editors and staff at Human Kinetics who have helped make this dream a reality for the two of us.

Finally, I'd like to thank my parents, Charles and Nancy Mueller, family, and friends for the unparalleled amount of support, love, and encouragement to *carpe diem* that they have provided as I have chased after my professional and athletic dreams.

—**Kimberly Mueller**

Helen Keller said, "Alone we can do so little; together we can do so much." I am grateful for the opportunity to have had an important role in the completion of this book and believe it will be a powerful reference for many. There are many people to thank and acknowledge for their work and insight. First, I thank the scientific community of professors and researchers who diligently work to discover the benefits of the many supplements addressed in this book. It is their dedication to ethical, unbiased science that enables us to find true understanding. Particularly, I'd like to thank the many professors of Florida State University and the University of Nebraska who invested their time and effort in me as a graduate and doctoral student, especially Dr. Wanda Koszewski from the University of Nebraska. Thank you to Dr. Jeff Stout, University of Central Florida, for his insightful review of the book, as well as to Dave Ellis and Lori Bestervelt. I'd like to thank Human Kinetics for the opportunity to coauthor this book and for the diligent work of their editors and staff. Thank you to my parents, Glenda and David Hingst, for their encouragement and support in all my professional endeavors. Finally, I acknowledge God, His son and my savior Jesus Christ, who shows His love for us in that while we are still sinners, Christ died for us.

—Josh Hingst

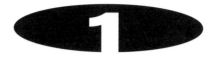

Understanding Supplements

The strongest thing I put into my body is steak and eggs. I just eat. I'm not a supplement guy. Steroids are not even a thought.

Jim Thome, professional baseball player

Jim Thome, a designated hitter and first baseman for the Minnesota Twins, hits a homerun with his quote. Balanced whole food nutrition is indeed the most important factor in fueling athletic performance. However, when every second faster, every ounce stronger counts, an athlete will often do everything possible to gain that competitive edge, from using specialized gear to the latest in sport nutrition. Combine this innate drive to succeed in sport with an interest in filling nutritional gaps and maintaining overall health and wellness, and you have serious fuel for the dietary supplement industry, making it one of the fastest-growing markets worldwide with an estimated $25 billion in yearly sales in the United States alone.

A dietary supplement, officially defined in the Dietary Supplement Health and Education Act of 1994, is a pill, capsule, tablet, powder, or liquid intended to supplement the whole food diet by providing any combination of the following nutritional ingredients: vitamins; minerals; herbs or other botanicals (excluding tobacco); amino acids; a dietary substance used to increase total dietary intake (such as carbohydrate and protein); and a concentrate, metabolite, constituent, or extract. Many of the sport nutritional supplements currently used by athletes are advertised as increasing testosterone levels in the body, similar to anabolic steroids (AAS), thereby enhancing the athlete's ability to build lean body mass. Other nutritional supplements are marketed as improving energy levels during workouts or competition or speeding recovery postworkout. There are supplements whose labels claim they facilitate body fat and weight loss, which is especially alluring to athletes competing in sports such as dance and gymnastics, where physique is spotlighted. Unlike steroids, however, which are only available in the United States with a doctor's prescription thanks to the list of known side effects, nutritional supplements can be purchased over the counter with relatively scant regulation on claims being made and safety for the consumer. Even so, data have indicated that some 70%-90% of collegiate and Olympic-level athletes supplement with at least one ingredient, hoping that the potential benefits of taking these substances outweigh any associated risks (Froiland et al., 2004; Burns et al., 2004).

With the growing popularity and use of nutritional supplements has come an alarming increase in the number of athletes, both amateur and professional, testing positive for banned substances, further raising concern from ethical and safety standpoints. In the late 1990s and early 2000s, Victor Conte and Bay Area Laboratory Co-Operative (BALCO) worked with chemists to develop tetrahydrogestrinone (the Clear), a formerly undetectable performance-enhancing steroid that was distributed to several high-profile sport stars in the form of so-called nutritional supplements. Agents of the Internal Revenue Service, Food and Drug Administration (FDA), San Mateo Narcotics Task Force, and United States Anti-Doping Association (USADA) eventually brought BALCO to justice, but the outcome left several athletes with tarnished images.

Perhaps in his quotation, Thome intended to share some of his frustration about the revelations from BALCO and later the 2007 Mitchell Report, which accused 89 fellow Major League Baseball players of using anabolic steroids, human growth hormone (HGH), or other performance-enhancing substances to drive their professional careers to another level, often a record-breaking level. From October 2000 until November 2001, the International Olympic Committee investigated 634 nonhormonal nutritional supplements such as vitamins, minerals, proteins, and creatine obtained from 215 suppliers; the investigation found 15% to be contaminated with banned substances, mainly steroidal substances or prohormones, that were not listed on the product labels and that would have caused an athlete using the supplement to test positive during a doping test (Geyer et al., 2004). The news hasn't improved much in recent years. An investigation of over 60 dietary supplements, for example, discovered 12.5% contained banned substances not declared on the labels, specifically anabolic steroids and ephedrine (Martello, Felli, & Chiarotti, 2007). Additionally, a popular nutritional supplement for weight loss was found to contain the beta2-agonist clenbuterol, which is banned by both the World Anti-Doping Agency (WADA) and the NCAA (Geyer et al., 2008). These cases demonstrate how easily an athlete may become the victim of inadvertent doping, not to mention experiencing a heightened health risk.

Perhaps the most captivating 2012 news was the charging of seven-time Tour de France champion, Lance Armstrong, by USADA for having used illicit performance-enhancing drugs during his professional career. This charge not only lead to all his titles since 1998 being stripped from him but also to a lifetime ban from competition in all sports that follow the WADA code. A ban from sport, a passion for most athletes, is a legitimate risk for any athlete choosing to use a banned drug or unregulated substance during a competitive season. This emphasizes the importance of being an educated consumer when making the decision to use nutritional supplements in coordination with balanced whole food nutrition to enhance health and performance.

The purpose of this chapter is to provide an in-depth look at the evolution and use of dietary supplements in sports; discuss the legalities and regulations that affect the supplement industry; and explain the keys to being an informed consumer, including how to decipher supplement labels, safety considerations, important supplement resources, and various supplement bans.

Nutrition, Dietary Supplements, and Performance: A Historical Perspective

It is well known that certain nutrients, specifically carbohydrates, fats, proteins, vitamins, minerals, and water, are essential for health and sport performance. As sport scientist Ronald Maughan puts it, "Without proper nutrition, the full potential of the athlete will not be realized, because performance will not be at its peak, training levels may not be sustained, recovery from injury will be slower, and the athlete may be more susceptible to injury and infection." The idea that various ingredients in food could enhance physical stature, health, and athletic performance is not a modern phenomenon; rather, it dates to over 4,000 years ago. The ancient Greeks were at the forefront of sport nutrition as they sought various ingredients they could use to optimize athletic prowess during competition. Warriors of the time were reported to use such foods as deer liver and lion heart, hoping that consumption would produce bravery, speed, or strength. Although in its infancy, the concept of ergogenic or work-enhancing nutrients and the sport nutrition market it produced was beginning to bloom. In modern times, the topic of sport nutrition has continued to evolve, with health scientists working overtime to isolate and define ingredients that could enhance various metabolic reactions important to health and athletic performance. Current research continues to build on these nutritional discoveries and further refine the correct dosing, form, and timing of administration of each nutrient to help athletes maximize their health and performance potential.

Vitamin and Mineral Supplementation

At the forefront of the discovery of vitamins and minerals was the ancient Greek physician Hippocrates, who once stated, "Let food be thy medicine and medicine be thy food." These famous words served as a launching point for a series of research studies evaluating the impact of food ingredients on the prevention of debilitating diseases such as scurvy, which is estimated to have afflicted and killed millions of prisoners, slaves, soldiers, orphans, and sailors over several hundred years before Doctor James Lind discovered in the mid-1700s that a diet rich in citrus juices, later known to be rich in vitamin C, helped combat the disease. Nearly two hundred years later, in 1912, the term vitamin was officially coined by Polish biochemist Casmir Funk while he was busy making the discovery that thiamine helped correct symptoms of beriberi, including muscle weakness and heart failure, in deficient pigeons.

Over the following 30 years, a total of 13 vitamins, 9 water-soluble and 4 fat-soluble, were isolated and named along with their associated deficiency conditions. Collectively, along with 7 major minerals and 10 trace minerals, vitamins are known as micronutrients, or substances considered essential for health and protection against deficiency symptoms. See table 1.1 for descriptions and examples of these micronutrients. Beyond playing an important role in energy production, hemoglobin synthesis, maintenance of bone health, adequate immune function, and protection of the body against oxidative damage, micronutrients assist with synthesis and repair of muscle tissue during recovery from exercise and injury.

The importance of micronutrients in protection against deficiency symptoms and debilitating disease lead the United States Food and Nutrition Board to establish the Recommended Dietary Allowances (RDA) in 1941. The purpose of the RDAs is to define the daily dietary intake level of nutrients, including vitamins and minerals, considered sufficient to meet the requirements of nearly all (97%–98%) healthy individuals in each life stage and gender group. There is still debate, however, as to whether the RDAs are sufficient to support the increased metabolic demands of an athlete. Intense exercise, in particular, can accelerate the turnover and loss of micronutrients from the body, thus supporting the concept of increased micronutrient requirements to support building, repair, and maintenance of lean body mass in athletes.

As early as the late 1930s, vitamin and mineral supplements were being used in athletics. Front-of-the-pack Tour de France cyclists reporting that they rode better after taking vitamin and mineral supplements. In fact, the multivitamin and multimineral supplement, introduced in the 1940s, has remained one of the most commonly used supplements by athletes. While a multivitamin can certainly serve as nutritional insurance for an athlete in combination with a balanced whole food diet, research has failed to support the correlation between supplementation and enhanced performance.

TABLE 1.1 Micronutrients

	Water-soluble vitamins	Fat-soluble vitamins	Major minerals	Trace minerals
Description	Requires the presence of water for absorption; are not stored in the body, making daily intake essential.	Stored within fat throughout the body and are difficult to excrete from the body, making toxicity symptoms plausible when supplementing with mega doses.	Needed in large quantities in the body to form bone structure, build proteins, and balance body fluids.	Needed in small quantities to aid enzyme formation, immune system function, and reproduction.
Examples	B_1 (thiamine) B_2 (riboflavin) B_3 (niacin) B_5 (pantothenic acid) B_6 (pyridoxine) B_7 (biotin) B_9 (folic acid) B_{12} (coblalamin) C (ascorbic acid)	A (retinol) D (calciferol) E (tocopherol) K1 (phylloqui none)	Calcium Chloride Magnesium Phosphorus Potassium Sodium	Iron Zinc Manganese Copper Fluoride Molybdenum Iodine Chromium Selenium

The only exception is when a known dietary or blood nutrient deficiency presents itself.

Athletes at greatest risk for poor vitamin and mineral status and who may benefit from vitamin and mineral supplementation include those who restrict energy intake or follow extreme weight-loss regimens, those who eliminate one or more of the major food groups from their diet, those with food allergies or nutrient absorption issues, those completing an extraordinary high volume of training, and those who eat mostly processed foods.

Carbohydrate Supplementation

In the 1920s, after making the connection that low blood glucose levels were associated with symptoms of fatigue, stupor, and inability to concentrate, collectively known as bonking, scientists started to explore the idea that carbohydrate supplementation could enhance performance. During the 1925 running of the Boston Marathon, for instance, it was discovered that athletes who ate a high-carbohydrate diet in the 24 hours leading up to the race and who supplemented with hard candy immediately prior to starting—as well as during—the race were able to maintain better blood sugar levels, thereby avoiding the bonk, and run faster thanks to more carbohydrate fuel left in the glycogen tank. This precipitated a series of studies further evaluating the role of carbohydrate in exercise, especially in endurance performance.

In the 1960s Swedish researchers demonstrated that consumption of a high-carbohydrate diet during endurance training improved performance (Ahlborg et al., 1967). In addition, it was found that carbohydrate supplementation during exercise helped delay the onset of muscle fatigue associated with depleted muscle glycogen stores, also known as hitting the wall. To determine the optimal amount of carbohydrate needed to maximize glycogen stores, researchers would manipulate the dietary carbohydrate intake of athletes in the week leading up to endurance performance. Physiologist Gunvar Ahlbord introduced the concept of glycogen super compensation, also known as carbo-loading, which became a mainstay practice among endurance athletes in the 1970s. It continues to be used by team sport athletes such as football, basketball, soccer, and hockey players, all in sports where the duration of high-intensity play can increase the risk for glycogen depletion and consequent performance decline.

The Ahlborg, or classic, method of carbo-loading entails an athlete training to exhaustion to deplete glycogen stores 1 week prior to race day and then ingesting a low-carbohydrate diet for 2-5 days before increasing carbohydrate intake to 70%-85% of total caloric intake, often upward of 600 g (2,400 calories), for 1-2 days to facilitate glycogen supercompensation. However, this method of carbo-loading left many athletes feeling irritable and unmotivated during the depletion phase and bloated with water weight and sluggish during the loading phase. The depletion phase is now discounted by health professionals. Current carbo-loading techniques instruct athletes to follow an appropriate taper in training starting 2-3 weeks out from race day while consuming 45%-65% of their caloric intake from carbohydrates. The final 72 hours precompetition constitute the loading phase, with athletes increasing dietary intake of carbohydrate by approximately 25%, or to a level equivalent to 3.6-5.5 g of carbohydrate/lb (8-12 g of carbohydrate/kg) of body weight.

Over the next 40 years, continued identification of the benefits of carbohydrate supplementation on muscle and liver glycogen stores and consequent performance during high- and low-intensity exercise spearheaded the creation of sport drinks; the first known sport nutrition product, Gatorade, was developed by researchers at the University of Florida in 1965 to help the performance of the Florida Gators football team. Gatorade, a mixture of glucose and sucrose in water at approximately a 6% solution, is essentially responsible for the profitable sport beverage and food market today, which includes products such as energy gels (Hammer, Powergel, Gu), energy chews (Clif Shot Bloks, Honey Stinger), and energy bars (Bonk Breaker, Pure Fit, PowerBar).

Current research continues to evaluate the effects of carbohydrate on exercise, with attention focused on the effects of using various types and combinations of carbohydrates on carbohydrate absorption and consequent muscle performance during exercise.

Protein Supplementation

Since ancient times, proteins and their building blocks, amino acids, have been consumed to support vigorous training and enhance athletic performance. It was once reported that the legendary, powerful Greek wrestler Milo of Croton ate upward of 20 lb (9.1 kg) of meat daily to support his training regimen. While on the excessive end of the spectrum, Milo may have had an inclination that higher protein intakes helped increase the free pool of amino acids essential for protein synthesis. A total of 20 amino acids, 8 of which are essential (must be obtained through the diet) in adults and 12 of which the body can synthesize from other metabolism products, combine in various ways to help develop muscles, bone, tendons, skin, hair, and other tissues as well as aid nutrient transportation and enzyme production.

Essential Amino Acids	Nonessential Amino Acids	
Isoleucine	Alanine	Histidine
Leucine	Arginine	Proline
Lysine	Asparagine	Serine
Methionine	Aspartic Acid	Tyrosine
Phenylalanine	Cysteine	
Threonine	Glutamic Acid	
Tryptophan	Glutamine	
Valine	Glycine	

Until the 1970s when protein supplements became more readily available, athletes would follow Milo's example, increasing protein intake through consumption of such protein-rich foods as beef, eggs, chicken, fish, dairy foods, soybeans, nuts, and legumes. The evolution of protein supplements began in the 1930s when a young pharmacist named Eugene Schiff developed a method of processing whey from milk for human consumption, leading to the development of Schiff Bio-Foods, a whey packaging company turned supplement company. Soon after, it was found that supplemental protein could facilitate increases in muscle mass and gains in strength, which lead to the introduction of protein powders in sports, including the whey protein created by Schiff. Bob Hoffman, who is considered the father of American weightlifting, referred to protein powder as a secret weapon for the athletes he trained for the 1954 World Weightlifting Championships.

While the current RDA for protein intake is 0.36 g/lb (0.8 g/kg) of body weight for the average American, there is conflicting evidence regarding the optimal dose for athletes. It is known that additional protein and essential amino acids, in conjunction with an energy-efficient diet, are critical for muscle growth, especially during the early stages of a strength-training program. It is also known that protein oxidation accelerates during cardiovascular exercise, thereby providing a reason for increased protein consumption by strength and endurance-oriented athletes. Consequently, leaders from the American College of Sports Medicine (ACSM), American Dietetic Association (ADA), and Dietitians of Canada (DOC) essentially doubled the daily protein recommendations for athletes. Endurance-focused athletes, such as runners, cyclists, and triathletes, were instructed to aim for a daily intake of 1.2-1.4 g/kg (0.54-0.63 g/lb) of body weight; strength-focused athletes, such as football players, target a range of 1.2 to 1.7 g/kg (0.54-0.77 g/lb) of body weight. Protein intake above these recommendations, especially at the expense of other valuable macronutrients such as carbohydrates, healthy fats, and nutrient-dense fruits and vegetables, can jeopardize an athlete's performance instead of enhance it.

Because most athletes consume plenty of protein from whole food intake to meet current recommendations, supplementation is rarely needed. However, supplements can be more practical in some settings to ensure athletes are getting adequate high-quality proteins needed before, during, or after training. In addition, there are special populations of athletes for whom protein supplementation is needed from a health and performance standpoint. For example, athletes following vegetarian or vegan diets may benefit from supplemental protein due to the relatively lower quality and digestibility of plant protein sources, with factors such as fiber reducing protein absorption by as much as 10%. Supplemental protein may also help preserve muscle mass in athletes who are restricting calories or trying to lose weight.

Herbal and Botanical Supplementation

Herbals, which are derived from the leaves, bark, berries, roots, gums, seeds, stems, or flowers of plants and are rich in naturally occurring substances called phytochemicals (known to have nutritive value), have been used to enhance health and performance for over 4,000 years. In China and Japan, for example, warriors and wrestlers along with other athletes were documented as using a variety of raw herbal concoctions and teas to help improve endurance and strength. An herbal practitioner by the name of Galen created the first classification system, pairing common illnesses with their associated herbal remedies in 200 AD and laying the groundwork for the use of herbals in the pharmaceutical world. In fact, several current medications are merely extracts of traditional herbs. Today, herbals can be consumed in teas and tinctures (as topical applications), in liquid forms such as energy drinks, and in pills and capsules.

It is estimated that 1 out of 5 athletes uses some form of herbal supplement, often in sport drinks or foods they are consuming. One of the biggest sellers worldwide is ginseng, which claims to have anabolic qualities among other ergogenic traits. Herbal supplements are often marketed to help increase energy, produce fat loss, promote muscle growth, or trigger other physiological or metabolic responses important for exercise performance. Unfortunately, the research supporting such ergogenic qualities is currently lacking.

Safety also seems to be a relevant issue as several herbal supplements have been detected with high levels of heavy metals. According to several studies, these metals include lead, which causes unhealthy blood levels that produce undesirable symptoms such as lethargy, abdominal pain, nausea, headaches, and in serious cases seizure and coma. Cadmium, hexavalent chromium, mercury, and arsenic are metals often seen in herbal supplements outsourced from China where the soil, water, and air run a greater risk of being contaminated. Furthermore, supplement purity is in question as a result of mislabeling. In 2010 an herbal weight-loss supplement was found to contain fenfluramine, a stimulant drug withdrawn from the U.S. market in 1997 after studies demonstrated that it caused serious heart valve damage; other potentially harmful pharmaceutical ingredients were also absent from the product label. Some believe more stringent regulation is needed as a result of such cases. Some countries, including Germany, regulate herbals like medicine; the United States currently regulates most herbal supplements as dietary supplements under the Dietary Supplement Health and Education Act; as a result, safety data collection and appropriate risk assessments have not been conducted on most herbal ingredients. This reality magnifies the importance of being an educated consumer when choosing to pair whole food intake with dietary supplements.

Supplement Trends for the Future

Over the past century, there has been quite a bit of progress in our understanding of how and why various food ingredients and dietary supplements may aid health and physical performance. Perhaps of greatest relevance to athletes, and a direct result of the information gathered from a variety of historical scientific studies, was the introduction of sport-specific food products such as energy gels, chews, bars, and sport drinks designed to address a wide variety of performance-limiting factors, including muscle cramping, glycogen depletion, muscle growth, and recovery. The recent explosion of sport nutrition programs offered at universities has generated a plethora of new studies that have evaluated how currently used and newly discovered ingredients can combat these factors through proper dosing and timing of intake.

In response to the dramatic increase in the numbers of athletes competing in endurance events such as marathons, triathlons, and century rides, look for a wave of new ingredient blends and products geared specifically toward endurance athletes. Customization will also be a hot trend for the future. Leading this trend are companies such as Infinit Nutrition (www. infinitnutrition.us) that custom-blends ingredients, including carbohydrate, protein, amino acids, caffeine, and electrolytes, to create sport drinks specifically catering to an athlete's unique health, training needs, and performance goals. Another company is You Bar (www.youbars.com), which allows athletes to custom-blend a variety of ingredients to form energy bars, trail mixes, protein shakes, and cereals. There are also several companies such as Vitaganic (www.vitaganic.com) that custom-blend vitamins, minerals, and herbals to create a once-a-day formula designed to address athletes' specific health concerns and goals.

An emerging field of study is nutrigenomics, which evaluates how foods affect our genes and how individual genetic differences can affect the way we respond to nutrients and other naturally occurring compounds in the foods we eat. Researchers at Kansas State University published an article exploring the role of specific nutrients in gene expression and how nutrients may affect the progression of disease as well as human performance (Getz, Adhikari, & Medeiros, 2010). It's believed that in the next 5-10 years, we will be able to visit our physicians to determine our genetic makeup and work with nutritional professionals to customize our diets based on our unique physiological needs and goals. Essentially, nutrigenomics will help transform the Western medical world, making food rather than drugs more of a mainstream treatment.

On the health front, in line with the new wave of thinking that the root of many health issues may be inflammation, a multitude of antiinflammatory ingredients (generally extracts from plants and food ingredients such as tart cherries) are being marketed for disease protection as well as athletic recovery. For example, in recent Olympic Games, several groups of athletes took 4 oz (.12 L) of tart cherry juice twice daily to help counter inflammation and aid recovery. Omega-3 fatty acids and fish oils continue to be touted as strong antiinflammatories and are among the most commonly used supplements. Quercetin, found naturally in apples and red onions, has also be shown to have strong antiinflammatory properties and has been included in several sport food products in the form of chews, capsules, and drinks. Continue to watch this trend grow over the next decade.

Of utmost concern to athletes and those working with them is the purity and safety of supplements, which is why many of the more reputable sport nutrition companies have invested in truth-in-labeling programs. Companies such as NSF Certified for Sport (www.nsfsport.com), which is recognized by the National Football League (NFL), National Football League Players Association (NFLPA), Major League Baseball (MLB), Major League Baseball Players Association (MLBPA), Professional Golfer's Golf Association (PGA), Ladies Professional Golf Association (LPGA), and the Canadian Center for

Ethics in Sports (CCES), ensure that participating sports supplement manufacturers provide confirmation of substance content and purity, compliance with regulations, and assessment of public safety and environmental concerns for products used by athletes. A link to NSF approved supplements can be found in the References and Resources file at www.humankinetics. com/products/all-products/Athletes-Guide-to-Sports-Supplements-The. NSF is a global, independent public health organization whose goal is to protect human health and safety worldwide. NSF is considered the gold standard of third-party testing. NSF wrote the only accredited American National Standard (NSF/ANSI 173) that verifies the health and safety of dietary supplements. Sports supplements must undergo rigorous testing and inspection to verify compliance with NSF/ANSI Standard 173, which includes

- banned substances screening (screens for more than 180 prohibited substances on the World Anti-Doping Agency's, NFL, and MLB prohibited substances lists);
- label claim review (confirms the label matches contents);
- toxicology review (certifies formulation);
- contaminant review (checks for undeclared ingredients or contaminants in the product); and
- facility audits (biannual good manufacturing practices audits at the manufacturing facility, plus an on-site inspection to check for banned substances).

With the increased concern regarding athletes testing positive for banned substances, it is likely more programs offering independent testing that ensures purity will exist in the future. Moreover, it is the hope that the products of all supplement companies will someday be mandated to undergo such testing prior to becoming available to consumers. According to USADA, in order for third-party testing to be credible, the following criteria should be met: (1) is free from conflicts of interest, (2) has external accreditations, (3) conducts an audit of the supplement company based on good manufacturing practices established by the US Food and Drug Administration (FDA), (4) evaluates the dietary supplement for overall safety and quality, and (5) has a validated and accredited method to test for prohibited substances.

Prevalence of Supplement Use

Dietary supplement use is widespread among U.S. adults aged 20 and over. The National Health and Nutrition Examination Survey (NHANES, 2011) reported that between 2005 and 2008, more than 50% of the U.S. population used at least one dietary supplement, including multivitamins, minerals, and herbs, and the multivitamin and multimineral supplement was the top choice among consumers. Dietary supplements are often perceived as band-aids for poor lifestyle choices, including imbalanced nutrition, lack of exercise, and deficient sleep patterns. While exercise may not be a problem for most athletes, there still remains a perception that dietary supplementation can help offset the consequences of a diet rich in nutritionally empty foods. This is not the case, yet the use of dietary supplements grew more than 10% between 1994 and 2002, though in more recent years (2005-2008), growth rates have subsided and even declined slightly.

With a growing number of athletes using dietary supplements, many sport governing bodies are laying down ground rules to minimize health and safety risks to athletes, maintain ethical standards, and reduce liability risks. For example, the Iowa High School Athletic Association discourages school personnel, including coaches, from supplying, recommending, or permitting the use of any drug, medication, or food supplement solely for performance-enhancing purposes. Even so, in an unpublished survey of their student-athletes in grades 9–12, it was discovered that 96% were taking some form of supplement, with the most popular being vitamin supplements, energy enhancing products (e.g., Red Bull), meal replacement bars and shakes, creatine (males only), and weight-loss products (females only). Friends, coaches, and parents were identified as top sources of information; doctors and registered dietitians surprisingly failed to be mentioned.

Similar results have been seen among college-aged athletes as well as professional athletes. Data indicate that some 80%-90% of collegiate athletes are using some type of sports supplement (Froiland et al., 2004; Burns et al., 2004). Female athletes commonly report using multivitamins, calcium, and vitamin D supplements, while males typically use amino acid and protein supplements. Interestingly, at the Olympic level, recent reports have shown the use of dietary supplements dropped by 8% over a 7-year period from 2002 to 2009 (Heikkinen et al., 2011), perhaps due to many athletes being stripped of their medals by the International Olympic Committee (IOC) after being busted by WADA for use of banned substances. At the professional level, surveys taken at the Olympic Games revealed 69% of athletes in Atlanta and 74% at the Sydney Games were using sports supplements though more recent reports have demonstrated decreasing numbers among this population of athletes, perhaps due to concern about supplement purity (Huang, Johnson, & Pipe, 2006; Heikkinen et al., 2011).

It's impossible to ignore the prevalence of dietary supplement use in athletics. Thus, it's important for athletes, coaches, and sport performance professionals to be educated on how supplements are regulated and what to look for in a dietary supplement. It's also important for them to have a resource providing credible evidence to support the benefits of a sports supplement.

Regulation of Dietary Supplements

According to the medical advisor for *Consumer Reports,* Dr. Orly Avitzur (as reported by CNN Health in 2011), "There is a false perception that supplements fall under the same regulatory umbrella as prescription drugs." In actuality, both historically and currently, dietary supplements have been treated much like foods in the United States. The regulatory power of the FDA and the Federal Trade Commission (FTC) was further limited and compromised under President Clinton with the signing of the Dietary Supplement Health and Education Act (DSHEA) in 1994. Prior to the DSHEA, the Congress was considering a couple of bills that would have strengthened the power of the FDA and FTC to combat health frauds. The proposed laws would have allowed the establishment of harsher penalties for the marketing of supplement products with unsubstantiated drug claims on labels and would have made it illegal to advertise nutritional or therapeutic claims on supplement labels.

Not surprisingly, the health food industry responded with a fury of outcries from retailers and consumers who were manipulated into thinking they'd be run out of business and lose their freedom to purchase dietary supplements. Of course, neither of these claims was true. The goal of the proposed laws was merely to protect consumers by ensuring supplement labels were accurate, ingredients were safe, and false health claims from manufacturers and distributors would be prevented. Interestingly, the results of several surveys reveal that most consumers want just that. They want the government to review safety data and approve dietary supplements prior to sale. They want the government to verify all health-related claims before they can be included in advertisements and on product labels. Yet, this is the opposite of what the DSHEA permits. And so the tide turned in favor of the dietary supplement market, allowing the industry to turn into one of the most profitable trades, especially with the increased availability of Internet and online mass marketing portals such as Facebook and Twitter.

As a result of the deregulation of dietary supplements by the DSHEA, athletes, coaches, and parents of athletes should understand the following three risks associated with dietary supplement use:

1. **Supplement purity:** Athletes often believe that because dietary supplements can be purchased at a store or over the Internet, they must be pure. Unfortunately, this is often untrue. A 2011 investigation by the California firm Anti-Doping Research, for example, revealed that 10 products purchased from the popular online store amazon.com contained illegal steroids that are known to have dangerous side effects such as liver toxicity (William Reed Business Media). A failed drug test can be devastating to an athlete and all parties involved, which is why it is critical to be informed prior to purchasing dietary supplements. Although the FDA has established quality standards for dietary supplements to help ensure their identity, purity, strength, and composition, there are many facilities that manufacture dietary supplements

that have yet to be inspected by the FDA. As a result, athletes should be aware that some dietary supplements may contain other ingredients not included on their labels as well as list inaccurate quantities of active ingredients. Fortunately, several independent organizations, including U.S. Pharmacopeia, ConsumerLab.com, NSF International, Informed-Choice, and Natural Products Association, offer quality testing that assures the product was properly manufactured, contains the ingredients listed on the supplement label, and is void of harmful levels of contaminants. Athletes choosing to add dietary supplements to their performance regimen should look for these stamps of approval, though they should also be aware that such approvals do not guarantee the safety or effectiveness of the product.

2. **Supplement safety:** It is often thought that if a substance is natural, it must be safe and beneficial. Under current regulations, unfortunately, this isn't always true. Dietary supplements, including herbals and such hormones as DHEA and melatonin, can be marketed and introduced on store shelves before manufacturers are even required to submit safety information to the FDA, which essentially leaves the consumer blind when it comes to potential health risks. Without immediate access to safety information, the FDA is forced to scramble for information regarding adverse events, product sampling, studies in scientific literature, and other sources of evidence of danger in an attempt to regulate the safety of dietary supplements. It is impossible for the FDA to keep up with the thousands of existing and new dietary supplements readily available in health stores, through sales reps, and on the Internet; thus, the safety of untested dietary supplements must be questioned. Weight-loss supplements have frequently been on the safety hot seat. In 2004, for example, as a result of adverse health effects such as heart attacks, strokes, and death, the FDA banned ephedrine alkaloids that were marketed for reasons other than asthma, colds, or allergies. Unfortunately, the ban was enacted after many had already experienced some of the negative consequences of ephedrine toxicity. Athletes should be aware that dietary supplements often contain active ingredients that can exert strong effects on the body and are likely to cause some side effects, especially when used as a replacement for, or in combination with, prescribed medications. In addition, contaminants such as heavy metals, pesticides, and microbiological toxins found within some dietary supplements are legitimate risks to the overall health of an athlete.

3. **Unproven supplement claims:** Supplement companies can make claims about products without supporting scientific evidence as long as they do not claim to prevent, treat, cure, or mitigate disease. Distributors of sports supplements have the ultimate leeway since claims are generally associated with some performance variable rather than a disease state. Often, the primary support for an ergogenic (performance-enhancing) claim is testimonial rather than science based. Furthermore, it is not uncommon to find advertisements suggesting that all athletes, including those consuming

a well-balanced diet, are at risk for nutritional deficiencies. This is a stretch from the truth. Even when science is involved, the research study design is often poor, the number of subjects small, or the research is funded by a company involved with the dietary supplement, making any valid indication of proof of claim virtually impossible. Therefore, athletes and coaches should always approach supplement claims with skepticism and remember the old adage, "If it sounds too good to be true, it probably is."

The regulation of dietary supplements is truly at a crossroads although there continues to be a battle between supplement industry leaders and the FDA. The supplement industry is fighting because more stringent regulation by the FDA, especially as it relates to safety, will make it harder to release and market various dietary supplements, thus having a potential negative impact on profit margins. The FDA is invested in protecting consumers from fraudulent marketing and potential health risks associated with ingestion of any supplement ingredient, including ingredients often not listed on the label. Many believe that the availability of supplements and the freedom of the consumer to access potential health- and performance-enhancing ingredients will be limited by FDA efforts to incorporate mandatory testing of all new ingredients prior to their market release. Dietary supplements should continue to be available to consumers, yet most health professionals believe the purity and safety of the ingredients need to be established first.

Concerns regarding supplement safety escaladed to an all-time high after the FDA's struggles to ban ephedra despite its several reported adverse side effects, including deaths. In direct response, the Dietary Supplement and Nonprescription Drug Consumer Protection Act was enacted in 2006, serving as a stepping stone in the right direction in regard to supplement safety. Under this Act, manufacturers of dietary supplements and nonprescription drugs are required to notify the FDA about serious adverse events related to their products, including deaths, life-threatening experiences, inpatient hospitalizations, persistent or significant disability or incapacity, birth defects, and the need for medical intervention to prevent any such problems. In addition, a telephone number or address is required on product labels so consumers can contact the manufacturer as needed.

In 2011, FDA dietary supplements chief Dan Fabricant introduced the framework for new dietary ingredients (NDI), defined as any dietary ingredient that was not sold in the United States as a dietary supplement before October 15, 1994. With the FDA's NDI notice, specific safety information for any dietary supplement containing a new dietary ingredient is required from the manufacturer prior to marketing. While safety information is yet to be required in advance for older dietary supplement ingredients, manufacturers still have to report any adverse effects to the FDA. Much like the increased regulatory suggestions made by the FDA in the early 1990s, the introduction of the NDI notice has stirred quite a bit of controversy, with dietary supplement industry leaders once again claiming that any gain of regulatory power by the FDA would be catastrophic, stifling new product development and threatening scores of products already on the market. This is likely not true, but such regulation will help ensure that the scores of new ingredients being discovered get a safety stamp of approval prior to being released to the marketplace.

Tips for Being a Supplement-Savvy Athlete

The battle for regulatory power is likely to be an ongoing one, but the hope for the future is a dietary supplement industry that provides more scientific, rather than testimonial-based, evidence for the claims being made, and more importantly, one that requires independent testing from a third party to ensure the purity and safety of the ingredients for consumers. This is especially relevant for the athlete wanting to avoid failing a drug test and potential ban from competition. In the meantime, the following tips offer advice for coaches, athletes, parents, and health professionals on how to be proactive and educated consumers by researching the legitimacy of claims as well as any reported risks associated with the ingredients in the supplement.

1. **Talk with your health care provider before making a decision.** A single online search of dietary supplements will lead to a plethora of information, often conflicting and usually generated by unqualified parties. A trip to the gym may lead to a sales pitch for a variety of supplements. Many fitness professionals are pressured to meet a specific sales quota for a supplement line the gym is carrying or are merely looking for additional income. There are even nutrition clinics sponsored by supplement companies that offer free nutrition coaching, but these are fancy ploys for their sales reps to sell products. Thus, it is important to be extremely selective about where and from whom you are gathering information. Athletes are encouraged to speak to a health care provider, such as a doctor or pharmacist, about dietary supplements being considered prior to using those supplements to establish potential benefits as well as safety risks. This is especially important for athletes with pending surgeries.

For more detailed nutrition and dietary supplement advice, athletes should speak with a registered dietitian (RD), who is the most credible source of nutrition information as a result of extensive schooling and continuing education, completion of a 6- to 12-month dietetic internship, and successfully passing a national examination. A registered dietitian can help customize a menu plan designed to meet the nutritional demands of training and competition. The RD can also help determine the safety and efficacy of dietary supplement use by

- assessing the nutritional status of the athlete to determine the likelihood of inadequate or excessive intake of vitamins and minerals;

- evaluating the potential benefit or harm of nutrient supplementation given an athlete's nutritional and health status;
- evaluating the safety of a nutrient supplement given the form, dose, and potential for interaction with food, other dietary supplements, and over-the-counter and prescription medications;
- educating athletes as to the potential benefit of receiving nutrients through conventional and fortified foods;
- recommending nutrient supplementation when food intake is inadequate;
- evaluating research regarding nutrient supplementation; and
- being aware of regulatory, legal, and ethical issues involved in recommending and selling nutrient supplements.

Fortunately, it is estimated that over 50% of university athletic departments as well as professional and amateur athletic teams have either an RD onsite or contract out with one. Many of these professional RDs are members of the Collegiate and Professional Sports Dietitians Association (CPSDA), have completed a secondary degree in exercise physiology or sport nutrition, have personal experience in sport, or are Board-Certified Specialists in Sport Dietetics (CSSD). The CPSDA has coined the term *sports RD* to identify those dietitians working in professional, collegiate, amateur, and military performance settings. The Commission on Dietetic Registration developed a certification in sport dietetics to identify RDs with documented practical experience and successful completion of an examination in sports nutrition. Because of sports RDs' involvement in these settings and experience in working with sports supplements, they are generally the best source for information. A list of sport-minded registered dietitians in the United States can be found at www.scandpg.org/search-rd.

2. **Become familiar with reputable online resources for supplements.** All parties involved with an athlete, including the athlete himself or herself, should be aware of the resources available. Table 1.2 provides a quick reference guide of credible websites for information on important issues involving dietary supplements.

3. **Look for clean supplements.** Independent testing by third-party labs can confirm the ingredients listed on supplement labels. Training the body for peak performance is not something that happens overnight. Athletes spend hours each day over several months to prepare for competition, and coaches and parents spend equal amounts of time in support of an athlete's performance endeavors. The last thing anyone wants holding him or her back is a failed drug test generated by a contaminated dietary supplement. Thus, any athlete thinking about using a dietary supplement should make sure that there has been a stamp of approval garnered from an independent testing lab.

Dietary supplements that have gone through independent testing via third-party organizations ensure

- the contents of the supplement actually match what is printed on the label,
- there are no ingredients present in the supplement that are not openly disclosed on the label, minimizing the risk that a dietary supplement or sport nutrition product contains banned substances, and
- there are no unacceptable levels of contaminants present in the supplement.

Table 1.2 provides a list of some of the independent testing laboratories that serve as resources for athletes looking for information on which supplement companies have had products tested for banned substances and purity.

TABLE 1.2 Online Resources for Dietary Supplements

Purity of dietary supplements	For the general public: Consumer Laboratory (CL), www.consumerlab.com US Pharmacopeial Convention, www.usp.org For athletes: NSF Certified for Sport Program, www.nsf.org Human Sports Performance (HSP), www.humansportsperformance.com Informed Choice, www.informed–choice.org Informed Sport, www.informed-sport.com
Safety of dietary supplements/ ingredients	Supplement Safety Now, www.supplementsafetynow.com
Dietary supplement regulation	Food and Drug Administration, www.fda.gov Federal Trade Commission, www.ftc.gov Council for Responsible Nutrition (CRN), www.crnusa.org Natural Products Association (NPA), www.npainfo.org
Nutrition and dietary supplement information	Office of Dietary Supplements (NIH), http://ods.od.nih.gov American Dietetic Association (ADA), www.eatright.org Australian Institute of Sport (AIS), www.ausport.gov.au/ais/nutrition Gatorade Sports Science Institute, www.gssiweb.com Sports, Cardiovascular, and Wellness Nutritionists (SCAN), www.scandpg.org Sports Oracle, www.sportsoracle.com Supplement 411, www.usada.org/supplement411
Drug testing and banned substances lists	National Collegiate Athletic Association (NCAA), www.ncaa.org United States Anti-Doping Agency (USADA), www.usantidoping.org World Anti-Doping Agency (WADA), www.wada-ama.org

Reading supplement labels	Council for Responsible Nutrition,
	  www.crnusa.org/pdfs/CRN_How_to_read_a_ds_label.pdf
	  www.crnusa.org/pdfs/DS-RegsLabel-061510.pdf

Research	Pub Med, www.pubmed.com, Sport Science, www.sportsci.org Journal of the International Science of Sports Nutrition, www.jissn.com International Journal of Sport Nutrition and Exercise Metabolism, http://journals.humankinetics.com/IJSNEM *Journal of Dietary Supplements,* http://informahealthcare.com/jds

Understanding Research Studies

While there are numerous scientific studies available, the majority provide less than valid results due to either poor study design or the small number of subjects. Therefore, when evaluating research associated with dietary supplements, it is important to look for studies that meet at least some of the following criteria:

- **Double-blind:** In this type of clinical study, both the subjects participating and the researchers are unaware of when the experimental medication or procedure has been given or followed.

- **Placebo-controlled:** In this method of research, an inactive substance (placebo) is given to one group of subjects (control group) while the treatment (e.g., dietary supplement) being tested is given to another group (experimental group). The results obtained from the two groups are then compared to see if the treatment being tested is more effective than the placebo. When conducted as a double-blind study, this type of research is considered the gold standard of clinical research.

- **Controlled randomized trial**: This is a study in which subjects are selected according to relevant characteristics and are then randomly assigned to either an experimental group or a control group.

- **Clinical trial:** This is an experimental study with human subjects. Gold-standard clinical trials are double-blind, placebo-controlled studies that use random assignment of subjects to experimental or control groups.

- **Large number of subjects:** In general, the larger the number of subjects, the more valid the research results.

- **Replicated research:** When results of a study have been replicated, they gain more clout.

- **Statistical significance:** A result is considered statistically significant when it has a p-value (probability value) of less than 5% ($p < 0.05$), which means that the result would occur by chance less than 5% of the time and is fairly common. However, more statistically compelling levels of significance are $p < 0.01$ and $p < 0.001$, meaning the result would occur by chance less than 1% of the time.

4. **Choose supplements that have scientific evidence of results.** While the purity of the dietary supplement can be established through independent testing, the efficacy of supplement claims cannot, which is why it is important for the athlete to opt for dietary supplements that have evidence of results from well-controlled and replicated scientific research.

5. **Learn how to read supplement labels.** The dietary supplement label (see figure 1.1) lists essential information about the product in the bottle. Prior to using any supplement, it is critical to always read the label and follow directions for use.

How do you read a supplement label?

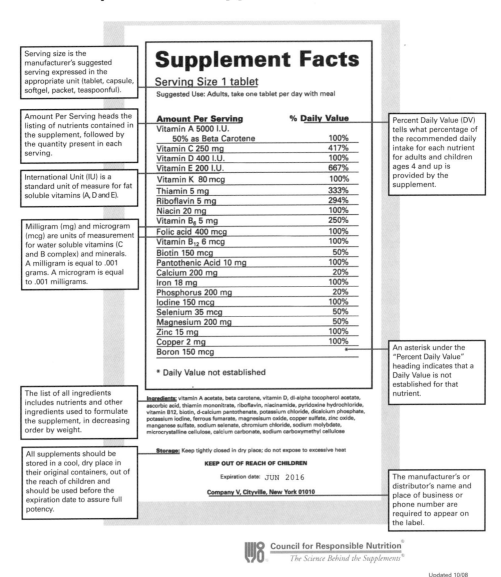

FIGURE 1.1 Before choosing a supplement, it's important to understand the information on the supplement label.

Used with permission from the Council for Responsible Nutrition www.crnusa.org.

6. **Know how to report fraudulent supplements or adverse reactions.** Any athlete who experiences an adverse reaction to a dietary supplement should immediately contact his or her health care provider after which the problem can be reported directly to the FDA by calling the FDA's MedWatch hotline at 1-800-FDA-1088 or submitting a report by fax to 1-800-FDA-0178.

Dangers of Supplement Contamination

Jessica Hardy, an Olympic swimming hopeful, tested positive in 2008 for clenbuterol. This positive test was later discovered to be the result of a contaminated supplement Jessica was taking leading up to the Beijing Olympic Games. Although Jessica unknowingly and negligently was taking a contaminated supplement, she was still required to serve a 1-year suspension. At the time a 1-year suspension would have disqualified Hardy from the 2012 Olympics as well. Fortunately, the American Arbitration Association and the IOC ruled it would be unfair to punish Hardy to this extent. She was allowed to compete in the London Games, where she earned a bronze medal in the 4 × 100 m freestyle relay and a gold medal in the 4 × 100 m medley relay. Hardy's situation should bring awareness to and cause concern in other athletes regarding the risks associated with sports supplements.

Summary

Over the past 100+ years, many nutritional ingredients have been discovered and found to play vital roles in health, well-being, and performance. The year 2012 marked the 100th anniversary of the official coining of the term vitamin, with Casmir Funk leading the way through his discovery of the B vitamin thiamine, which helps offset symptoms of beriberi (a nervous system disease caused by a thiamine deficiency in the diet). Soon after, vitamin supplements made their way into athletics based on the idea that enhanced performance might be an end benefit. In the 1920s scientists determined that inadequate carbohydrate intake was associated with an inability to concentrate, as well as premature muscle fatigue or hitting the wall. This led to the theory that carbohydrate supplementation may help enhance performance. In the 1930s protein supplements were introduced and were later thought to be a secret weapon for weightlifters. Most ingredients are herbals, which have been used to enhance health and performance for over 4,000 years in Asian culture. However, the full benefits of supplementation with nutritional ingredients have yet to be proven, with research still in its infancy. Even so, several recent surveys of athletes demonstrate a majority use at least one supplement ingredient for performance or health purposes.

Unfortunately, a legitimate risk to an athlete is a failed doping test due to use of contaminated nutritional supplements, despite ongoing efforts to improve relatively ineffective or nonexistent regulatory and manufacturing guidelines. Reviews of supplements available via online shopping have revealed that many products are laced with steroids and stimulants, which are prohibited for use in sports. Although it has been suggested that athletes avoid dietary supplements all together, this approach is unrealistic and unnecessary. There are a variety of legitimate reasons for an athlete to use supplements in coordination with a well-balanced diet. Furthermore, over the past decade, there has been an influx of data from clinical trials demonstrating a variety of health- and performance-oriented benefits with the use of a handful of dietary supplements. Fortunately, more supplement manufacturers are having their products rigorously tested by third-party testing facilities to minimize risks. Athletes choosing to pair their performance diet with dietary supplements are encouraged not only to choose supplements that are tested by facilities such as NSF, but also to speak to a doctor, pharmacist, or registered dietitian about the use of supplements prior to implementation.

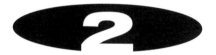

Keys to
Peak Performance

The will to win, the desire to succeed, the urge to reach your full potential . . . these are the keys that will unlock the door to personal excellence.

Eddie Robinson, legendary football coach

Tapping into athletic potential and unlocking the door to peak performance require a dedicated focus on a myriad of cardiovascular, muscle, psychological, and health-centered variables that are largely influenced by smart physical training and proper nutrition. To gain a competitive advantage, athletes often go beyond training and whole food nutrition and use dietary supplements marketed to address specific components of performance such as muscle strength or anaerobic endurance, which are important for athletes' success in their respective sports. The purpose of this chapter is to discuss the science behind the variables that generate the claims made about popular dietary supplements today.

Each performance variable, including related subcomponents, is assigned a symbol that will serve as a quick reference tool in the A-to-Z supplement guide presented in chapter 3.

Performance variable	Components included	Symbol
Fuel usage		
Cardiovascular function	Aerobic capacity Anaerobic endurance	
Muscular function	Strength Power Speed and strength endurance	
Psychological function	Concentration and focus Motivation	
Hydration status	Fluid balance Electrolyte balance	
Recovery	Short term: Glycogen repletion Rehydration Long term: Immunity Joint, tendon, and muscle health	
Weight and body composition	Lean body mass gains Body fat losses	

Fuel Usage

Watch an image of an athlete in motion, and it is easy to see how dynamic the human body is. Each intricate movement is driven by billions of microscopic units, each with its unique function, fueled by a molecule called adenosine triphosphate (ATP). The human body carries enough ATP energy within the muscles (~100 g) to support 1-4 seconds of intense activity before needing to tap into its triple-line system of energy production to fuel sport performance. All lines of the energy system work together, yet the intensity of sport activity dictates the proportion of energy supplied by each (see table 2.1).

ATP-Creatine Phosphate Energy System

The smallest fuel tank, called alactic or ATP-CP, operates without oxygen and uses creatine phosphate (CP) in the muscles to generate ATP for 5-10 seconds of explosive activity, making it a commonly used, important fuel

TABLE 2.1 Primary Metabolic Demands of Various Sports

Sport	Phosphagen system	Anaerobic glycolysis	Aerobic metabolism
Baseball	High	Low	--
Basketball	High	Moderate to high	--
Boxing	High	High	Moderate
Diving	High	Low	--
Fencing	High	Moderate	--
Field events	High	--	--
Field hockey	High	Moderate	Moderate
Football (American)	High	Moderate	Low
Gymnastics	High	Moderate	--
Golf	High	--	--
Ice hockey	High	Moderate	Moderate
Lacrosse	High	Moderate	Moderate
Marathon	Low	Low	High
Mixed martial arts	High	High	Moderate
Powerlifting	High	Low	Low
Skiing:			
Cross-country	Low	Low	High
Downhill	High	High	Moderate
Soccer	High	Moderate	Moderate
Strength competitions	High	Moderate to high	Low
Swimming:			
Short distance	High	Moderate	--
Long distance	--	Moderate	High
Tennis	High	Moderate	--
Track (athletics):			
Short distance	High	Moderate	--
Long distance	--	Moderate	High
Ultra-endurance events	Low	Low	High
Volleyball	High	Moderate	--
Wrestling	High	High	Moderate
Weightlifting	High	Low	Low

Note: All types of metabolism are involved to some extent in all activities.

Reprinted, by permission, from N.A. Ratamess, 2008, Adaptations to anaerobic training programs. In *Essentials of strength training and conditioning,* 3rd ed., by National Strength and Conditioning Association, edited by T.R. Baechle (Champaign, IL: Human Kinetics), 95.

system for athletes engaged in sports that incorporate quick, all-out bursts of energy (e.g., jumping, sprinting, blocking). Because creatine is stored in limited capacity (~120 g), creatine supplements have become popular among power- and speed-oriented athletes wanting to enhance performance.

Anaerobic-Lactate Energy System

More sustained, moderate- to high-intensity efforts lasting up to 3 minutes (e.g., 800 m dash) or repeated explosive periods of activity (e.g., boxing) rely on the midsize fuel tank, called anaerobic-lactate (AN-LA) or the lactic acid energy system, which, in the absence of oxygen, breaks down glucose (carbohydrate) through a series of enzymatic reactions into pyruvic acid to help generate ATP energy. This metabolic process is called anaerobic glycolysis; it results in the formation of fatigue-inducing lactic acid as well as hydrogen ions that impair muscle contraction through a number of mechanisms. Several popular supplements claim to buffer lactic acid and hydrogen ions, thus helping to offset muscle fatigue caused by acidosis, allowing an athlete to perform longer with greater power and speed.

Aerobic Energy System

The final and largest energy tank, called aerobic, breaks down carbohydrates (stored in the body as glycogen), fats, and at times protein in the presence of oxygen to generate a plentiful amount of ATP energy; it plays an important role during endurance sport activity as well as aiding recovery between periods of heightened exertion (e.g., interval training). Unlike anaerobic metabolism, where lactic acid and hydrogen ions can build up and potentially limit performance, the byproducts of aerobic metabolism, carbon dioxide and water, are easily disposed of through respiration or breathing, making it easier to sustain an aerobic effort for a longer time.

During aerobic metabolism, glucose (carbohydrate), stored as glycogen in limited amounts within the liver and muscles, is broken down via glycolysis. The human body is capable of storing enough carbohydrate energy to fuel up to 2 hours of moderate- to high-intensity training before depletion is inevitable, and the onset of low blood sugars (known as "hitting the wall") and muscle-fatigue ensue. This is why use of carbohydrate supplementation from sources like sport drinks, energy gels, bars, and chews becomes a crucial practice for athletes during endurance events, such as a marathon, lasting longer than a couple of hours as well as team sports involving higher-intensity exercise for prolonged durations, including basketball, football, soccer, and hockey. In addition, athletes may taper training volume while increasing dietary intake of carbohydrate, often with the help of carbohydrate supplements, for 3 days prior to competition to facilitate increased storage of carbohydrate, a practice known as carb-loading.

When glycogen (i.e., carbohydrate) depletion occurs, training intensity must be reduced to facilitate increased oxygen consumption needed to break down fat, which is stored as triglycerides in large amounts within adipose tissue throughout the body. Like glucose, triglycerides can be broken down to form free fatty acids, which undergo a process called beta oxidation to produce ATP. One of the primary physiological goals of an aerobic training program is to increase the reliance on fat metabolism, even when generating more power or speed, thus helping to spare glycogen stores and extend endurance. Several nutritional ingredients, including caffeine, have been explored for their potential role in boosting fat metabolism, thereby helping to spare muscle glycogen and enhance endurance performance.

As the last-resort source of energy, protein can be broken down into amino acids (building blocks of protein) and converted into either glucose or other metabolic intermediates such as acetyal coenzyme A to generate ATP. While most aerobic activity uses minimal amounts of protein for energy, during times of low glycogen availability, such as in the later stages of an endurance event such as the Ironman triathlon, protein can contribute as much as 18% of total energy requirements, thus having implications for recovery. This is one reason protein supplementation has been researched as a plausible addition to intense or high-volume training regimens. The use of protein supplements, taken pre-, during, and posttraining, has been explored by sport scientists for its potential role in sparing muscle glycogen, thereby enhancing endurance performance, stimulating protein synthesis, preventing protein breakdown, and aiding recovery from sport activity.

Cardiovascular Performance

All athletes, regardless of sport, depend on the ability of the heart, blood vessels, and lungs to supply oxygen and energy to working muscles. During training and competition, these demands grow, causing the heart to beat more rapidly and with greater force, the rate of blood flowing through the heart and to the muscles to increase up to 20-fold, and the lungs to fill up with more oxygen. Cardiovascular performance is limited by the ability to keep up with these increased demands and, more specifically, the body's ability to consume oxygen. The need for oxygen is dependent on two key physiological parameters: (1) maximal aerobic capacity and (2) anaerobic threshold.

Maximal Aerobic Capacity

Maximal aerobic capacity, also known as $\dot{V}O_2$max, is defined as the highest rate of oxygen consumption attainable during exhaustive exercise. This rate is supported by the maximum pumping capacity of the heart as well as the ability of the muscles to resist fatigue. Because the body requires oxygen to convert food into energy, the ability to consume large amounts of oxygen facilitates increased energy production for enhanced speed and endurance. Therefore, having a high $\dot{V}O_2$max is like being equipped with the powerful engine of a race car. $\dot{V}O_2$max provides a foundation for overall aerobic potential, making it an important performance variable for endurance sports such as the triathlon, cycling, rowing, distance running, cross-country skiing, and swimming as well as team sports requiring endurance such as soccer, basketball, and hockey.

$\dot{V}O_2$max is often expressed as an absolute rate in liters of oxygen per minute but is more accurately represented as milliliters of oxygen per kilogram of body weight per minute, especially when evaluating differences between men and women. Values of aerobic capacity vary greatly between individuals and even between athletes competing in the same sport due to such factors as genetics, age, training status, sex, and body composition. Male athletes tend to have $\dot{V}O_2$max values 15%-30% higher than female athletes, likely due to differences in body composition since research shows aerobic capacity to decrease with increased body fat. Depending on baseline fitness, physical training can boost aerobic capacity by as much as 20%. Genetics, alone, has been shown to account for 25%-50% of the variance in $\dot{V}O_2$max seen between individuals.

$\dot{V}O_2$max numbers typically range between 2.5 and 6.0 L/min, or 25-94 ml/kg/minute with untrained females and trained elite male endurance athletes falling on the low and high end of the spectrum, respectively. The highest $\dot{V}O_2$max ever recorded was by elite male Nordic skier Bjorn Daehlie at 94 ml/kg/dL, which towers over the average athlete's $\dot{V}O_2$max by 30%-40%. The highest $\dot{V}O_2$max recorded for a female was by a Russian Nordic skier with a measured $\dot{V}O_2$max of 77 ml/kg/min. Table 2.2 displays the aerobic capacities of athletic groups based on sex.

$\dot{V}O_2$max is affected by altitude. Even after allowing for full acclimatization, athletes living, training, or competing at an altitude of sea level to 5,000 feet (1,524 m) should expect about a 5%-7% loss in aerobic capacity; for every 1,000 feet (305 m) of elevation gain above 5,000 feet (1,524 m), expect another 2% drop.

Improving Aerobic Capacity

Athletes wanting to improve maximal oxygen aerobic capacity should focus on increasing the rate of oxygen delivery to and consequent uptake by the muscles. It is well known that training has a profound impact on both. Recently, several nutritional ingredients and supplements, often marketed as oxygen enhancers, have shown promise in providing additional benefit. Research evaluating the impact various nutritional ingredients have on oxygen consumption, both via delivery and uptake, generally looks at one or several of the following five variables:

1. **Cardiac output:** During exertion, an athlete's heart becomes a powerful pump, allowing for more blood, oxygen, and nutrients to be delivered to the working muscles and aiding the elimination of carbon dioxide, lactate, and other metabolic waste products that can exacerbate muscle fatigue and negatively affect performance. The actual amount of blood pumped by the heart each minute is known as cardiac output and is influenced by both stroke volume (the amount of blood that the heart pumps each time it beats) and heart rate (the number of times the heart beats in a minute).

TABLE 2.2 $\dot{V}O_2$max (ml/kg/min) in Various Athletic Groups

Sport	Age (years)	Males	Females
Baseball/Softball	18-32	48-56	52-57
Basketball	18-30	40-60	43-60
Canoeing	22-28	55-67	48-52
Cycling	18-26	62-74	47-57
Football	20-36	42-60	
Gymnastics	18-22	52-58	36-50
Ice hockey	10-30	50-63	
Jockey	20-40	50-60	
Orienteering	20-60	47-53	46-60
Racquetball	20-35	55-62	50-60
Rowing	20-35	60-72	58-65
Skiing, alpine	18-30	57-68	50-55
Skiing, Nordic	20-28	65-94	60-77
Ski jumping	18-24	58-63	
Soccer	22-28	54-64	50-60
Speed skating	18-24	56-73	44-55
Swimming	10-25	50-70	40-60
Track and field, discus	22-30	42-55	
Track and field, running	18-39	60-85	50-75
	40-75	40-60	35-60
Track and field, shot put	22-30	40-46	
Volleyball	18-22		40-56
Weightlifting	20-30	38-52	
Wrestling	20-30	52-65	

Adapted, by permission, from J.H. Wilmore and D.L. Costill, 2005, *Physiology of sport and exercise*, 3rd ed., Champaign, IL: Human Kinetics, 95.

At rest, cardiac output for adults averages about 5-8 L/min, but for elite-level endurance athletes competing in cross-country skiing, this can increase to an amazing 40 L/min.

Nutrition and Cardiac Output

Athletes following healthy diets that are low in saturated fats and rich in whole grains, fruits, and vegetables can help protect against plaque buildup in the arteries that leads to blockages and restricted blood flow that negatively affect cardiac output. In addition, several ingredients, such as nitric oxide found in beetroot, can help dilate the blood vessels and allow for greater blood flow to the working muscles during exercise.

2. **Blood volume:** Defined as the total volume of fluid, including red blood cells and plasma that circulates through the heart, arteries, and capillaries, blood volume is closely regulated by the kidneys. A boost in blood volume, naturally seen with physical training and further enhanced with heat and altitude acclimatization, occurs as a result of increases in antidiuretic hormones, aldosterone, and the plasma protein albumin. The primary benefits are enhanced oxygen transport abilities and consequent improvements in endurance performance and muscle recovery. A typical adult maintains a blood volume of 4.7-5 L, with blood levels for females slightly lower. An elite-level endurance athlete may have blood levels as much as 30% higher than those of the average adult.

Banned Substance Alert

EPO (erythropoietin and plasma expanders, which help boost blood volume and red blood cell production, are prohibited substances in athletic competitions worldwide. Testing positive would immediately disqualify the athlete and lead to a temporary ban from competition.

3. **Hemoglobin:** This is a protein in red blood cells that carries oxygen. Healthy levels fall between 13.8 and 7.2 gm/dL for men and between 12.1 and 15.1 gm/dL for women. Slightly lower levels in athletes, especially those engaged in endurance training and competition, are common and generally are caused by a phenomenon known as sport anemia, or pseudoanemia. The expansion of plasma volume resulting from aerobic training reduces the concentration of red blood cells that carry hemoglobin. Despite a reduced concentration of red blood cells, the rise in plasma volume actually aids oxygen delivery to the muscles. Levels significantly lower than the norm, however, may indicate excessive fluid intake or a nutritional deficiency in iron, folate, vitamin B_{12}, or vitamin B_6, all of which can negatively affect cardiovascular performance.

4. **Mitochondrial density and enzyme levels:** Deep inside muscle fibers are microscopic structures called mitochondria, also known as powerhouses due to the role they play in energy production. The number of mitochondria present within the muscle, or mitochondrial density, increases in response to calcium ion levels rising during muscle contraction and ATP levels failing to keep up with demands in skeletal muscle cells during exercise. Training, especially endurance-focused activity, not only helps to improve mitochondrial density but also facilitates an increased number of oxidative enzymes available to break down glucose, fat molecules, and certain amino acids before combining with oxygen to produce ATP energy for muscle contraction and other cellular functions. This adaptation in trained muscle allows for more

fats to be used to generate ATP, thereby helping to spare muscle glycogen, critical for reaching peak endurance potential.

5. **Capillary density:** Improving capillary density, the number of tiny blood vessels within each muscle cell, aids the distribution of oxygen- and nutrient-rich blood to the muscles; doing so also aids the clearance of lactate from the fast-twitch (Type IIa and Type IIb) muscle fibers and into the slow-twitch (Type I) muscle fibers for processing fuel, thereby reducing muscle fatigue, aiding muscle recovery, and maximizing endurance potential.

Anaerobic Endurance

Thought to be a better predictor of performance than aerobic capacity, anaerobic endurance refers to the ability of an athlete to sustain a maximum level of work in the absence of or with limited amounts of oxygen. Anaerobic endurance is a relevant performance variable for stop-and-go sports requiring intense bursts of energy: soccer, basketball, football, tennis, boxing, and hockey, among others; it also applies to certain styles of weightlifting when the goal is to keep the time between sets as short as possible. It becomes a relevant factor for endurance athletes competing in events such as a cycle or running race where a response to an opponent's attack needs to be quickly countered (e.g., sprint to the finish line).

During anaerobic activity, which involves rapid contraction of fast-twitch muscle fibers, the demand for oxygen and fuel exceed the rate of supply, triggering a shift of focus from aerobic to anaerobic metabolism. For the first 10-20 seconds of anaerobic activity, energy is generated from stored ATP and the creatine phosphate (CP) energy system; beyond that, muscle glycogen breakdown and glycolysis provide additional energy. Unlike the aerobic fuel tank, however, whose energy supply can last hours, the anaerobic fuel tank can only supply enough energy for physical exertions lasting up to a few minutes before the fuel runs out or clearance of fatigue-inducing byproducts, specifically lactate, fails to keep up with their production, a state known as lactate or anaerobic threshold (LT).

Nutrition and Anaerobic Endurance

There are several dietary supplements that have demonstrated promise in aiding anaerobic endurance, including creatine, which helps build total body creatine stores, and buffering agents such as bicarbonate, phosphate, and more recently beta-alanine. These ingredients can help increase cellular and blood pH by countering the effects of hydrogen ion accumulation and consequent muscle fatigue during high-intensity training and competition.

Recreational athletes typically hit their LT near 65%-80% of their $\dot{V}O_2max$, whereas elite and world-class endurance athletes tend to peak at 85%-95%

of their $\dot{V}O_2$max. This allows professional athletes such as Haile Gebrselassie to hold a strong pace for longer distances, including the marathon.

Improving Anaerobic Endurance

To improve anaerobic endurance, an athlete should focus on increasing (1) the amounts of ATP and CP on hand, (2) the amount of glycogen available for breakdown, and (3) lactate tolerance and clearance ability of the muscle. These can be achieved through incorporation of interval training (e.g., 100 m sprint repeats) into any exercise or training program. Such high-intensity efforts help improve the activity of glycolytic enzymes such as phosphofructokinase (PFK) and hexokinase (HK), important for better muscle-force generation and sustained contractions during exertion.

Muscle Performance

Many sports require an athlete to be explosive and powerful. Athletes are required to accelerate and decelerate rapidly, change direction quickly and efficiently, jump maximally, swing or throw as hard as possible, and maintain this maximal performance for an extended period. Strength, power, and work capacity are key variables that can influence an athlete's ability to perform all of these tasks.

Strength, Power, and Hypertrophy

Muscle strength can be defined as the maximal amount of force that a muscle or muscle group can generate. It is not to be confused with muscle power, which is a product of both force and the speed or velocity at which force can be generated. A common misconception is the idea that the strongest athlete will be the fastest or most explosive. While this is not the case, it is true that a physically stronger athlete will be a faster and *more* explosive athlete. Therefore, developing strength is an essential performance variable. Many athletes engage in structured weight-training programs in the off-season that target maximizing strength before the competitive season begins.

Power is the ability to generate a large amount of force quickly. As the speed of movement increases, the amount of force that the muscle is capable of producing decreases. As the speed of movement slows, the muscle is capable of producing more force, and maximal force is produced at slower speeds. This is the disconnect between strength, or maximal force, and power. A sprinter has only 0.15-0.18 seconds to apply as much force as possible to the ground while running. If the muscle isn't well trained to apply force as quickly as possible, it will be difficult for training to carry over into the event. Strength and power are developed through physiological and neurological changes to the muscle. Physiologically, through training, the entire muscle can increase in size, including the cross-sectional area of the muscle and the density of muscle fibers within. A larger, denser muscle results in an improvement in strength and power. These changes are largely influenced by the endocrine system. During exercise, a cascade of hormonal events takes place. Amounts of stress and catabolic hormones—those that induce the breakdown of larger molecules into smaller ones (cortisol, epinephrine, and norepinephrine)—increase to meet the demands of the training event. Cortisol, epinephrine, and norepinephrine act catabolically to break down carbohydrate, fat, and protein stores; they also act on the nervous system to increase motor unit and muscle fiber recruitment. A motor unit simply refers to a motor neuron and the muscle fibers it connects. Activation of more motor units, and consequently more muscle fibers, will increase the number of active fibers contributing to the development of muscle contraction and force. Build-up of these catabolic hormones is followed by a response of anabolic hormones, including testosterone, growth hormone, and IGF1 (insulin-like growth factor 1) that act on the muscle to initiate anabolic muscle-building and recovery responses. Anabolic hormones spark increases in the rates of protein synthesis, or muscle building. This process of creating a larger, denser muscle is known as hypertrophy, and these changes elicit improvements in the muscle's strength and power capabilities. Hypertrophy is a common goal for bodybuilders, who are trying to create the best, biggest, and most aesthetic-looking muscles. The development of sports supplements has been strongly influenced by bodybuilding, and although many sports supplements are targeted toward bodybuilders, they are also used by other athletes hoping to build lean body mass.

Another common misconception is that the only way to have stronger and more powerful muscles is for them to get bigger. The majority of changes in strength and power are actually the result of neurological changes. The body is complex and requires many muscle fibers and motor units working together to produce force. Each muscle is made up of thousands of muscle fibers and several motor units. Various muscle fibers are grouped together to make up a motor unit. The speed at which these motor units are activated, the number of muscle fibers innervated within each motor unit, and the synchronization of motor units within the same muscle and other muscles working together all affect muscle performance. Some of the neurological changes that take place through training include the following:

- An increase in the number of muscle fibers that contract simultaneously. Based on neurological signals, your brain recruits and activates more muscle fibers to contract. By applying resistance and requiring the muscle to develop more force, the body will adapt neurologically and signal more muscle fibers to contract.

- Increase in the rate of contraction of muscle fibers. The faster the muscle is able to contract and develop force, the more power it will produce.

- Improved efficiency and synchronization of firing muscle fibers. Through adaptation to training, the muscle fibers become more efficient and operate in sync.
- Decreased inhibition of antagonistic muscle fibers. During a leg extension where the quadriceps are the primary moving muscle, the hamstrings contract and inhibit leg extension. Training lessens this degree of inhibition.
- Improved efficiency of stretch reflexes controlling muscle tension. You've probably heard the analogy that your muscles are like a rubber band: The farther they are stretched, the faster and more forcefully they contract in the opposite direction. This stretch reflex can be trained, improving its efficiency and the amount of force and speed at which muscle fibers contract.
- Improved conduction velocity and excitation threshold of nerve fibers. This involves the speed at which neural signals activate motor units and the amount of muscle fibers activated with each signal.

A muscle function icon will be used in chapter 3 to identify certain sports supplements that target improving these neurological functions and produce gains in power and strength.

Speed and Strength Endurance

Athletes who engage in sports requiring repetitive periods of maximal effort, such as sprinting to defend a goal, sliding defensively in a basketball game, or resisting an opponent in a wrestling match, require anaerobic endurance. Most athletes understand the concept of specificity of training, which centers on training the body as specifically as possible for the demands of a particular sport. An athlete's ability to sprint repeatedly during a football game or soccer match requires metabolic efficiency and fitness. Athletes must be capable of clearing the fatigue-inducing byproducts of high-intensity muscle contraction, such as lactate and hydrogen ions, during recovery sessions and rest periods. In addition, athletes require a well-trained neuromuscular system that is capable of resisting fatigue and maintaining the muscles' ability to develop peak force and power. Lowered muscle glycogen levels negatively affect the neuromuscular system, which requires athletes in prolonged strength and power sports to maximize glycogen before competition and prevent its depletion during competition to ensure peak performance. Dietary supplements such as caffeine and the amino acids taurine and tyrosine are thought to prevent neuromuscular fatigue and improve speed and strength endurance.

Psychological Function

When evaluating the dynamics of sport performance, the focus is often on the cardiovascular and muscle systems. Yet it's the athlete's brain that acts as the control center for many of the body processes that propel performance, making the brain an essential component of athletic success. Athletes must make quick decisions on the field and have mind-muscle connection in order to optimize performance. Feeding the brain with specific nutrients and supplements can help enhance reaction time, balance, dexterity, focus, visual acuity, speed, strength, endurance, and confidence. For example, a current supplement energy drink called Nawgan is described as an alertness beverage and is advertised as "what to drink when you want to think." It contains an ingredient known as citicoline, which contains a combination of cytidine and choline. Choline has a role in the production of acetylcholine, an important neurotransmitter that affects the peripheral nervous system (muscle contraction) and the central nervous system (arousal and sensory perceptions). Other dietary supplements such as ginkgo biloba (see entry in chapter 3) also claim to improve cognitive performance. The mechanisms of ginkgo are less understood but may involve a neural protective effect on the central nervous system. Tyrosine, which is a nonessential amino acid, may also affect the central nervous system and the brain's perception of fatigue and motivation. For sports requiring a high level of hand-eye coordination and quick decision making, including baseball, basketball, and tennis, these types of supplements are appealing and potentially offer a competitive advantage.

Hydration

When it comes to performance decline in athletes, dehydration, defined as the excessive loss of body fluid, including both water and electrolytes, is a common culprit. With 60%-70% of total body mass and 70%-75% of muscle mass comprised of fluid, it is not hard to understand why. Maintenance of fluid balance is key to optimal cardiovascular, thermoregulatory, central nervous system, and metabolic functioning as disruptions can alter physical performance by reducing blood volume, decreasing skin blood flow, decreasing heat dissipation, increasing core body temperature, and increasing the rate of muscle glycogen use. A mere 2% loss of body weight can start to negatively affect performance with such symptoms as cessation of sweating, muscle cramps, nausea, vomiting, lightheadedness, weakness, heart palpitations, and decreased urine output, with urine color a dark yellow to burnt orange.

How this translates with respect to athletic performance was clearly defined in a research study evaluating the impact dehydration at levels up to 2% has on running speed for 1,500, 5,000, and 10,000 m (Armstrong et al., 1985). Just a 1% change in body mass correlated with adding 0.17, 0.39, and 1.59 minutes to 1,500, 5,000, and 10,000 m finish times. A 2% decline in body mass lead to a further reduction in speed ranging from just over 3% for the 1,500 m to well over 6% for the 5,000 and 10,000 m in comparison to performance when the runners were in a state of fluid balance. As losses start to approach and then exceed 5%, the capacity for work can decrease by as much as 30%. Dehydration becomes life threatening when 10%-20% of body weight is lost. While endurance athletes and team sport athletes engaged in training and competition for 2 or more hours are at greatest risk for the performance detriments associated with dehydration, there is evidence that the capacity to perform high-intensity exercise of short duration (e.g., sprinting) can drop by as much as 4%-5% with prior dehydration equivalent to only 2.5% of body weight (Sawka et al., 1985). The cumulative impact of dehydration can be devastating for any athlete, but is especially relevant for athletes competing in several short-duration events over a period of several hours to several days. Imagine reaching the 100 m final of an important track meet only to experience a 45% decline in performance capacity!

Monitoring Hydration

It is estimated that during exertion, the average athlete will lose 1-2 lbs (0.45-0.90 kg) of body weight each hour. During exertion in extreme environmental conditions, such as heat and humidity, sweat rate can easily double. To protect against performance and health declines associated with disturbances in important physiological functions, athletes should target drinking fluids at the rate losses occur via sweating. Unfortunately, research has shown that the volume of fluid that most athletes choose to drink voluntarily during exercise replaces less than one-half of their fluid losses, making dehydration, especially during prolonged training and competition, a legitimate concern for athletes as well as the team of coaches, trainers, and parents supporting them. Furthermore, extreme environmental conditions may produce a rate of loss that exceeds what is tolerated by an athlete or physically absorbed by the body. Nonetheless, by calculating sweat rate (see figure 2.1), the athlete's team of coaches and trainers can devise a drinking protocol to help minimize the health and performance detriments of dehydration.

Preventing Dehydration

Continual access to fluid during training and competition can sometimes present a challenge and certain environmental factors—heat, humidity, and altitude—can increase fluid needs to a level beyond what the body can often physically absorb. As a result, many athletes practice heat acclimatization and use nutritional strategies to help maximize fluid uptake, improve hydration status, and protect against the undesirable performance and health declines of dehydration.

Heat Acclimatization

Consistent exposure to heat and humidity through training or living promotes several physiological adaptations that can be extremely advantageous to

---

Testing Protocol

1. Measure preexercise nude weight.
2. Measure fluids consumed during exercise.
3. Measure urine volume in ounces (if possible) during exercise.
4. Measure postexercise nude weight.
5. Make note of total exercise time in hours (e.g., 0.5 hour, 1.5 hours) and any other relevant data such as exercise intensity and environmental conditions.

Calculation

1. Subtract postworkout weight from preworkout weight (in pounds) and multiply by 16 ounces.
2. Subtract total volume of urine (ounces).
3. Add total volume of fluids (ounces) consumed during exercise.
4. Divide by exercise time to determine hourly sweat rate in fluid ounces.

An online calculator is available at www.triharder.com/THM_SwRate. aspx, which can be used with English or metric measurements.

FIGURE 2.1 Sweat-rate calculation.

the athlete as well as comforting to parents and coaches who may be concerned about an athlete's risk for heat injury. These positive adaptations include a boost in blood volume, which assures that the body can meet the demand for blood supply by the muscles and skin, and enhanced sweating ability, which includes a faster onset of sweating, greater distribution of sweat over the body, and an increase in sweat rate. To help conserve fluid, the body also becomes more efficient in retaining sodium, thereby lowering the concentration of the mineral in sweat. Full acclimatization takes time to complete, about 10-14 days, although some benefits are seen as soon as 4-5 days.

Nutritional Strategies

Enhancing fluid uptake is dependent on the rate at which fluid is emptied from the stomach into the small intestine for absorption into the bloodstream. Carbohydrates and electrolytes are two key ingredients that help increase fluid uptake, which is one reason health professionals often recommend sport drinks as a better fluid choice than water during longer training sessions and competition. The concentration of carbohydrates, however, is important, with optimal levels for uptake at 4%-6%; this means that the drink should contain approximately 15-20 g of carbohydrate/8 oz (15-20 g of carbohydrate/240 mL). The inclusion of electrolytes, especially sodium and potassium, facilitates intestinal absorption of water. Finally, the osmolality, or the total concentration of particles or nutrients in a sport drink, including carbohydrate and electrolytes, plays a role in fluid uptake. Levels that are equal (isotonic) or marginally lower (hypotonic) than that found in blood (275-299 milliosmoles/kg), are ideal for fluid uptake. Some sport drink companies, like Infinit Nutrition (www.infinitnutrition.com), even provide an osmolality calculator to help an athlete create a custom blend that is optimal for fluid uptake and performance.

When leading up to as well as during competition, especially when battling heat or humidity, many athletes follow a nutritional practice known as salt loading, using liquids such as broth or pickle juice with electrolyte supplements to bring in more sodium. The goal is protection against the muscle cramping and fatigue associated with dehydration. One study found that supplementation with a highly concentrated sodium beverage prior to running to exhaustion at 70% of $\dot{V}O_2$max in a hot environment helped athletes maintain a higher blood volume, lower core body temperature, and lower level of perceived exertion than when they consumed a low-sodium beverage before running (Sims et al., 2007). Because sodium affects the osmolality of a solution, extremely high levels of sodium are generally not recommended for consumption during training and competition. Salt-loading protocols for precompetition entail consuming from 0.5 to 1 g of sodium per hour with fluids in the 2-3 hours prior to starting training or an event. (Note that it is important not to consume 2 g in one acute dose.) This can easily be achieved through high-sodium food or sipping on a sport drink with added electrolytes prior to competition.

A final practice used by many athletes to aid hydration during competition is hyperhydration, most commonly done through an intake of large volumes of fluid in the days and hours leading up to competition. While taking in large volumes of fluid does indeed speed the release of fluid from the gut into the small intestine for absorption, this practice can backfire if fluids consumed beyond absorption start to alter the normal balance of electrolytes, sodium in particular, in the body. Low blood sodium, also known as hyponatremia, most commonly affects female endurance athletes; symptoms initially manifesting themselves as headache, muscle weakness, confusion, nausea, vomiting, irritability, and drowsiness.

Short- and Long-Term Recovery

Training for strength and endurance athletes involves stressing the body through planned training, allowing recovery and adaptation of the body. Various types of stress are used to elicit specific adaptations such as changes in strength, power, speed, lactic acid threshold, or oxidative capacity. While the actual training or stress is important, the often overlooked aspect is rest and recovery. Without adequate recovery the body is unable to adapt to the training stress; the athlete does not improve and ultimately becomes overtrained—a state all athletes must work hard and train smart to avoid. Many sports supplements are designed to either enhance or shorten the window of time needed for recovery. The recovery process is complex and involves many body systems working together, including the neuromuscular, metabolic, endocrine, immune, and antioxidant defense systems. Some sports supplements include one or two active ingredients that target a specific system while others might include five or more active ingredients, with claims that they assist many systems in the recovery process. Many types of supplements can be used for short- and long-term recovery. Some focus on the early window of recovery immediately postworkout (1-4 hours) while others target shortening the longer-term recovery windows of 48-72 hours. Additionally, labeling may suggest the supplement can improve sleep quality and enhance muscle recovery during sleep.

- **Neuromuscular system:** The functioning of this system affects strength and power, making adequate recovery of this system essential. Of all the systems involved in recovery, this system might be one of the least understood. Communication between the central nervous system and the peripheral nervous system signals muscle contraction and movement. The number of muscle fibers and motor units recruited, in addition to the speed of contraction and amount of force the muscle can produce, are dependent upon adequate recovery of this system. There are ways to measure neuromuscular function, but research has been limited related to the impact that nutritional supplements or other nonnutrition recovery modalities may have.

- **Metabolic system:** The production of ATP is influenced by the form of exercise an athlete engages in as well as the availability of energy substrates such as phosphocreatine and glycogen stores. The number of energy systems used for sports make it clear that the availability of substrates such as creatine phosphate and muscle glycogen are needed to provide ATP and allow the muscle to function at peak performance. Restoration of these substrates is another key piece for optimal recovery. Muscles also undergo depletion of fuel stores; those stores must be restored before adequate performance can be ensured in the next training session or event. For anaerobic, or strength and power, athletes these stores include creatine phosphate and glycogen. Carbohydrates or glycogen stores are the only fuels that can be used anaerobically by muscle; therefore, sports that require lots of high-intensity (e.g., sprinting, jumping, those that involve changes of direction) will tap into and quickly deplete glycogen and creatine phosphate. Muscle glycogen is also important for the endurance athlete as low glycogen stores consistently prove to limit performance. Certain supplements are claimed to enhance the restoration of muscle glycogen and creatine phosphate stores, therefore speeding recovery. Supplements containing special formulations and types of carbohydrates are becoming popular; in addition, many supplement companies manufacture specialized formulations of creatine that the companies claim are superior to those of other competitors.

- **Endocrine system:** The endocrine system is a complex system of glands that secrete a variety of hormones in response to exercise and in periods of recovery following exercise. Hormones such as cortisol, epinephrine, norepinephrine, testosterone, growth hormone, and IGF-1 (insulin-like growth factor 1) are all included in this complex system. The catabolic hormones (cortisol, epinephrine, norepinephrine) drive the breakdown of fat, glycogen stores, and protein. These hormones allow the body to respond to the stressful demands of exercise. More stressful exercise or training sessions will elicit greater release of these catabolic hormones. Anabolic hormones (testosterone, growth hormone, and IGF-1) are also released during exercise and throughout the recovery phase following exercise. These anabolic hormones can initiate protein synthesis, begin the restoration of carbohydrate stores, and signal the adaptation of muscle and the neuromuscular system to training. The balance between these catabolic and anabolic hormones is an important concept for athletes to understand. Constant exposure to stressful training (high volumes of work at high intensities) will drive up a catabolic response. If an appropriate period of recovery is not allowed, these catabolic hormones will dominate and push the body into an overtrained state in which increased risk of injury and poor performance persists. However, if adequate nutrients, sleep, and rest are provided, the anabolic response will dominate, giving the body time to recover; adapt to the training stress; and become stronger, more powerful, or develop greater resistance to fatigue. Supplements such as branched-chain amino acids, protein powders, and specialized carbohydrates are claimed to affect muscle recovery in the early recovery window (1-4 hours) following training. Others, including amino acids arginine and ornithine, herbal supplements, icariin, ecdysteroids, chrysin, and astralagus are claimed to naturally increase levels of anabolic hormones. Another group of minerals that includes zinc and amino acids (e.g., melatonin, GABA) are claimed to improve the quality of sleep and recovery during sleep. Some supplements are claimed to enhance the release of anabolic hormones during sleep or improve neuromuscular recovery during sleep.

- **Immune system:** Within the past 20 years, it has become evident that the immune and antioxidant defense systems play a role in development, recovery, and health of athletes. In general, exercise in moderate duration and intensity enhances immune function. However, exercise of longer duration and higher intensity negatively affects and suppresses immune function. As a result, athletes must do everything possible to limit immune suppression and keep the immune system functioning. Colds, flu, and upper respiratory tract infections will hinder an athlete's progress, negatively affect training, and result in poor performance. In addition, the immune system has a role in the recovery process of muscle. Proteins of the immune system, known as cytokines, assist in the antiinflammatory and healing process of muscle, providing another reason for athletes to do everything possible to maintain healthy immune function. A variety of herbal ingredients, vitamins, minerals, and amino acids are promoted as strengthening or providing support to the immune system.

• **Antioxidant defense system:** Antioxidants are another group of nutrients that have been given much media attention in recent years. All types of stress, exercise included, produce free radicals. Free radicals damage healthy cells throughout the body. Antioxidants are the nutrients that neutralize and dispose of free radicals before they can damage cells. Fortunately, our bodies are equipped with built-in antioxidant defense systems. A common misconception is that dietary sources of antioxidants are the only defense against free radicals. This is not true; in fact, our most powerful defenses are naturally built into the cell. The added physical stresses of training will expose athletes to higher levels of free radicals, and supplements are marketed to protect athletes against them. Vitamins A, E, and C; minerals such as selenium and zinc; and natural components in foods and spices such as resveratrol, quercetin, curcuminoids, ginger, and cinnamon are all touted as powerful antioxidants thought to further protect athletes and their cells from free radicals.

• **Joint support:** Maintaining healthy joints and avoiding chronic joint pain or injury is important for athletes of all ages. Nothing can disrupt training and alter improvements in performance more than chronic pain or a lingering injury that prevents an athlete from training at 100%. One of the most common minor injuries seen in athletes is arthritis, or joint inflammation. Athletes involved in sports requiring repetitive throwing or swinging—baseball, softball, and tennis, among others—often experience arthritis of the elbow, shoulder, or wrist; athletes in sports requiring lots of running and changes of direction often experience inflammation of the knees or hips. A branch of the sports supplement industry has targeted this concern of athletes, the aging, and the inactive, all of whom commonly experience arthritis. Triple Flex, SomaFlex, and Move Free are current names of supplements that target this issue. Degeneration of the connective tissues, or cartilage, within joints is a common cause of inflammation that can result in joint pain. Promotional materials for popular supplements such as chondroitin and glucosamine suggest these nutrients can assist in preserving cartilage and prevent degeneration, limiting pain and dysfunction. Unique forms of proteins that comprise joint tissue are often bottled and packaged as supplements, focusing on the belief that ingesting these components will improve the production of tissue within the joint. The supplements hyaluronic acid and glycosylated undenatured type II collagen (UC-II) are examples. In addition, foods, particularly healthy fats and fatty fish or fish oil supplements, are proving to provide some powerful antiinflammatory effects that are postulated to benefit joint pain and potentially provide relief. Nutrients found in fruits, vegetables, herbs, and spices also have antiinflammatory power. Bromelain (a component of pineapple), the Indian spice turmeric, and ginger root are just a few examples. Many of these nutrients are being bottled in pill and powdered form and sold as dietary supplements. The protection of healthy joints is multifaceted and requires athletes to train smart: avoid overtraining, eat right, and optimize rest and recovery.

Weight and Body Composition

If a group of athletes were asked what they would most like to change about themselves to improve performance, chances are one of the most popular answers would involve losing body fat or improving body composition. However, a common misperception of athletes is that leaner or leanest is always best. All athletes are genetically different in terms of body types and body composition. There is not a single equation for body composition. Altering body composition is dependent on energy and calorie intake. Athletes must train when in an energy- or calorie-restricted state to tap into body fat stores and change body composition. For some athletes, severe calorie restriction is required to reach and maintain a lean body composition. This type of restriction will negatively affect performance. Athletes must be wise about making attempts to alter body composition. Body composition should be a focus during off-season training when peak performance is not required.

Athletes are motivated to alter or improve body composition for a number of reasons. It is a simple thought, but a decrease in body fat essentially means that an athlete will be running, jumping, swimming, and changing direction with less mass or weight to move. For example, a male athlete who weighs 165 lbs (74.8 kg) and has 10% body fat carries 16.5 lbs (7.5 kg) of adipose tissue, or body fat. If the athlete reduces his body fat to 7%, he has lowered his fat mass to approximately 11.5 lbs (5.2 kg); his body can move more efficiently with less body fat. Athletes whose movement is more efficient or economical will accomplish the same objective with less energy. A leaner athlete moving with less body fat will be more efficient and expend less energy doing the same task as someone who is carrying more body fat. In addition, athletes such as high jumpers or sprinters want to maximize strength:mass ratios in order to optimize their performance. Maintenance of strength and power is key while minimizing body weight or mass. If strength is lost along with mass, improvements in performance will not be realized.

The desire for athletes to be leaner, along with a need for many nonathletes to lose weight, has created an explosion of fat-burning and weight-loss supplements. These supplements are one of the most popular types of products on the market. A recent search of a popular online sports supplement store found nearly 200 names and brands of so-called fat burners available for purchase. Unfortunately, fat burners and weight-loss supplements are also some of the most dangerous: They often contain potent stimulants much more powerful than caffeine that can affect cardiovascular function and result in death. Extreme caution should be used when choosing these products. Another concern is that these supplements are often adulterated and tainted with ingredients or pharmaceutical drugs not listed on labels that may have powerful (often harmful) effects on the body.

Most fat burners and weight-loss supplements can be assigned to one of three categories:

- Stimulant based: These contain stimulants such as caffeine, epineph-rine, synephrine, guarna, and many others. Product claims include the ability to speed up resting metabolic rate and burn fat.

- Appetite suppressants: These include *Hoodia gordonii* and others that assist in controlling appetite and limiting calorie intake.

- Fat malabsorptive: These ingredients limit the amount of fat absorbed during digestion, resulting in lowered calorie intake. Chitosan, which is a structural element found in the shell of crabs, shrimp, and lobster, is a popular ingredient found in weight-loss supplements due to its speculated ability to bind fat and prevent its absorption. These types of products can have some undesirable side effects such as loose stools and diarrhea. In addition, their use will also limit the absorption of fat-soluble vitamins, healthy fats, and essential fatty acids need for optimal function.

Summary

Each performance variable must be optimized for an athlete to reach his or her potential. Balancing and managing these variables through proper train-ing, rest and recovery, nutrition, and the use of appropriate sports supple-ments when recommended is key. Chapter 3 addresses the supplements available to athletes. This information will assist athletes in understanding how each supplements works to enhance the performance variables dis-cussed in this chapter.

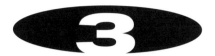

A-to-Z
Supplement Guide

The supplement entries use the symbols listed in the following table to easily identify the supplements that have been proven to be beneficial or possibly beneficial for the corresponding performance variables. If a supplement has been proven to be beneficial for a particular performance variable, the supplement entry is marked with a black symbol; if the research shows that a supplement is possibly beneficial, the entry is marked with a gray version of the corresponding symbol.

Performance variable	Components included	Symbol
Fuel usage		
Cardiovascular function	Aerobic capacity Anaerobic endurance	
Muscular function	Strength and power Speed and strength endurance	
Psychological function	Concentration and focus Motivation	
Hydration status	Fluid balance Electrolyte balance	
Recovery	Short term: glycogen repletion rehydration Long term: immunity, Joint, tendon, and muscle health	
Weight and body composition	Lean body mass gains Body fat losses	

Aaron's Rod

(see *Rhodiola rosea*)

Acai Berry

aka *Euterpe olearacea, açaï d'Amazonie, acai extract, acai fruit, acai palm*

What it is: Containing approximately 70 calories per 3.5 oz (99 g) serving, acai is a small, reddish-purple berry found on a breed of palm tree called *Euterpe oleracea* that grows in Central and South America. Acai contains phytonutrients called anthocyanins that have antioxidant properties and, like other fruit, are a good source of dietary fiber. Touted as a superfood that promotes weight loss, enhances immune function, and reduces inflammation, acai is commonly sold in the consumer market as frozen pulp or juice, as well as added to beverages, smoothies, and foods available in supplement form.

How it works: Acai's mechanism of action is unclear, but it is thought that the antioxidant qualities of anthocyanin play a role in limiting the production of unstable molecules called free radicals. This protects the body's cells from damage during heightened periods of stress, including exercise stress, and may lend the athlete protection against excessive inflammatory stress and immune breakdown that can put a damper on performance.

Performance benefit: It is purported that acai may help reduce inflammation and enhance immune function, thereby helping an athlete maintain his or her health during intense cycles of training. When consumed as part of a diet rich in fruits and vegetables, acai may help support weight loss as well.

Research: While the antioxidants in acai are thought to provide some of its beneficial qualities, it is estimated that less than 5% of the anthocyanins contained within the acai berry are actually absorbed into the human body. A human trial demonstrated an improvement in absorption rate when acai was consumed in pulp or juice form, but the small subject size makes the validity of the results questionable (Mertens-Talcott et al., 2008). Interestingly, some animal evidence has attributed the immune-boosting qualities of acai to its polysaccharide (chains of sugar found within the plant) content rather than its anthocyanin content (Holderness et al., 2011). It is evident that more well-designed research on human subjects should be conducted to confirm a mechanism of action and produce any valid recommendations for use. Indeed, the current consensus by health experts is that beyond including the berry as part of a diet rich and fruits and vegetables, there is no unbiased scientific evidence to support the notion that supplementation with acai in any form will promote weight loss, reduce inflammation, or do anything significant to enhance the health or performance of humans.

Common usage: Antioxidants within the pulp and juice of the acai plant are absorbed better by the body and can be included as part of a healthful diet rich in fruits and vegetables. Supplements are currently not recommended due to lack of scientific support.

Health concerns: Acai berry, consumed in whole fruit form, is likely safe though the long-term safety of supplement use has yet to be confirmed.

Acetate Replacing Factor

(see *alpha-lipoic acid*)

Acetyl-L-Carnitine (ALC or ALCAR)

What it is: Acetyl-L-carnitine (ALCAR) is a derivative of the amino acid L-carnitine. It is produced naturally in the brain, liver, and kidneys and is known to facilitate the uptake of acetyl CoA into the mitochondria during fatty acid oxidation, enhance acetylcholine production, and stimulate protein and membrane phospholipid synthesis (Scafidi, 2010).

How it works: The ergogenic application of ALCAR supplementation for athletes is unknown. No studies have evaluated the effectiveness of ALCAR in a healthy population of athletes. Despite limited research ALCAR is commonly found in a wide variety of nutritional supplements targeted toward athletes. ALCAR claims to provide a wide range of benefits, including enhancing energy production, increasing testosterone levels, improving mood and cognitive function, and increasing fat oxidation. ALCAR is speculated to improve energy production in the muscles via its facilitation of acetyl CoA uptake. ALCAR may have a neuromuscular mechanism related to its enhancement of acetylcholine production and ability to reduce oxidative stress of the neuromuscular system ("Acetyl-L-Carnitine Monograph," 2010).

Performance benefit: For athletes, supplementation may improve energy production through enhanced mitochondrial energy production. Additionally, ALCAR may have the ability to enhance neuromuscular function and recovery from training. Neuronal benefits could improve strength, force, and power production for all athletes. Lastly, ALCAR could help reduce the oxidative stress associated with exercise and speed recovery.

Research: There are no scientific studies evaluating any of these proposed benefits. The only research studies available are related to the effectiveness of ALCAR in disease states. Results of these experiments are generally positive. ALCAR has been able to slow the progression and deterioration of cognitive function in those suffering from Alzheimer's (Kobayashi et al., 2010). ALCAR is beneficial in treating some of the severity and symptoms associated with peripheral neuropathy, a condition experienced by diabetics

>*continued*

Acetyl-L-Carnitine (ALCAR) >*continued*

as well as cancer patients receiving chemotherapy and HIV patients using various drugs for treatment ("Acetyl-L-Carnitine Monograph," 2010)

Common usage: Studies in disease-state populations have used a dosage of 1-3 g of ALCAR daily. Multiple strategies, including 500 mg provided 2 times daily and 1,000 mg provided 3 times daily, have been employed; divided dosages are recommended. A best or most effective approach to supplementation has not been found; however, 1 g appears to be the minimum and 3 g the maximum recommended ("Acetyl-L-Carnitine Monograph," 2010).

Health concerns: ALCAR is considered safe, even with long-term supplementation (i.e, 1 year). Noted adverse reactions include agitation, nausea, and vomiting ("Acetyl-L-Carnitine Monograph," 2010).

Acetylcysteine

aka *N-acetylcysteine, NAC*

What it is: A derivative of the amino acid L-cysteine, which is produced naturally by the body, acetylcysteine (NAC) is marketed as an antioxidant that may protect an athlete against skeletal muscle fatigue.

How it works: Production of reactive oxygen species (ROS), often called free radicals, during muscle contraction is associated with muscle fatigue and damage in the short term as well as favorable adaptive responses, specifically a stronger natural antioxidant defense system, in the long term. However, this positive adaptation may not be great enough to offset the accumulation of ROS during heavy periods of training and competition, especially for athletes just returning to training or the weekend warrior who accumulates the bulk of training over 1-3 days, ultimately leading to diminished performance capacity. It is thought that supplementation with acetylcysteine increases the body's antioxidant capacity, and in particular an antioxidant compound called glutathione, within the muscles, thereby preventing against muscle fatigue and damage that can otherwise hurt performance and recovery.

Performance benefit: Athletes may benefit from enhanced protection against muscle fatigue, helping extend endurance during both high- and low-intensity training and competition. An acute dose of 1,800 mg has been shown to reduce respiratory fatigue during high-intensity exercise, helping to extend endurance.

Research: There are conflicting views on the efficacy of antioxidant supplementation, especially at high doses over the long term, for trained athletes who have natural antioxidant defense systems that are thought to be sufficient to offset the potential detriments of ROS. However, short-term supplementation may present some benefit across the fitness spectrum.

A randomized, placebo-controlled study evaluating the impact of short-term (7 days) supplementation with a daily total of 1,200 mg of NAC showed that untrained subjects benefitted from significant improvements in maximal oxygen uptake ($\dot{V}O_2$max) and total antioxidant capacity as well as reduced lactate production and levels of muscle fatigue during a graded exercise test compared to a control group (Leelarungrayub et al., 2011). Similarly, a 6-day supplementation protocol with NAC was shown to maintain higher levels of performance in recreationally trained men during repeated periods of intermittent exercise; this result led study investigators to conclude that NAC may benefit athletes during short-term competitive situations when adaptation is inconsequential, such as tournament play or track and field events when an athlete is engaged in multiple performances over a few days (Cobley et al., 2011). Acute supplementation may also aid the performance of well-trained athletes, according to a small, double-blind, crossover study that found an intravenous infusion of NAC extended exercise time to exhaustion by 26.3% compared to the placebo (Medved et al., 2004). These results, however, were refuted in a study of similar design with an acute oral dose of 1,800 mg of NAC demonstrating no significant impact on $\dot{V}O_2$ kinetics and exercise time to exhaustion during heavy cycling exercise in well-trained athletes as compared to a placebo (Wicker et al., 2008). Additional research is needed to establish the merit of NAC supplementation for highly trained athletes as well as the ideal duration of use during a competitive season.

Common usage: Available in tablet and capsule form as well as in solutions at a potency of 10%-20%, NAC is generally supplemented at doses of 600 mg taken 1-3 times daily. Research suggests a short-term supplementation protocol of up to 14 days is preferable over long-term use.

Health concerns: Nausea, vomiting, diarrhea, rashes, and headache have been reported with oral delivery of NAC. Additionally, while rare in occurrence, formation of cysteine stones in the kidneys have occurred.

Supplement Warning

Loading the cell with high doses of antioxidants, especially over the long term, may interfere with the positive adaptation effects of exercise training and hinder important ROS-mediated physiological processes, including vasodilation that helps enhance oxygen and blood flow to working cells and insulin signaling that promotes the uptake of glucose into muscles for energy use.

Acetylformic Acid

(see *pyruvate*)

African Ginger

(see *ginger*)

Agaricus Blazei Murill

(see *medicinal mushrooms*)

AKBA-3-O-Acetyl-11-Keto-β-Boswellic Acid

(see *Boswellia serrata*)

Albumin

(see *egg protein*)

α-Linolenic Acid

(see *omega-3 fatty acids*)

Allium Sativum

(see *garlic*)

Alpha-Keto Acid, Alpha-Ketopropionic Acid

(see *pyruvate*)

Alpha-Lipoic Acid

aka *thiotic acid, lipoic acid, lipolate, dihydrolipoic acid, acetate replacing factor, pyruvate oxidation factor*

What it is: A naturally occurring compound found within the body and also derived from consumption of such foods as organ meats, spinach, and yeast, alpha-lipoic acid plays a key role in the conversion of nutrients, especially glucose, into energy. It also has antioxidant qualities of potential benefit to the endurance, strength, and immunity of an athlete.

How it works: Animal research has demonstrated alpha-lipoic acid to activate GLUT4, a protein important for the uptake of glucose by muscles, as well as a molecule called PGC1alpha, which seems to enhance the cell's ability to synthesize more mitochondria. Both are key factors in enhancing muscle endurance. GLUT4 also serves as a proposed mechanism of action because of its apparent ability to increase uptake of creatine by the muscles, which may facilitate gains in muscle strength. Additionally, as an antioxidant that is both water and fat soluble, alpha-lipoic acid protects all the cells of the human body; in particular, it can help dispose of increased metabolic waste products produced during exercise that may otherwise damage cells and hurt overall immune function and recovery from intense training.

Supplement Fact

Alpha-lipoic acid occurs in nature in two mirror image forms, labeled R and S, with only the R form being used by the body. Look for supplements containing the R label versus the R/S label.

Performance benefit: Athletes may benefit from enhanced muscle endurance and strength as well as improved recovery times.

Research: Much of the current research evaluating alpha-lipoic acid is animal focused and has yielded mixed reviews. One study of rats demonstrated a 45% increase in glucose uptake by muscles after 15 days of supplementing with 30 mg of alpha-lipoic acid/kg of body weight (Saengsirisuwan et al., 2004). When supplementation was combined with 60 minutes of treadmill running, glucose uptake by the muscles increased an impressive 124%, signaling the profound impact training has on glucose uptake dynamics. Nonetheless, supplementation with alpha-lipoic acid did significantly enhance this effect. Because the study was conducted on obese animals, however, it is difficult to draw conclusions for a fit, athletic human population. One human study did determine that a daily supplementation protocol with 600 mg of alpha-lipoic acid over 8 days reduced oxidative damage in the muscles of healthy trained and untrained men after completing a weighted exercise test, suggesting potential applications from a recovery perspective (Zembron-Lacny et al., 2009). Yet another study found that prolonged daily supplementation with 1.6 g of alpha-lipoic acid in combination with 1,000 IU of vitamin E/kg of body weight over 14 weeks produced a detrimental impact, significantly reducing training-induced mitochondrial increases in the muscles of both trained and untrained rats (Strobel et al., 2011). While conclusions are difficult to draw due to the combined supplementation protocols, there are a sprinkling of preliminary results such as those found in this study that imply long-term antioxidant supplementation may negatively interfere with the body's natural antioxidant defenses.

Common usage: Alpha-lipoic acid, available in capsule form, should be taken on an empty stomach at a research-supported dose of 200 mg taken 2-3 times/day.

Health concerns: Though infrequent in occurrence, reported side effects include allergic skin reactions such as rashes, hives, and itching as well as gastrointestinal disturbances such as stomach aches, nausea, vomiting, and diarrhea.

>continued

Alpha-Lipoic Acid >*continued*

Additional performance benefit: Alpha-lipoic acid, likely as a result of its positive impact on insulin sensitivity and fat metabolism, has been shown to decrease food intake and increase energy expenditure; therefore, it may have promising applications for athletes interested in dropping body fat.

Alpha-Tocopherol, Alpha-Tocotrienol

(see *vitamin E*)

Amanita Muscaria, Amavadine

(see *vanadium*)

American Ginseng

(see *ginseng*)

Ananas Comosus, Ananase

(see *bromelain*)

Anhydrous Caffeine

(see *caffeine*)

Antiberiberi Vitamin

(see *thiamine*)

Antiscorbutic Vitamin

(see *vitamin C*)

Arctic Root

(see *Rhodiola rosea*)

Arginine

What it is: Arginine is a conditionally essential amino acid. Our bodies are capable of synthesizing and making arginine. However, in certain conditions such as disease, trauma, or extreme stress, our bodies cannot produce sufficient quantities, making dietary sources of arginine essential (Campbell, La Bounty, & Roberts, 2004). Arginine is naturally found in foods such as nuts, seeds, beans, fish, and chicken. Typically we consume 3-6 g of arginine daily from food (Paddon-Jones, Borsheim, and Wolfe 2004).

How it works: Arginine plays a number of roles in the body. It can be metabolized into glucose for energy during exercise and is important in the production of nitric oxide and creatine. Arginine is also known to stimulate growth hormone, a powerful anabolic hormone (Campbell, La Bounty, & Roberts, 2004).

Performance benefit: Arginine is speculated to benefit athletes because of its role in the production of growth hormone, synthesis of creatine, and production of nitric oxide. Growth hormone is capable of promoting protein synthesis, which is critical for muscle recovery and building; it is also lipolytic, promotes the burning of fat, and can improve body composition. Nitric oxide is a vasodilator, which dilates the arteries and capillaries, allowing improved blood flow to the muscles. Increased blood flow allows superior delivery of oxygen and other nutrients enhancing performance. The potential impact of arginine on growth hormone and nitric oxide production would make it beneficial for strength and power as well as endurance athletes.

Research: A 2009 study (Liu et al.) found a 6 g arginine supplement was not effective in promoting nitric oxide production in well-trained athletes. A 2010 study (Bloomer et al.) of a variety of preworkout nitric oxide–stimulating supplements found none capable of producing any beneficial effects on performance or nitric oxide production. Some studies have produced conflicting results, but many of these studies have used disease-state populations such as those with cardiovascular disease. Conflicting results have also been found in relation to the effects of arginine on the stimulation of growth hormone. In 2008 one study by Kanaley suggested that 9 g of arginine would be best to increase the resting level of growth hormone and possibly stimulate growth hormone production by 100%. Other researchers have been unable to repeat these effects, making the claim that arginine can increase levels of growth hormone speculative at best. A 2010 study (Camic et al.) found that both a 1.5 g and a 3 g dose of arginine before exercise were capable of preventing neuromuscular fatigue. More research is needed to verify a potential ergogenic benefit of arginine in the prevention of neuromuscular fatigue as similar studies have not shown improvements in anaerobic performance. Thus, any definitive conclusions about the benefits of arginine for athletes related to nitric oxide production, growth hormone production, or athletic performance are difficult to make.

Common usage: Single or multiple doses totaling 2-9 g per day are most often used.

Health concerns: The observable safe limit for arginine intake is 20 g/day (Alvares, 2011).

Ascorbate, Ascorbic Acid

(see *vitamin C*)

Ashwagandha

(see *Withania somnifera*)

Aspartates

aka *aspartic acid, aspartate salts, L-aspartic acid, L-amino succinate*

What it is: As salts of the amino acid aspartic acid, aspartates are commonly bound to the minerals magnesium, potassium, calcium, and zinc in dietary supplements to facilitate enhanced absorption. Beyond being naturally produced in the body, thus nonessential in nature, aspartate can be obtained from the diet through sugar cane, molasses, dairy, and meat. Ties to human performance originated in the late 1950s when human trials demonstrated magnesium and potassium aspartate supplements reduced muscle fatigue, helping to extend endurance in athletes.

How it works: During physical training, especially that of high intensity, the exhaustion of high energy molecules within the muscles (called ATP) during contraction causes lactate and ammonia levels to rise; increases in these levels are postulated to contribute to the onset of muscle fatigue and reduced endurance capacity in athletes. It is thought that aspartates reduce muscle fatigue by accelerating the conversion of ammonia to urea, thereby lowering levels of ammonia in the muscles and allowing more ATP energy to be produced for enhanced endurance. Furthermore, it is hypothesized that aspartate salts promote a faster rate of glycogen resynthesis during exertion, helping to protect against the fatigue-inducing glycogen depletion commonly known in sports as hitting the wall and bonking.

Supplement Fact

Closely related to aspartic acid is asparagine, a nonessential amino acid first isolated from asparagus juice back in the early 1800s. Together, asparagine and aspartate play a role in the production of oxaloacetic acid, which helps produce energy within the mitochondria as a key intermediate in the Kreb's metabolic cycle.

Performance benefit: Athletes may benefit from reduced fatigue during training and competition, resulting in enhanced endurance.

Research: While preliminary research favored aspartate supplementation for enhanced endurance, these studies were primarily animal based and used aspartate bound to other nutrients such as magnesium and potassium or arginine, making it hard to draw conclusions regarding what percentage, if any, impact was due to the aspartate salt and if applications could be made to a human population (Olney, Labruyere, & de Gubareff, 1980; Colombani et al., 1999; Abel et al., 2005). In fact, human data have not been favorable on the performance front. A 2007 double-blind study of 15 trained athletes, for example, failed to demonstrate any metabolic benefit (glycogen sparing) or improved endurance performance in trained athletes taking an isolated amino acid blend containing 7 g of asparagine and 7 g of aspartate before completion of an exercise-to-exhaustion test compared to a placebo (Parisi et al.). Thus, it is evident that additional large-group human studies using an isolated supplementation protocol are needed before any recommendations can be made for use in athletics.

Common usage: Not enough sound scientific data is available to establish dosing recommendations though supplement manufacturers often recommend 4-5 g of aspartates, available in capsule or powdered form, in the 24-hour period leading up to competition as a means of providing a boost to performance. To reduce fatigue, daily doses of 250 mg of both potassium and magnesium aspartate have been indicated.

Health concerns: L-aspartate is currently listed on the U.S. Food and Drug Administration (FDA) Generally Recognized as Safe (GRAS) list. Adverse effects have not been reported for doses of up to 10 g of aspartates over 24 hours. Doses above this may cause gastrointestinal irritation, including diarrhea.

Additional performance benefits: Aspartates may stimulate the immune system, helping athletes stay healthy during training and competition.

Astragalus

aka *astragalus membranaceus, astragalus mongholicus, huang qi, Radix astragali (RA)*

What it is: An herbal plant native to China, astralagus is also known as *huang qi,* meaning "yellow" leader to describe its yellow root. Astralagus is purported to provide a wide array of medicinal benefits especially relating to immune function. While over 2,000 species of astragalus exist, *Astragalus membranaceus* and *Astragalus mongholicus* are the types primarily used. They are often found in soups, teas, extracts, and capsules or in combination with other herbs such as ginseng and echinacea.

How it works: Intense physical training can suppresses immune function and increase an athlete's risk of contracting an infection, especially in the

>*continued*

acute period postcompetition. Astragalus contains antioxidants, which help protect cells, including those important to immune function, against damage caused by free radicals. In addition, studies have shown astragalus to carry antiviral properties, stimulating the immune system and thereby helping to protect against illness such as the common cold and upper respiratory tract infections.

Performance benefit: Astragalus may help support and enhance immune function, thereby protecting against illness that can sideline an athlete from competition.

Research: Preliminary evidence suggests astralagus taken in isolation or with other herbs may aid immune function, though well-designed trials on humans, in particular on athletic or healthy populations, are minimal. One animal study found a combined herbal concoction favoring astragalus at a dose of 12 or 24 g/kg (9.6-19.2 g/kg *Astragalus membranaceus*) over 28 days offset symptoms of chronic fatigue syndrome through added immune support, helping to enhance the swimming endurance capacity of rats (Liu, Zhang, & Li, 2011). Similarly, a small double-blind study of healthy humans identified a supplementation protocol using *Astagalus membranaceus* at a dose of 2 g taken twice daily along with three medicinal mushrooms over 6 weeks that elicited a favorable immune response, significantly lowering the incidence of colds, influenza, or secondary infections in comparison to a placebo (Clark & Adams, 2007; Clark 2007). Additional human trials are needed to confirm these benefits.

Common usage: For immune function, a daily dose of 1-25 g of astragalus, generally split into 2-4 doses throughout the day, has been used.

Health concerns: Use of astragalus is considered safe for most adults, but because it is commonly used in conjunction with other herbal concoctions, possible secondary side effects are currently unknown.

Additional performance benefits: There is some evidence astragalus, as part of an herbal blend, may help increase uptake and use of oxygen, thereby helping to fight fatigue and extend endurance in athletes (Chen et al., 2002).

Avocado Soybean Unsaponifiables (ASU)

aka *piascledine*

What it is: Avocado soybean unsaponifiables (ASU) are natural components of avocado and soybean oils. ASU has become a popular addition to many joint supplements that promise to relieve pain and improve the symptoms of arthritis. The two types of saponifiables from avocado and soy appear to work synergistically in a ratio of 1:2 (Altinel et al., 2007). In France ASU is prescribed as a pharmaceutical drug known as Piascledine.

How it works: ASU has been shown to inhibit the inflammatory promoting cytokine interleukin (IL)-1β and its negative effects on synovial cells and chondrocytes, thereby preventing joint degeneration and improving joint function and health. ASU can also stimulate the growth of and prevent catabolism (breakdown) of cartilage. These powerful mechanisms can prevent inflammation and degeneration of connective tissue in healthy joints.

Performance benefit: Athletes commonly experience joint injuries resulting in pain, inflammation, and degeneration. ASU could prevent these negative effects, thereby lessening chronic joint strain and improving recovery from injury.

Research: ASU has not been studied extensively, and the majority of research trials have used in vitro methods and animals. Research trials on dogs in 2007 and 2009 found ASU to inhibit production of TGF-β and stimulate healing of chondrocytes (Altinel et al., 2007; Boileau et al., 2009) This finding is in line with other animal trials and in vitro studies. Some trials have used human subjects. A 2008 meta-analysis reviewed the results from four randomized control trials (RCTs) in humans using ASU in the treatment of osteoarthritis. The manufacturer of Piascledine, the pharmaceutical drug prescribed for the treatment of osteoarthritis in many countries, supported all four trials. Results of the meta-analysis were positive, showing reductions in pain and improved joint function as assessed by the Lequesne index, a validated questionnaire commonly used in research studies on arthritic conditions (Christensen et al.). The only long-term study found supplementation of 300 mg daily for 2 years resulted in no significant intergroup differences (Lequesne et al., 2002). While positive evidence exists, more research from multiple scientific labs is needed to further clarify benefits (Ernst, 2003).

Common usage: A dose of 300 mg taken once daily is recommended. The benefits of ASU are not improved with higher doses. Further scientific trials should continue to clarify best-use supplementation strategies.

Health concerns: Reported adverse drug reactions related to ASU are rare, and its use appears safe and nontoxic.

B

Baking Soda

(see *sodium bicarbonate* and *sodium citrate*)

B-Alanine

(see *beta-alanine*)

Balatan Cherry

(see *tart cherry*)

B-Complex Vitamin

(see *thiamine*)

Beetroot

aka *table beet, red beet, garden beet, beet, beetroot juice*

What it is: Containing powerful antioxidants called anthocyanins that contribute to its distinctive reddish-purple flesh and skin, beetroot is a plant in the amaranth family whose root and leaves can be served raw, baked, steamed, pickled, or as a juice. Beetroot has been touted as a natural source of potentially performance-enhancing dietary nitrates, containing nearly 300 mg of those nitrates per 100 g (~4 oz) serving.

How it works: Once ingested, dietary nitrates from beetroot are converted into nitric oxide in the body. Nitric oxide serves as a vasodilator, opening up the blood vessels to allow more blood and oxygen to be delivered to the muscles, thereby lowering the oxygen cost of exercise and making aerobic exercise less tiring for the athlete.

Supplement Fact

The physiological effects of beetroot kick in 30 minutes postconsumption with activity peaking after 90 minutes and staying elevated for approximately 6 hours. Overall health and performance benefits may last as long as 2 weeks postconsumption

Performance benefit: Athletes will benefit from reductions in the oxygen cost of exercise, improving endurance and tolerance to high-intensity training.

Research: Scientists at the University of Exeter in England have published a series of well-designed studies evaluating the effects of a 500 mL (~16 oz) dose of organic beetroot juice on overall performance in healthy men. The initial study, conducted in 2009, found that a 6-day supplementation protocol with beetroot juice extended cycle-to-exhaustion time by 92 seconds, representing a 2% decline in the time needed to cover a set distance, compared to a placebo control beverage of black currant juice (Bailey et al.). The same 6-day supplementation protocol helped reduce the oxygen consumption in trained runners during moderate- and high-intensity running, thereby extending their time to exhaustion by 15% (Lansley et al., 2011b). A follow-up study looking at the impact that beetroot juice has when taken 2.5 hours before both a 4 km and a 16.1 km time trial, separated by 3 days, replicated the initial results with trained male cyclists improving performance by 2%-3% compared to the placebo trials (Lansley et al., 2011a). The benefits of beetroot, however, seem to diminish a bit over longer-distance time trials: A small 2012 study failed to demonstrate a significant benefit to performance during a 80 km bike time trial for trained cyclists who consumed the same 0.5 L dose of beetroot juice 2.5 hours before beginning (Wilkerson et al.).

Common usage: The research-supported dose for performance benefits is 500 mL (~16 oz) of juiced beetroot taken 2.5 hours before a short, high-intensity period of exercise.

Homemade Beetroot Juice

Ingredients: To yield the research-recommended dose of 500 mL, eight small or four large beetroots will be needed.

Step 1: Clean the beetroots. Cut off green tops as needed. Scrub any dirt off the outside of the beets with a produce brush and rinse. Leave the skin intact for added nutrition.

Step 2: Cut the beetroots into halves or quarters and throw into a juicer. Because beetroots are a very hard vegetable, be sure to allow some time for juicing to occur.

Tip: Add other fruits and vegetables to adjust the flavor to desired taste.

Health concerns: There have been a few reports of abdominal cramps, diarrhea, and a temporary and harmless purple coloring of the urine known as beeturia with use of beetroot. Of special note, the World Health Organization (WHO) has an established daily upper limit of 222 mg for dietary nitrates and nitrites due to previous links to gastrointestinal cancer and blood disorders in infants. This limit well surpasses the research-supported performance dose of beetroot juice. However, as refuted in research by registered dietitian Norman Hard of Michigan State University, these detrimental effects are associated with the dietary intake of nitrates and nitrites from processed meat and well water, not from vegetables such as beetroot (Hord et al., 2009).

Beta-Alanine

aka *3-aminopropanoic acid, B-alanine*

What it is: Beta-alanine is an amino acid that is naturally synthesized in the body and thus not an essential component of the diet. It does not play a role in the biosynthesis of any major proteins or enzymes as many amino acids do, but it does aid the synthesis of carnosine, a dipeptide found within both Type I (slow-twitch) and Type II (fast-twitch) muscle fibers. Many scientists believe this role to be the primary contributing factor to beta-alanine's ergogenic qualities: Studies have shown increased intramuscular levels of carnosine to be associated with reductions in muscle fatigue and enhancements of overall work capacity.

How it works: The bulk of research on beta-alanine has evaluated its impact on intramuscular levels of carnosine (B-alanyl-L-histidine), a dipeptide essential for maintaining an optimal pH within the muscle. During exertion, especially during high-intensity efforts, the breakdown of ATP for energy production triggers an increase in hydrogen ions and consequent drop in muscle pH. This process is scientifically known as acidosis, commonly expressed in athletes as a burning sensation that leads to extreme muscle fatigue, reduced power output, and eventual muscular failure. Carnosine serves as an effective buffer, naturally absorbing hydrogen ions, allowing the muscle to continue firing, and enabling overall strength and endurance to remain at peak levels.

Performance benefit: Purported benefits of beta-alanine supplementation include a boost in explosive muscle strength and power as well as increases in anaerobic endurance and aerobic capacity, thus allowing an athlete to train harder for longer.

Research: Randomized, controlled trials have confirmed that supplementation with beta-alanine has the potential to significantly increase carnosine levels within the muscle, especially in Type II fibers, which provides an efficient buffering system for fatigue-inducing hydrogen ions that can negatively impact anaerobic endurance, especially in performances lasting from 60 to 240+ seconds (Hobson et al., 2012). For example, daily supplementation by elite rowers with 5 g of beta-alanine over 7 weeks corresponded with a 45.3% and 28.2% increase in carnosine levels within the soleus and gastrocnemius muscles, respectively. This result yielded a 4.3-second improvement over 2,000 m of rowing (Baguet et al., 2010). Furthermore, a 2012 meta-analysis of 15 published manuscripts including a total of 360 subjects completing 57 measures within 23 exercise tests using 18 supplementation regimens confirmed a median performance improvement of 2.85% with a median daily total intake of 179 mg of beta-alanine (Hobson et al.). The impact of beta-alanine, however, hasn't consistently yielded favorable results, especially when the effects are evaluated across all sport activities. Indeed, Smith-Ryan and colleagues (2012) failed to discover any performance benefit when evaluating the effect of 2×800 mg beta-alanine taken three times daily on anaerobic running capacity or total time to run exhaustion for short bursts at 90%-110% peak velocity or speed lasting 1.95-5.06 minutes. Many sport scientists also remain skeptical about the benefits that beta-alanine has on aerobic capacity and muscle strength, especially in highly trained athletes. Thus, it appears that more research is needed to confirm the potential buffering and consequent anaerobic endurance benefits of specific doses of beta-alanine for athletes engaged in various sports.

Common usage: To achieve the research-supported increase in muscle carnosine levels, between 3.2 and 6.4 g of beta-alanine/day are recommended for up to 12 weeks; performance benefits begin occurring in as little as 2 weeks with more dramatic results occurring after 4 weeks of continuous supplementation. Taking beta-alanine in coordination with carbohydrate may facilitate a quicker performance response, likely due to an increase in insulin, a hormone responsible for transporting amino acids such as beta-alanine, into cells. It is also theorized that timing beta-alanine intake immediately before and after a workout may facilitate increased uptake of beta-alanine into the muscles, likely due to increased blood flow during exertion. In addition to supplementation, beta-alanine can be obtained from such dietary sources as chicken, beef, pork, and fish.

Health concerns: Supplementation with the research-supposed dose of beta-alanine for up to 12 weeks appears to be safe, but there have been reports of skin irritation, flushing, and tingling with doses above 10 mg/kg of body weight. In addition, there is concern that high doses, especially taken for 4 or more weeks, can interfere with taurine uptake and negatively affect cardiac function.

Beta-Carotene

aka *provitamin A*

What it is: Beta-carotene, which readily converts to vitamin A when needed by the body to support normal growth and development, immune function, and vision, belongs to a class of red, orange, and yellow pigments called carotenoids. Beta-carotene is found in abundance in many fruits and vegetables containing these colors. As a fat-soluble antioxidant, beta-carotene helps protect the integrity of cell membranes. It is stored in the liver and fatty tissues.

How it works: Intense physical training triggers an increase in the production of free radicals and other reactive oxygen species (ROS), often at rates that surpass the strengthened antioxidant defenses of even the fittest athletes.

>*continued*

Beta-Carotene >*continued*

This can lead to irreparable damage to lipids in cell membranes as well as the genetic material in cells, causing a plethora of health and performance concerns for the athlete. In particular, the inflammatory response brought on by lipid peroxidation, a type of free radical reaction, can suppress immune function, increasing an athlete's susceptibility to infection, especially of the upper respiratory tract. Beta-carotene is capable of fighting off free radical reactions within the cell membrane, thereby making the cells less vulnerable to viral attack; it may further strengthen immunity by increasing the number of T-helper cells and stimulating the activity of natural killer cells.

Performance benefit: Beta-carotene may help protect athletes, especially those engaged in ultraendurance events, from nagging illnesses that can put a damper on training and hinder performance. There is some evidence that beta-carotene's role in protecting the cell membrane from damage induced by lipid peroxidation may be effective for reducing symptoms associated with allergies and asthma, especially those symptoms that are exercise induced, as well as other inflammatory-based conditions such as osteoarthritis.

Research: While there is an abundance of well-designed studies confirming a positive relationship between supplemental and whole-food intake of beta-carotene and plasma levels of the antioxidant, results evaluating its impact on markers of oxidative stress and immune function are conflicting, especially within an athletic population. For instance, a small study on elite kayak paddlers demonstrated that enhanced blood levels of beta-carotene along with several other antioxidants did little to protect the athletes against the detriments of exercise-induced lipid peroxidation and inflammation (Teixeira et al., 2009b). However, another placebo-controlled, double-blind study demonstrated that a 7-day supplementation protocol with a popular antioxidant cocktail containing 18 mg of beta-carotene, 900 mg of vitamin C, and 90 mg of vitamin E significantly enhanced plasma antioxidant levels as well as neutrophil enzyme activity after trained athletes completed a 2-hour aerobic run (Robson, Bouic, & Myburgh, 2003). Tauler and colleagues (2006) also found significantly elevated plasma levels of vitamin C, vitamin E, and beta-carotene and consequent blood cell antioxidant enzyme defenses in amateur trained athletes after daily supplementation with 500 mg/day of vitamin E and 30 mg/day of beta-carotene with 1 g/day of vitamin C added for the final 15 days. This response, however, is likely due to vitamin C rather than beta-carotene according to previous research evaluating the impact of a similar antioxidant mix on upper respiratory infections in ultramarathoners (Peters et al., 1994). Some studies have shown that beta-carotene, when taken exclusive of other antioxidants at daily doses of 15-50 mg, can significantly increase the number of T-helper cells and boost natural killer cell activity in healthy individuals of a wide age spectrum, suggesting immunosupportive qualities (Ross, 2012; Wood et al., 2000). However, a 2012 meta-analysis that included 78 randomized trials with 296,707 participants (73% were healthy or without disease) concluded that supplementation with beta-carotene, especially over a prolonged duration, may actually increase the risk for mortality (Bjelakovic et al.).

Common usage: The research-supported daily dose of beta-carotene for general health is currently 15-50 mg (25,000-83,000 IU) with water-based supplements generally being recommended over oil-based for optimal absorption.

Health concerns: There are some reports of skin discoloring (turning a yellow-orange hue) at doses above 100,000 IU or 60 mg per day. Expectant mothers should take extra precautions as large doses of beta-carotene can be harmful to the fetus.

Beta-D-Ribofuranose

(see *D-ribose*)

β-Ecdysterone

(see *ecdysteroids*)

Beta Glucan

aka *beta 1,3/1,6 glucan, beta1,3/1,4 glucan, oat bran, oat-derived beta glucan, yeast-derived beta glucan*

What it is: A polysaccharide or complex chain of glucose molecules that is often regarded for its immunostimulant properties, beta glucan can be derived from a variety of sources, including whole grains (especially oat and barley); certain fungi such as baker's yeast; and the medicinal mushrooms reishi, maitake and shitake. The chemical makeup often dictates the biological activity of the compound.

How it works: Intense physical training can challenge the immune system as much as it does the athlete, with declines in such key immune markers as neutrophils, natural killer cells, T cells, and B cells often culminating in upper respiratory tract infections (URTI). Beta glucan activates key immune cells to help trap and consume various viral, bacterial, protozoan, and fungal invaders that can cause infection.

Performance benefit: For up to 2 weeks after intense exercise, especially endurance exercise or event, an athlete is at heightened risk for infection, which can slow the recovery process and cause unwanted physical and mental stress. Beta glucan may provide a boost to immune function and help an athlete stave off infection as well as sustain the energy levels and vigor needed to train and compete at peak.

>continued

Beta Glucan >*continued*

Research: One placebo-controlled, double-blind study discovered a significant reduction in URTI-related symptoms such as sore throat, stuffy or runny nose, and cough as well as better overall health and a more positive mood in runners who followed a daily supplementation protocol of either 250 mg or 500 mg of yeast-derived beta-glucan for 4 weeks after completing a marathon (Talbott, S. & J. Talbott, 2009). The higher dose provided only a slightly greater protective effect, signaling the fact that more isn't necessarily better. In fact, another placebo-controlled, double-blind study determined the lower dose of yeast-derived beta glucan, 250 mg, enhanced immune activity in recreational athletes via improved monocyte concentrations and cytokine levels both pre- and postexercise after only 10 days of supplementation (Carpenter et al., 2012). Additionally, Bobovcak and colleagues (2010) showed a mere 100 mg dose of a mushroom-based beta-glucan (*Pleurotus osteratus*) each day for 2 months was essentially able to eliminate the decrease in natural killer cell activity and the overall natural killer cell count seen in elite athletes after intensive exercise, thereby supporting immune system integrity. Where the beta glucan is derived, however, may play a role in purported immunobenefits as daily supplementation with an oat-derived beta-glucan over 18 days failed to alter resting- or exercise-induced changes in immune function or URTI incidence in trained cyclists completing a 3-hour cycle test at 57% maximal watts (Nieman et al., 2008).

Common usage: According to research, a range of 100 to 500 mg of beta glucan taken daily throughout a heavy training cycle is an effective dose for enhanced immune protection. To aid absorption, beta glucan should be taken on an empty stomach. Beta glucan derived from yeast or mushroom seems to yield the most promising benefits for immune function.

Health concerns: The Food and Drug Administration (FDA) has given beta glucan the GRAS (Generally Recognized as Safe) rating, meaning there are no known side effects or adverse reactions associated with its intended use.

Additional performance benefit: Increasing macrophage and immune cell activity promotes the breakdown and removal of damaged tissue; thus, supplementation with beta glucan may aid recovery from athletic injury and facilitate faster wound healing.

Betaine

aka *trimethylglycine, TMG, glycine betaine*

What it is: Betaine is a derivative of the nonessential amino acid glycine and is synthesized naturally within the body as well as obtained from such dietary sources as wheat, beets, spinach, and shellfish. While traditionally used as a dietary supplement for animals, betaine has recently appeared as a sports supplement with the thought it may help facilitate hydration, increase strength gains, enhance endurance, and improve recovery.

How it works: Betaine has several physiological functions of potential benefit to athletic performance, one of which is its role as an osmolyte, helping to increase water retention by cells and thereby protecting against dehydration. In addition, betaine has been shown to enhance vascular health, helping to increase circulation and consequent blood and oxygen flow to working tissue, which may benefit endurance as well as strength gains. It is also hypothesized that betaine can enhance strength and power performance by increasing skeletal muscle creatine concentration.

Performance benefit: Athletes may benefit from better hydration status during training and completion as well as achieve enhanced strength and endurance gains. There is some evidence that supplementation with beta-ine enhances fat metabolism, which could spare muscle glycogen and aid endurance performance.

Research: The potential benefits of betaine as it relates to athletic performance appear to be multifaceted though results of well-designed human studies have been mixed to date. For example, a well-designed study found supplementation with 2.5 g of betaine mixed into 500 ml of Gatorade sport drink and taken daily over 14 days to elicit a moderate, though statistically insignificant, improvement in muscle endurance as indicated by increases in total repetitions and total volume load in the bench press protocol compared to a placebo (Trepanowski et al., 2011). On the other hand, a similar protocol consisting of 2.5 grams of betaine taken in 2 split doses along with 300 mL of Gatorade sport drink over 14 days yielded significant increases in the vertical jump power and isometric squat force of trained males compared to presupplementation test results (Lee et al., 2010). However, there were no performance improvements reported for jump squat power or the number of bench press and squat repetitions. In another study, the same split protocol taken with 240 mL of a sport drink significantly increased the number of repetitions performed by recreationally trained athletes at 90% or greater of peak power in a squat exercise protocol after 1 and 2 weeks of supplementation as compared to the placebo (Hoffman et al., 2009). Of particular interest to athletes when both anaerobic and aerobic endurance are employed, Armstrong and colleagues discovered that rehydration with fluids containing betaine (water with 5 g of betaine/L of fluid or 6.5% carbohydrate-electrolyte solution with 5 g of betaine/L of fluid) significantly improved the plasma volume, oxygen consumption, plasma lactate concentration, and thermal sensation of runners completing a 75-minute aerobic treadmill test followed by a sprint to exhaustion compared with a comparable placebo of either water or sports drink (2008). While the benefits to sprint performance to exhaustion after the aerobic run were statistically insignificant and likely irrelevant for the recreationally trained athlete, the result may equate to the ability to outsprint a competitor for a score in an important game or secure a podium spot during a championship race for the elite-level athlete. Nonetheless, with inconsistent and often statistically insignificant results, it is evident further human studies are warranted before valid conclusions for use of betaine as an ergogenic aid can be made.

>*continued*

Betaine >*continued*

Common usage: Manufactured as a byproduct of sugar beet processing, betaine supplements are available in powder, tablet, and capsule form. The doses supported by research range from 2.5 to 5 g of betaine taken daily, generally in split doses, for up to 2 weeks precompetition.

Health concerns: Reported side effects are generally mild and include stomach upset, nausea, and diarrhea. Athletes with cardiovascular risk factors should be aware that betaine has been shown to increase total cholesterol levels.

Beta1, 3/1, 4 Glucan

(see *beta glucan*)

Beta-Tocopherol, Beta-Tocotrienol

(see *vitamin E*)

Bifidobacterium

(see *probiotics*)

BioPerine

(see *piperine*)

Bitter Orange

(see *synephrine*)

Blackcurrant Seed Oil

(see *gamma-linolenic acid*)

Black Ginger

(see *ginger*)

Black Pepper

(see *piperine*)

Borage Oil

(see *gamma-linolenic acid*)

Boron

aka *boric acid, boron oxide*

What it is: Boron, which was found to be present in plants in 1857, is a trace element. In the late 1800s, it was used as a food preservative until a German scientist found that high doses resulted in disturbances in appetite. It was later concluded that 4,000 mg/day was the upper limit for intake (Nielsen, 2008).

How it works: Initially, it was believed that boron had no specific or vital functions in humans; however, in the 1980s, boron-deprived diets fed to animals resulted in bone disturbances. This lead to more scientific research and our current understanding that boron has roles in bone growth, cognitive performance, inflammatory response, and the immune system. The exact mechanisms are unclear. Many scientists believe the impact of boron on health is similar to that of omega-3 fatty acids, carotenoids, and other nutrients: Higher intakes promote optimal health but are not necessarily essential or life supporting. Boron is found abundantly in food and drinking water. Fruits and vegetables are the densest sources of boron, and amounts found in drinking water vary based on geographic location. Apples, grapes, tomatoes, celery, almonds, broccoli, and bananas are excellent sources of boron (Devirian & Volpe, 2003).

Performance benefit: Boron is speculated to benefit athletes through its ability to promote the growth and development of bone, improve cognitive performance, and provide protection against inflammation induced by injury or naturally resulting from the stress of training. Additionally, it has been claimed that boron raises testosterone levels, suggesting that it may be a natural alternative to steroids.

Research: In scientific studies boron deprivation has been shown to decrease bone volume and the number of osteoblast (bone forming) cells in bone (Nielsen, 2008). In animal studies, adequate boron intakes are associated with improved responses to antigen-induced arthritis. Boron depravation has also been shown to impact inflammation-regulating cytokines and chemokines. Thus, research confirms that boron has important roles in bone formation, cognitive function, and inflammatory and immune responses. It has also been speculated that boron can affect levels of testosterone and could serve as a natural alternative to steroids. Interestingly, a recent study found supplementation with 11.6 mg of boron decreased proinflammatory cytokines and increased levels of free testosterone after 1 week of supplementation (Nanghii et al., 2011). This is in contrast to a 1993 study that found 2.5 mg of boron supplementation for 7 weeks did not produce changes in lean body mass, strength, or testosterone in body builders (Ferrando & Green, 1993). Further research is needed to clarify the benefits of boron for athletes.

>continued

Boron >*continued*

Currently, it seems as if the benefits are only experienced in boron-deficient states induced via intakes of .045-.062 mg/day. The estimated mean intake of boron for the United States is .86-1.13 mg/day, ranging from a low of .35 mg/day to a high of 3.25 mg/day. Because boron is found so abundantly, inducing deficiency is difficult and rare.

Common usage: Most supplements sold contain 1.5-11.6 mg.

Health concerns: Intakes of 1-13 mg of boron/day are considered to be within an acceptable, safe range (Nielsen, 2008).

Boswellia Serrata

aka *frankincense, olibanum, AKBA -3-O-acetyl-11-keto-β-boswellic acid*

What it is: *Boswellia serrata* (BS) is a species of deciduous tree commonly found in India and Arabia. The gum resin of BS has a long history dating back to biblical times. It has a wide variety of uses, including for medicinal purposes, religious ceremonies, and perfume production.

How it works: The gum resin of BS contains boswellic acids (BAs). BAs have antiinflammatory properties ("Boswellia serrata," 2008). As a result, BS has been used as a beneficial treatment for various inflammation-related diseases such as bronchial asthma, Crohn's disease, and arthritis (Ernst, 2008).

Performance benefit: Antiinflammatories, such as ibuprofen, are commonly used by athletes to limit inflammation and pain resulting from muscle injury, arthritic joints, or muscle soreness (delayed-onset muscle soreness, or DOMS) from heavy, intensified training. Because of its antiinflammatory effects, BS is a likely supplementation candidate for athletes looking for an alternative to nonsteroidal antiinflammatories (NSAIDS) such as ibuprofen.

Research: Clinical studies involving BS are encouraging, showing it to be effective in inhibiting 5-lipoxygenase as well as TNF-α, a known proinflammatory cytokine ("Boswellia serrata," 2008). It also shows promise in the treatment of inflammation-related diseases such as osteoarthritis and rheumatoid arthritis. While these studies show promise, they are not extensive, are limited in subject number, and are commonly found in complementary medicine journals, which rarely publish negative results. No research to date has evaluated the effectiveness of BS in limiting inflammation and pain related to muscle injury or DOMS in athletic populations. Studies related to osteoarthritis of the knee have found BS to be effective in reducing pain and improving function compared with a placebo (Sengupta et al., 2011). The gum resin of BS contains boswellic acids (BAs), of which, 3-O-acetyl-11-keto-β-boswellic acid (AKBA) is the most potent antiinflammatory ("Boswellia serrata," 2008). Unfortunately, most gum resins of BS only contain 2-3% AKBA. The bioavailability of BS is also poor and known to be a limiting factor. Currently, scientists are looking to improve the effective use of BS by increasing the concentration of AKBA and improving its bioavailability.

Common usage: The common usage for BS is 600-3,000 mg/day (Ernst, 2008).

Health concerns: No serious or irreversible adverse effects have been noted when using BS in a range of 600-3,000 mg/day ("Boswellia serrata," 2008).

Bovine Colostrum (BC)

(see *colostrums*)

Branched-Chain Amino Acids (BCAAs)

aka *leucine, isoleucine, valine*

What it is: Branched-chain amino acids (BCAAs) include the amino acids leucine, isoleucine, and valine. All three are considered essential amino acids; they cannot be made in the body and must be consumed in the diet from protein-rich foods. BCAAs account for 35% of the essential amino acids found in muscle proteins. BCAAs are unique in that they can be oxidized in skeletal muscle, whereas other essential amino acid are mainly catabolized, or broken down, in the liver (Shimomura et al., 2004).

How it works: BCAAs and especially leucine are key stimulators of protein synthesis or muscle building and also play a role in the prevention of muscle breakdown. BCAAs are unique from other amino acids in that they can be oxidized in the muscle for fuel. As a result, it is thought that BCAAs can be used as fuel during exercise, producing performance benefits especially in longer-duration endurance sports.

Performance benefit: Because of the role BCAAs have in the regulation of protein synthesis and protein breakdown, it is believed that they can be used to prevent the catabolic effects of exercise when supplemented before or during training and used to enhance muscle building or protein synthesis when supplemented postexercise. In addition, many believe that BCAAs can have performance-enhancing effects due to their ability to be oxidized and used for fuel by the muscles. This belief has prompted many endurance athletes to supplement with BCAA before and during competition or training.

Research: There is a significant amount of evidence that BCAAs can prevent protein breakdown and muscle damage during exercise. Many studies

>continued

Branched-Chain Amino Acids (BCAAs) >continued

have revealed that BCAAs supplemented before training can decrease markers of muscle damage such as creatine kinase and lactate dehydrogenase for both endurance- and resistance-trained athletes (Shimomura, 2010; Jackman, 2010; Coombes & McNaughton, 2000; Koba et al., 2007). Interestingly, it appears that this effect is less consistent for older athletes versus younger athletes. Supplementation with BCAAs after exercise also produces beneficial effects by stimulating muscle building and recovery. Research related to the performance-enhancing effects of BCAAs for endurance athletes is less promising, and most studies show no additional benefit from consuming BCAAs (Negro et al., 2008; Watson, Shirreffs, & Maughan, 2004). While immediate performance improvements are not seen, the benefits of decreased muscle damage and improved rebuilding or recovery after exercise could produce performance improvements over time. In addition, BCAAs appear to limit immune suppression resulting from exercise. BCAAs limit reductions of serum glutamine, an important nutrient for immune health often lowered as a result of intense and prolonged training (Negro et al., 2008). Questions still remain in terms of the effectiveness of BCAAs over the use of whole proteins. Since whole proteins, most notably whey protein, contain sufficient quantities of BCAAs, and in particular leucine, it does not appear that supplementation with BCAAs before or after training provides additional benefits if adequate amounts of high-quality whole proteins are consumed. A relatively new application of BCAAs in athletes is during recovery from injury. Early research appears positive that BCAAs can limit muscle wasting or atrophy associated with immobilization and decreases in physical training (Bajotto et al., 2011).

Common usage: A variety of supplementation protocols have been used with BCAAs. Most protocols use a higher dosage of leucine and smaller dosages of valine and isoleucine. Protocols have ranged from 6 to 14 g of BCAAs per day in a ratio of leucine:valine:isoleucine of 2 or 3:1:1.

Health concerns: No adverse effects of BCAA toxicity have been reported in relation to exercise and sport. Single doses of 10 g of BCAA/kg of body weight have been used in mice and did not result in death. No toxic effects of BCAAs have been observed from a 3-month intake of 2.5 g/kg of body weight/day or 1.25 g/kg of body weight for 1 year (Shimomura et al., 2004).

Bromelain

aka *Ananas comosus, bromelainum, ananase*

What it is: A proteolytic (protein-digesting) enzyme derived from the stem and juice of the pineapple plant, bromelain quickly gained popularity as a natural antiinflammatory and pain killer upon its release as a therapeutic supplement in 1957. It is currently used by many to help reduce edema, bruising, and healing time following trauma, including sport injuries and surgery.

How it works: Swelling and inflammation, which manifest as redness, heat, bruising, and pain, trigger a fibrous reaction in the body, causing collagen fibers to form adhesions that can inhibit muscle lengthening and consequent functionality of the injured tissue. Without treatment, the injury can lead to time away from training, decreased fitness, and poor performance. Bromelain's proteolytic characteristics facilitate the breakdown of adhesions in the circulatory system and in other connective tissue, such as the muscles; improve the delivery of nutrients and oxygen-rich blood to the injured tissue; and remove metabolic waste that can exacerbate inflammation. Additionally, it has also been proposed that bromelain halts the production of bradykinin, a chemical responsible for mediating the inflammatory response, and controls the number of white blood cells that accumulate within the blood vessels at the site of inflammation. Similar to other nonsteroidal antiinflammatory drugs (NSAID) such as Aspirin, Motrin, Aleve, and Celebrex, bromelian inhibits COX-2, an enzyme responsible for inflammation and pain.

Performance benefit: The antiinflammatory and pain-killing qualities of bromelain are purported to help aid the recovery of sore, inflamed muscles and joints after training and facilitate the healing of athletic injuries, especially those involving heavy bruising and hematomas. Bromelain may also provide relief for other inflammation-based conditions such as asthma, sinusitis, osteoarthritis, ulcerative colitis, and irritable bowel syndrome.

Research: While double-blind, placebo-controlled research evaluating the impact of bromelain over the past 50 years has confirmed significant decreases in edema, inflammation, and pain in a variety of clinical cases involving trauma and surgical procedures, the evidence as it relates specifically to muscle injury and recovery is either lacking or inconsistent (Mauer, 2001; Fitzhugh et al., 2008; Muller et al., 2012). For example, one small double-blind, placebo-controlled study failed to confirm the benefit of bromelain for treating DOMS with no improvements being found in pain levels, range of motion, or overall functionality of the muscle (Stone et al., 2002). On the favorable end, another small randomized, placebo-controlled study found a mixed supplement cocktail containing 5.83 g of three proteolytic enzymes—bromelain, papain, and fungal proteases—consumed daily over 21 days helped reduce the damaging impact of downhill running and reduce muscle strength losses by regulating leukocyte (white blood cell) activity and inflammation; however, it's hard to draw conclusions due to the combined supplementation protocol (Buford et al., 2009).

Common usage: Recommended therapeutic doses of bromelain range from 200 to 2,000 mg depending on the type and severity of the condition. For traumatic injuries, a dose at the high end of the spectrum, 2,000 mg, is recommended; it should be split into 4 doses and consumed on an empty stomach. For joint inflammation and pain, a range of 500 to 2,000 mg can be taken in 2 split doses on an empty stomach as well. As a digestive aid, however, a lower dose of 500 mg split into 4 doses and taken with meals is recommended.

>*continued*

Bromelain >continued

Health concerns: The most commonly reported side effects include indigestion, nausea, and diarrhea. Less frequently reported are vomiting, increased heart rate, drowsiness, and heavier bleeding during menstruation. Those with an allergy to pineapple may develop breathing problems, tightness in the throat, hives, rash, or itchy skin. Women who are pregnant or nursing, children under 18 years old, individuals with kidney or liver dysfunction, and those taking blood thinners and other medications should check with a physician before supplementation.

C

Cacao

(see *cocoa*)

Caffeine

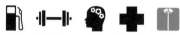

aka *theine, anhydrous caffeine, caffeine citrate*

What it is: First discovered by a German chemist in 1819, caffeine is a chemical compound found in over 60 species of plants, including coffee beans, tea leaves, cocoa beans, gaurana, and kola nuts. It remains one of the most well researched and used ergogenic aids in the world, providing beneficial effects for both physical and mental performance.

How it works: Caffeine is absorbed within the stomach and intestine. Blood levels of caffeine peak 45-60 minutes postingestion, triggering a number of physiological responses in the body that may aid performance for as long as 4 hours. Through its stimulant effects on the brain and central nervous system activity, caffeine allows an athlete to feel more alert with a clearer flow of thought, increased focus, and better general body coordination. Through its metabolic activity, caffeine mobilizes fatty acids from fat tissue in the bloodstream and increases fat oxidation, thereby helping to spare muscle glycogen and protect the athlete against premature muscle fatigue known as hitting the wall.

Performance benefit: Athletes may be able to better sustain exercise intensity as well as cognitive abilities, including concentration, focus, reaction time, and tactical decision making, throughout competition.

Research: There is an abundance of solidly designed studies demonstrating a wide spectrum of performance benefits associated with caffeine ingestion. The current available evidence suggests caffeine ingestion at a dose of 1.3-4.0 mg/lb (1.3-4.0 mg/.45 kg) of body weight provides significant enhancement of endurance exercise performance, with studies demonstrating a 20%-50% increase in exercise time to fatigue in cyclists and runners (Cox et al., 2002; Hogervorst et al., 2008; Burke, 2008; Ganio et al., 2009). Early research attributes this effect, in part, to an approximate 30% increase in fat oxidation during exercise and thus a desirable glycogen or carbohydrate sparing effect (Costill et al., 1978; Ivy et al., 1979). Other mechanisms of action, mainly as they relate to central nervous system fatigue, have been explored and shown to play a role in reducing ratings of perceived effort and pain intensity, thwarting fatigue, and enhancing the physical and mental performance of athletes. For instance, male soccer players who consumed a total of 3.7 mg of caffeine/lb (1.68 mg/.45 kg) of body weight in the form of a sport drink taken 1 hour before and in 15-minute intervals during a

>*continued*

90-minute exercise protocol not only improved sprinting performance and countermovement jumping ability but also enhanced subjective experiences (i.e., made the workout less painful) more so than consumption of a noncaffeinated isocaloric sports drink (Gant et al., 2010). Similarly, consumption of a caffeine-containing energy drink in a dose equivalent to 1.36 mg/lb (1.36 mg/.45 kg) of body weight 60 minutes preexercise increased the ability to repeatedly sprint the distance covered during a simulated soccer game at a high intensity; it also enhanced the height at which the players were able to jump, a result of merit considering how often team sport athletes are up in the air competing for a ball (Del Coso et al., 2012).

Common usage: Most research has demonstrated positive performance effects at caffeine doses of 1.3-4.0 mg/lb (1.3-4.0/.45 kg) of body weight; however, doses as low as 0.45 mg/lb (0.45 mg/.45 kg) of body weight have shown to be beneficial as well, signaling the fact that more is not necessarily better. Caffeine doses can be split so that some is taken pre- and some during competition, or the caffeine can be taken all at once. Because an athlete can develop a tolerance to caffeine, the most beneficial impact on performance is likely to be seen preceding a washout period of 7-10 days when no caffeine is consumed. Withdrawal symptoms, such as headaches, can be avoided by slowly reducing caffeine consumption leading up to the washout period.

Food and Drink Caffeine Content

12 oz (.35 L) cola	35-55 mg
12 oz (.35 L) iced/flavored tea	25-30 mg
8 oz (.24 L) brewed tea	40-60 mg
8 oz (.24 L) green tea	15 mg
8 oz (.24 L) hot cocoa	15 mg
8 oz (.24 L) drip coffee	115-175 mg
8 oz (.24 L) brewed coffee	80-135 mg
8 oz (.24 L) instant coffee	65-100 mg
2 oz (.06 L) espresso	100 mg
8 oz (.24 L) energy drink	80-300 mg
Caffeinated energy gels	25-50 mg

Health concerns: Caffeine ingestion may increase urine formation within an hour after consumption; however, moderate levels (<300 mg) do not seem to have a detrimental impact on hydration status during exercise, likely due to adrenaline blocking caffeine's effect on the kidneys. Exceeding 300 mg of caffeine, however, can interfere with hydration status as well as increase heart rate, impair fine motor control, interfere with sleep patterns, and irritate the stomach, all of which can impair athletic performance and compromise health. The lethal dose of caffeine has been indicated at 70-90 mg/lb (70-90 mg/.45 kg) of body weight, or the equivalent of approximately 80-100 cups of coffee.

Supplement Fact

The NCAA banned substance list (found in the References and Resources file at www.humankinetics.com/products/all-products/Athletes-Guide-to Sports-Supplements-The) lists several stimulants, including caffeine over a certain limit. Because caffeine is a common ingredient in foods and drinks, the NCAA allows an upper limit of 15 mcg/mL of urine tested. For reference, it is estimated that over a 2- to 3-hour period, a 100 mg dose of caffeine (~1 cup of coffee) will yield a urine caffeine concentration of 1.5 mcg/mL. The International Olympic Committee removed caffeine from the banned list in 2004.

Calcidiol (25-Hydroxy-Vitamin D), Calcifidiol (25-Hydroxy-Vitamin D), Calcitriol (1,25 dihydroxy-vitamin D)

(see *vitamin D*)

Calcium (Ca)

aka *calcium carbonate, calcium citrate, calcium gluconate, calcium lactate, calcium phosphate*

What it is: Calcium has long been known as an important mineral for the development and maintenance of strong bones. While its importance in bone structure is well known, its other functions in muscle contraction, vasodilation, nerve transmission, and hormone secretion are critical to support life. These functions require a constant concentration of calcium be present in the blood (National Institute of Health, 2012). Bones represent a reservoir of stored calcium that can be called on to raise calcium levels when needed. The development of calcium deposits in bone or bone mineral density peaks around 17-23 years of age, with women peaking 2-3 years before men. Many have speculated that calcium supplementation can aid in achieving optimal peak bone mineral density and its maintenance throughout life. Ironically, calcium supplementation has also been implicated in weight loss and the prevention of obesity.

>continued

How it works: Aside from calcium intake, other diet and lifestyle choices such as inactivity, smoking, and excessive caffeine or alcohol intake will negatively affect development of bone mineral density (Patel, 2011). The aging process, especially for women following menopause, will exacerbate calcium losses from bone. There is some evidence to suggest that calcium intake can affect body composition and fat mass. High-calcium diets have been shown to increase lipid oxidation and decrease fat absorption in the GI tract. There is speculation that calcium can influence appetite, decreasing food intake.

Performance benefit: Calcium supplementation for athletes could provide protection against the development of stress fractures and improve body composition.

Research: Studies on the effectiveness of calcium supplementation alone and in combination with vitamin D on losses in bone mineral density and risk of fracture have produced mixed results. In 2011 a meta-regression, which reviewed results from 15 randomized, placebo-controlled trials involving calcium with or without vitamin D supplementation, concluded that calcium does affect the risk of fracture; however, this reduced risk is not the result of improved bone mineral density (Rabenda, Bruyere, & Reginster, 2011). Mixed results have also been found related to weight loss. In 2009 researchers found calcium and vitamin D supplementation (1,200 mg/day of calcium and 10 mcg/day vitamin D) decreased fat mass and assisted in appetite control (Major). Interestingly, these researchers found supplementation was only effective in those with low dietary calcium intake (<600 mg/day). A 2012 study found calcium supplementation of 1,050 mg/day with 300 IU/day of vitamin D did not produce weight loss; however, it did decrease abdominal fat (Rosenblum et al., 2012). At present it appears that calcium supplementation is beneficial in promoting optimum body composition and in some cases weight loss; however, benefits are most strongly seen in those with suboptimal dietary calcium intake. Calcium is also beneficial in the prevention of stress fracture risk, but many other nutritional and lifestyle choices have significant impacts as well.

Common usage: The RDA for calcium ranges from 1,000 mg/day to 1,300 mg/day for men and women between the ages of 4 and 71+. Peak absorption is achieved in doses under 500 mg; therefore, it is recommended that calcium be supplemented 3 times daily in 300-400 mg doses totaling 1,000-1,200 mg daily. Types of calcium supplements include carbonate, citrate, gluconate, lactate, and phosphate. Calcium carbonate is most effectively absorbed with food, whereas citrate forms can be absorbed with or without food. Food sources rich in calcium include milk, yogurt, cheese, fish such as salmon and sardines, and some vegetables including kale, bok choi, and broccoli. Calcium is also commonly fortified in fruit juices and cereals.

Health concerns: In some cases individuals may experience GI tract side effects, including constipation, bloating, or gas. Recently, a Women's Health Initiative study found a relationship between calcium supplementation and an increased risk of heart attack. Reanalysis concluded that the risk was only seen in those who were not taking calcium supplements before the study began. These recent findings have created some debate about the health claims and safety of calcium supplements (Bolland et al., 2011).

Calcium Ascorbate

(see *vitamin C*)

Calcium Pantothenate

(see *pantothenic acid*)

Calcium Pyruvate, Calcium Pyruvate Monohydrate

(see *pyruvate*)

Capric Acid, Caproic aAcid, *Caprylic Acid*

(see *medium-chain triglycerides*)

Capsicum

aka *cayenne, capsaicin, chili pepper, hot pepper, sweet pepper, red pepper, green pepper*

What it is: A plant widely known for the hot pungent properties of its fruits and seeds, capsicum, which in Greek means *to bite,* is not only used for culinary purposes but also is a common ingredient in athletic balms because of its apparent ability to provide temporary relief from muscle and joint pain associated with arthritis, backache, strains, and sprains when applied topically.

How it works: The fruit of the capsicum plant contains an active ingredient known as capsaicin at an estimated potency of 0.1%-1.5%. Long-term exposure to capsaicin, generally via topical application, has been shown to decrease the activity of transient receptor potential vanilloid 1 (TRPV1), or capsaicin receptors. This effect helps desensitize nerve endings and ultimately provides a natural treatment for nerve-focused pain as well as pain associated with the inflammatory response of damaged tissue common with athletic injury and osteoarthritis. Furthermore, capsaicin promotes circulation, helping to increase the flow of nutrients to damaged tissues, thereby facilitating recovery.

Performance benefit: Athletes might benefit from reduced pain with topical application.

>continued

Research: Topical capsicum has proven clinical benefit for a wide array of pain conditions, including those associated with athletic injury. One randomized, double-blind study found application with a cream containing 0.05% capsaicin to reduce subjective measures of pain associated with soft tissue damage by 30% or more initially and by 49% after 3 weeks of treatment, a significant improvement as compared to the placebo trial (Chrubasik, Weiser, & Beime, 2010). Subjects with chronic back pain also saw significant improvements in subjective measures of pain compared to the placebo. Patches at a potency of 8% capsaicin are clinically available with trials demonstrating pain relief up to 3 months with a 30-minute treatment, relevant data for athletes with lingering pain at the peak of competition (Armstrong et al., 2011). Capsicum plasters have also been shown to be effective in providing pain relief and facilitating quicker introduction of rehabilitation after painful orthopedic surgery procedures (Kim et al., 2009).

Common usage: The fruit and seeds of capsicum can be dried and ground into powder to provide a culinary kick to foods. For treatment of pain, application of a cream containing 0.025%-0.075% capsaicin concentration 3-4 times daily over a period of 2 or more weeks is indicated. Additionally, the use of capsicum-containing patches at 8% concentration or plasters providing 11 mg of capsaicin per plaster can be applied once daily and left in place for 4-8 hours.

Health concerns: Topical application of capsicum on skin is considered safe for most adults but may produce skin irritation, burning, and itching. Athletes with sensitive skin should test the product on a small patch of skin before using liberally. Capsicum should not be applied around the eyes, nose, or throat. Oral administration is also considered safe although acute symptoms may include stomach irritations, sweating, flushing, and runny nose. Athletes undergoing surgery should avoid oral use as capsicum has been shown to increase bleeding.

Additional performance benefit: There is some evidence that capsaicin helps increase fat burning through activation of the sympathetic nervous system, (Snitker et al., 2009). Another compound called capsinoids found with the capsicum plant has shown some promise in providing a boost to energy metabolism. More human data are needed before practical recommendations for use can be made.

Carbohydrate (CHO)

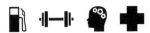

aka *sugars, saccharides (mono-, di-, poly-, oligo-)*

What it is: Put simply, carbohydrate is sugar (saccharides) and starch found naturally in such foods as fruits, vegetables, dairy, legumes, and grains as well as in manufactured products such as sport drinks, energy bars, energy chews, and energy gels that fuel the athlete much like gasoline fuels a race car. Carbohydrate provides 4 calories of energy per gram. See descriptions of the common carbohydrate types and sources in table 3.1.

How it works: Upon digestion, carbohydrate is broken down into glucose and oxidized at various rates for immediate energy use or stored as glycogen in the liver and muscles for later energy use. Athletes who balance out their meals with 45%-65% carbohydrate while meeting daily energy demands will store enough carbohydrate energy to fuel up to 3 hours of moderate-intensity exercise. Failure to consume adequate calories and carbohydrate to support training, commonly seen among athletes who are dieting and those with heavy training loads, and inadequate supplementation with carbohydrate during endurance training and racing more than 90 minutes increase the risk for glycogen depletion, otherwise known as bonking or hitting the wall.

TABLE 3.1   Common Carbohydrate Sources in Sport Foods

Carbohydrate type	Carbohydrate description	Oxidation rate
Fructose (F)	A monosaccharide found naturally in fruits and honey.	Slow
Galactose (G)	A monosaccharide that, together with glucose, makes up lactose, the sugar found in milk.	Slow
Isomaltulose (I)	Also known as Paltinose, isomaltulose is a natural constituent of honey and sugar cane and is manufactured from sucrose.	Slow
Trehalose (T)	Also known as mycose, trehalose is made up of unique chemical bond of two glucose molecules.	Slow
Amylose (A)	An unbranched chain of glucose found in plants that along with amylopectin make up starch.	Slow
Glucose (GL)	Also known as dextrose or grape sugar, glucose is a monosaccharide produced commercially from several forms of starch, including corn, rice, and wheat.	Fast
Sucrose (S)	Also known as table sugar, sucrose is a disaccharide made up of glucose plus fructose.	Fast
Maltose (M)	A disaccharide made up of two units of glucose.	Fast
Maltodextrin (MD)	A polymer of glucose that can enzymatically be derived from any starch, generally corn and wheat.	Fast
Amylopectin (AP)	A highly branched chain of glucose molecules that are found in plants and of which together with amylose, make up starch.	Fast
Waxy Maize Starch (WMS)	Comprised primarily of amylopectin, WMS is a highly branched starch derived from corn.	Fast

>continued

carbohydrate (CHO)   79

Carbohydrate (CHO) >continued

Bonking refers to depletion of liver glycogen stores that causes a shortage of glucose or energy being sent to the brain and consequent symptoms of dizziness, lethargy, and confusion. Hitting the wall refers to depletion of muscle glycogen stores and is marked by symptoms of muscle cramping, extreme fatigue, and reduced performance. Consuming carbohydrate postworkout is essential for optimal immune function and recovery.

Performance benefit: Athletes will benefit from increased endurance during both high- and low-intensity training and competition as well as improved recovery times.

Supplement Fact

Merely rinsing the mouth with any type of carbohydrate during high-intensity exercise of short duration (<60 minutes) may benefit performance.

Research: Since it is well established that carbohydrate can enhance the performance and recovery of an athlete, modern-day research has focused on specifics, evaluating the best type, blend, and quantity of carbohydrate for the most efficient delivery of energy to an athlete's working muscles (i.e., fast rate of oxidation). Two categories of carbohydrate exist: those that are oxidized at fast rates (up to 1 g/min) and those that are oxidized at slow rates (up to 0.6 g/min). Oxidation rates of the di- and polysaccharides sucrose (S), maltose (M), and maltodextrin (MD) along with the monosaccharide glucose fall on the fast side of the spectrum, whereas fructose and galactose are oxidized at slow rates. Additionally, a series of studies has shown carbohydrate oxidation rates can increase another 20%-30% to values of 1.7 g/min when a combination of carbohydrate, namely those such as glucose (GL) and fructose (F) that use different intestinal digestion and transport systems, are used (Jeukendrup, 2004; Currell & , Jeukendrup, 2008). A 2011 meta-analysis of 73 well-designed studies, for example, confirmed these findings and also discovered a blend of MD plus F at a dose of approximately 0.32 and 0.09 g/lb (0.32 and 0.09 g/0.45 kg) of body weight, respectively, taken each hour in an incremental fashion yields the most favorable effect on exercise time to exhaustion (Vandernbogaerde & Hopkins, 2011). The recovery benefits of the MD plus-F carbohydrate combination have also been shown to be significant, with a dose of 70 grams taken in a 2:1 ratio within 1 hour postworkout doubling rates of liver glycogen compared to a calorie-matched MD-GL combination (Decombaz et al., 2011).

Common usage: The most common carbohydrate supplements used by athletes include sport drinks (both liquid and powder form), energy gels, energy chews, and energy bars. For high-intensity training and competition lasting longer than 1 hour, merely rinsing the mouth with a carbohydrate solution can enhance endurance. For high-intensity events lasting 1-3 hours, ingestion of quickly oxidized carbohydrates (see table 3.1) at a rate of 30-60 g/hour is recommended. For prolonged training and competition over 3 hours, multiple carbohydrates should be used at a rate of 60-90 g/hour; based on current research, the following combinations are recommended: glucose, maltodextrin, amylopectin, or waxy maize starch (60 g/hour) plus fructose (30 g/hour); glucose, maltodextrin, amylopectin, or waxy maize starch (60 g/hour) plus sucrose (15 g/hour) plus fructose (15 g/hour) (see table 3.2).

Health concerns: Because the amount of carbohydrate transporters in the gastrointestinal tract is limited, and oxygen availability for digestion and absorption is low during exercise, consuming too many carbohydrate calories, especially from one type of sugar, can overwhelm the metabolic pathway being used. Doing so delays emptying of fuel from the gut and increases the risk for such unpleasant gastrointestinal symptoms as bloating, nausea, cramping, and diarrhea.

Additional performance benefits: Increasing the intake of carbohydrate (3.6-5.5 g/lb BW or 10-12 g/kg BW) for the final 72 hours leading up to endurance competition, a practice known as carbo-loading, can increase muscle glycogen stores by as much as 40%, especially when training volume is reduced in conjunction. This practice helps delay the onset of muscle fatigue, also known as the wall (Sedlock, 2008). Using multiple sources of carbohydrates will produce better results compared to using a single source.

TABLE 3.2 Carbohydrate Intake Recommendations

	Dosing recommendations	Preferable carbohydrate sources
Daily intake	2.7-4.5 g/lb body weight (2.7-4.5 g/.45 kg/bw)	Whole grains, legumes, fruits, vegetables, yogurt, milk
Precompetition	1-1.5 g/lb body weight (1-1.5 g/.45 kg/bw) in the 2-3 hours leading up to start	Easy-to-digest low-residue (low-fiber) carbohydrates: plain bread, pretzels, potatoes, white rice, cream of rice cereal, pasta, pulp-free juices, sports drinks
During competition	<1 hour: carbohydrate rinse 1-3 hours: 30-60 g/h >3 hours: 60-90 g/h	GL, S, MD, M, AP, WMS GL, S, MD, M, AP, WMS Multiple Sources: MD + S, MD + F, MD + GL + F
Postcompetition	0.5-0.7 g/lb body weight (0.5-0.7 g/.45 kg/bw) within 30 minutes + every 2 hours for 4-6 hours or until calorie deficit is replenished	Immediate: MD + S, MD + F, MD + GL + F Long-term: whole grains, legumes, fruits, vegetables, yogurt, milk

Casein

aka *milk protein*

What it is: Casein is a type of protein found in milk. Milk contains two main proteins: casein and whey. Roughly 80% of protein found in milk is casein, which is considered a complete protein because it contains all the essential amino acids. Essential amino acids are those that cannot be produced by the body and therefore must be consumed in the diet. The amino acid profile of casein is similar to whey, although not completely identical.

Supplement Fact

Milk is naturally a good source of both casein and whey protein. Consuming milk either before or after training can provide a mix of casein and whey proteins. Whey is removed from cheese during the production process used to make various cheeses, including cottage cheese; as a result, these cheeses are excellent natural sources of casein.

How it works: Casein, unlike whey, is much more slowly digested and releases amino acids into the blood at a slower and more prolonged rate. Protein acts similarly to high- and low-glycemic carbohydrates, which can raise blood sugar at different rates.

Performance benefit: Because of its ability to release amino acids into the blood at a slower and more prolonged rate, casein is thought to be beneficial especially at night before bed as well as in combination with fast-digesting proteins either before or after exercise. Supplying the body with a slow and prolonged release of amino acids at night during sleep is thought to improve muscle recovery.

Research: To date, few studies have examined the effects of consuming casein either at night or in combination with fast-acting proteins before or following exercise. Most research suggests that fast-acting proteins such as whey are most beneficial for stimulating protein synthesis and muscle recovery following exercise and are superior when compared to casein or soy protein alone. However, no studies to date have examined if whey protein in combination with casein provides additional benefits immediately following exercise or long-term over the span of a 6- to 12-week training cycle. One study found that milk, a whey and casein combination, was superior to soy protein isolate in stimulating protein synthesis following exercise; comparisons with whey alone have not been done (Wilkinson et al., 2007). More recently, another study was the first to evaluate the impact of consuming 40 g of casein 30 minutes before bed in a group of 16 men using resistance training. The casein supplement was shown to stimulate protein synthesis by roughly 22% and increase amino acid availability throughout the night. Casein did not reduce markers of protein breakdown; however, its positive impact on protein synthesis led to an overall positive effect on protein balance (Res et al., 2012). Future research is needed to establish optimum amounts of casein and determine if casein is superior to other types of complete proteins.

Common usage: Typically, 20-40 g of casein proteins are used in combination with whey proteins either before or following exercise or at night before bed.

Health concerns: High-protein diets (less than 3 g/kg of body weight) do not appear to pose any health concerns; however, athletes must understand that excessive intakes of protein at the expense of other important nutrients such as carbohydrate, healthy fat, and those found in nutrient-dense fruits and vegetables can negatively affect performance.

Cat's Claw

aka *vincaria, vinicol, Uncaria tomentosa, Uncaria guianensis*

What it is: Cat's claw is a thick woody vine native to the Amazon and tropical areas of South and Central America. The plant has been used for thousands of years for medicinal and sacred purposes. The name is derived from the hook-like thorns that grow along the vine in a pattern that resembles the claws of a cat. Several species of the plant exist; however, *Uncaria tomentosa* is preferred for use in dietary supplements because of its higher alkaloid content. In Germany and Austria cat's claw can only be dispensed with a prescription. Cat's claw is believed to strengthen the immune system, inhibit inflammation, and suppress tumor growth and the replication of viruses (Erowele et al., 2009).

How it works: Cat's claw contains a variety of components that are believed to be responsible for its positive impact on health. These include a variety of alkaloids, glycosides, triterpenes, and steroids. Specifically, quinovic acid, β-sitosterol, and stigmaterol have been isolated in the plant. The exact mechanisms for all of cat's claws beneficial effects are unclear, but recent research suggests its antiinflammatory properties are related to the inhibition of nuclear factor kappa beta (NF-kB) (Erowele et al., 2009).

Performance benefit: Cat's claw is most commonly marketed for its antiinflammatory effects, especially for relief of osteoarthritic conditions in joints. These effects could benefit athletes needing to treat inflamed tissues. It may also help prevent immune system suppression resulting from heavy training.

>*continued*

Research: There are not a significant number of well-controlled research trials for cat's claw, although in vitro studies and animal studies are positive (Carvalho et al., 2006). One study found that treatment of knee osteoarthritis in 45 patients with 100 mg of cat's claw capsules improved pain associated with activity verses a placebo. (Piscoya et al., 2001) This is the only known study using cat's claw alone for treatment. Other studies have used a combination of cat's claw and other herbal remedies, making it difficult to distinguish benefits exclusive to cat's claw (Miller et al., 2006; Miller et al., 2005). There are also no studies on athletic populations, nor research related to a beneficial impact on immune suppression during prolonged intense exercise. Therefore, real-life evidence to support cat's claw's use in athletes is lacking.

Common usage: Unfortunately, the lack of scientific studies preformed on human subjects makes it difficult to conclude a best-use strategy. Most dietary supplements are sold in 500-1,000 mg doses in either capsule of liquid form. Athletes should also proceed with caution as the nutritional components of herbal dietary supplements can vary depending upon growing and harvesting conditions as well as plant parts included and extraction methods.

Health concerns: The use of cat's claw appears to be safe, and few adverse events have been reported. Some possible adverse effects include GI tract distress, diarrhea, and increased risk of bleeding. Athletes with bleeding disorders or those taking drugs such as Warfarin should proceed with caution when using cat's claw.

Cayenne

(see *capsicum*)

Centella Asiatica

(see *gotu kola*)

Cevitamic Acid

(see *vitamin C*)

Chia Seeds

aka *Salvia hispanica*

What it is: Naturally derived from the desert plant *Salvia hispanica,* chia seeds are a valuable source of omega-3 fatty acids, dietary fiber, protein, antioxidants, and minerals. Historically, they were used as a key fuel source by the Tarahumara, also known as the running people, during ultraendurance journeys across tough Mexican terrain. Claims that just a small amount can provide the energy to cover long distances have made the seed quite popular among endurance athletes.

How it works: Chia seeds, which contain gummy fibers known as mucilage, form a gel-like substance when mixed with water. Scientists believe this also occurs in the gut, allowing a barrier to form between digestive enzymes and carbohydrate that works to slow the breakdown of carbohydrate and help maintain better blood sugar control, an attractive feature for athletes competing in events such as ultramarathons. It is also thought that the hydrophilic (water loving) nature of chia seeds, which can absorb 10 times their weight in water, may allow an athlete to stay better hydrated during competition, another critical component to endurance and overall performance.

Performance benefit: Athletes may benefit from more stable blood sugars and extended endurance when using chia seeds before and during events lasting longer than 90 minutes.

Research: There is limited scientific data regarding the efficacy of chia seed use beyond the scope of general health; however, increased interest and use by endurance athletes has led sport science researchers at a few universities to start collecting data. One completed crossover study, conducted by the Human Performance Labs at the University of Alabama, failed to discover any added performance benefit when providing a small group of highly trained athletes a calorie-matched carbohydrate-loading treatment consisting of 50% chia and 50% sport drink (Gatorade) versus 100% sport drink in preparation for a 1-hour aerobic treadmill run followed by a 10K time trial on a track. A 2-week washout period separated each trial. While the chia seeds provided no performance advantage, there were no detriments either, which lead the scientists to conclude that chia seeds may provide a viable option for reducing dietary intake of sugar during a carbo-loading protocol (Illian, Casey, & Bishop, 2011).

Common usage: To form a gel for use leading up to as well as during athletic competition, mix 2 tbsp of seeds into 16-ounce (.47 L) solution containing 50% sports drink and 50% water. For health benefits, chia seeds can also be eaten raw, ground, roasted, or baked; they are commonly served on top of cereal, yogurt, and salads and added to smoothies and baked goods.

Health concerns: The high dietary fiber content of chia seeds may cause digestive issues, including bloating and gas, especially when consumed before or during competition.

Additional performance benefits: Rich in omega 3-fatty acids, chia seeds may help promote better recovery by reducing the chronic inflammation associated with high-intensity and high-volume sport training.

Chili Pepper

(see *capsicum*)

Chinese Caterpillar Fungus

(see *Cordyceps sinensis*)

Chitosan

What it is: Chitosan is produced from chitin, which is a structural element in the shell of crustaceans such as crabs, shrimp, and lobster. It is commonly made into supplement form and sold as a weight-loss product.

How it works: Chitosan can bind dietary fats and bile acids giving it potential as a weight-loss supplement and for treating high cholesterol.

Performance benefit: Chitosan assists with weight loss by binding fat consumed in the diet and limiting its absorption in the small intestine. As a result, calorie intake is reduced, resulting in weight loss. It's important that athletes realize that dietary fat is essential for many functions of the body, and decreasing its absorption might have a negative impact on performance. Fat provides essential fatty acids, aids in the absorption of fat-soluble vitamins, and is an important component of cell membranes.

Research: Research related to chitosan is relatively limited. Most studies have used nonathlete overweight or obese populations. These studies have looked strictly at chitosan's ability to reduce body weight compared with a placebo. Most studies suggest chitosan is mildly effective at reducing body weight and body fat. A 2006 study of overweight adults found that 3 g of chitosan per day for 60 days reduced body weight by 2.8 lb (1.3 kg) compared to a .8 lb (.4 kg) gain in body weight for a placebo group (Kaats, Michalek, & Preus). These results are similar to those of three other studies (Egras, 2011). Meanwhile, 2005 and 2008 reviews of chitosan concluded that effects were minimal and unlikely to be clinically significant (Mhurchu et al., 2005; Jull et al., 2008). Data are still limited, and conclusive recommendations cannot be made at this time. In addition, it is unknown if athletic performance or recovery is negatively affected as a result of binding essential fatty acids or limiting absorption of fat-soluble vitamins.

Common usage: Chitosan is typically supplemented in 1,500-3,000 mg dosages and should be taken in either two 1,500 mg doses before the two biggest meals of the day or in three separate 1,000 mg doses before meals.

Health concerns: Chitosan should be avoided by anyone with a shellfish allergy. Otherwise, chitosan appears to be safe and well tolerated. However, adverse effects such as constipation, flatulence, increased stool bulkiness, bloating, nausea, and heartburn have been reported. A recent meta-analysis on chitosan found that 1.2-6.75 g of chitosan per day reduced total cholesterol by 11.5 mg/dL, suggesting its cholesterol lowering effects are modest.

Choline

What it is: Choline is a member of the B-vitamin family. Choline was discovered in 1864, but it was only in 1998 that choline was classified as an essential nutrient by the Food and Nutrition Board of the Institute of Medicine. Choline is derived from the Greek word *chole,* which means bile. Like bile acids, choline was identified when scientists discovered its ability to prevent fatty build up in the liver.

How it works: Choline has a number of significant roles in the body, including neurotransmitter synthesis, cell membrane signaling, lipid transport, and homocysteine metabolism (Sanders & Zeisel, 2007). Most important for athletes is choline's role as a precursor in acetylcholine (a neurotransmitter) synthesis with a vital role in muscle contraction.

Performance benefit: Acetylcholine is released at the neuralmuscular junction and binds to receptors on muscles. The binding activates muscle contraction. The interest in choline and acetylcholine began in the 1990s when scientists discovered that levels of choline were significantly reduced in marathon runners after completion of the 26.2 mi (42.2 km) run and required 48 hours to return to normal (Conlay, Saboujian, & Wurtman, 1992). In addition, choline is an important precursor to phosphatidylcholine, which is a phospholipid with an important role in cell membrane structure and signaling.

Research: Studies have provided evidence that only strenuous, prolonged exercise decreases choline levels significantly. Exercise must be longer than 2 hours in duration and at intensities greater than 70% to significantly decrease choline (Penry & Manore, 2008). Supplementation with choline is not beneficial unless choline levels are significantly depleted. Sandage and colleagues have conducted one of the few studies examining the potential use of choline during prolonged, choline-depleting exercise. They found that 2.8 g of choline supplemented 1 hour before and halfway through a 20 mi (32.2 km) run improved finish times (1992). A few studies have examined whether supplementation with choline above normal concentrations can improve physical performance; however, no benefits were found (Buchman, Jenden, & Roch, 1999; Burns, Costill, & Fink, 1988; Deuster & Cooper, 2002; Warber et al., 2000). More research is needed, especially in team sports such as football, basketball, and soccer. Currently, choline has potential benefit; however, this applies only during prolonged, high-intensity exercise.

>continued

Choline >*continued*

Common usage: Scientists have used fluids containing 2.43-2.8 g of choline consumed 1 hour before exercise and another 2.43-2.8 g dose provided during exercise as a means of preventing choline depletion. The AI (adequate intake) for choline is 425 mg/day and 550 mg/day for adult women and men, respectively. Higher-fat meats such as beef liver and eggs are excellent sources of choline. One whole egg contains 113 mg of choline. Chicken, milk, and soybeans also contain relatively high amounts of choline, followed by cauliflower and spinach.

Health concerns: The tolerable upper limit of choline as established by the National Academy of Sciences is 3-3.5 g for men and women.

Chondroitin

What it is: Chondroitin is a large gel-forming molecule that is a constituent of hyaline cartilage. Hyaline cartilage covers the bones of synovial joints such as the knee, hip, and shoulder. Cartilage is important because it absorbs shock and reduces friction during movement. Chondroitin is commonly supplemented orally in the form of chondroitin sulfate made from extracts of cartilaginous tissues in fish, birds, cows, or pigs (Black et al., 2009).

How it works: As a constituent of hyaline cartilage, chondroitin is beneficial in preventing the degeneration of joints such as the knee, hip, ankle, shoulder, and spine. It is hypothesized the availability of chondroitin is a limiting factor in the synthesis of different components of cartilage.

Performance benefit: Many athletes experience chronic joint pain as a result of training. The physical demands of sport and daily training place a significant amount of stress on joints. In addition, many athletes must overcome injuries to joints resulting in surgery or joint reconstruction. Recovery from these types of surgeries can result in changes to the joint, and chondroitin could have a positive effect on recovery.

Research: The majority of research on chondroitin has focused on elderly populations suffering from osteoarthritis of the knee or hip. In a healthy joint there should be minimal narrowing of the space between bones. As cartilage is lost, joint space narrows and increases the likelihood of developing osteoarthritis, resulting in pain and loss of function. Chondroitin's ability to improve joint pain and function is less clear, with some but not all studies showing mild improvement. Long-term supplementation is most effective. In some cases chronic supplementation for over 1 year is required before structural changes in the joint are observed. Chondroitin is commonly supplemented in combination with another popular joint supplement, glucosamine sulfate. Research shows mixed results relative to improvements when combining these supplements versus using them alone. The Glucosamine/Chondroitin

Arthritis Intervention (GAIT) conducted by the U.S. National Institutes of Health is one of the largest studies ever done related to chondroitin. The results of this study found neither chondroitin, glucosamine, nor the combination to significantly relieve pain compared to a placebo. However, patients suffering from higher levels of pain (moderate to severe) did show improvements in pain scores from a combination of chondroitin and glucosamine (Sawitzke, 2010). Another meta-analysis of chondroitin research in 2009 concluded that chondroitin was mildly effective in preventing joint space narrowing or degeneration of the joint over time; however, over 2 years of supplementation were required before effects were realized (Ho Lee et al.). More research is needed before conclusions can be made related to chondroitin's effectiveness in speeding recovery from joint reconstructive surgeries.

Common usage: Typically, 800-1,200 mg of chondroitin sulfate are supplemented daily in either 1 large dose or 2-3 smaller doses throughout the day. There is no evidence to suggest that multiple doses consumed throughout the day are more effective than one large dose. Chondroitin is commonly supplemented in combination with glucosamine sulfate, SAMe (S-adenosylmethione), or MSM (methylsulfonylmethane).

Health concerns: Chondroitin appears to be safe. It has been used in many short- and long-term research studies without any adverse health effects reported.

Chromium Picolinate

What it is: Chromium picolinate is made from the trace mineral chromium and picolinic acid. Only small amounts of chromium are needed for optimal health. Chromium can be found in a diverse selection of whole foods such as meats, whole grains, fruits, and vegetables. Broccoli, grape juice, whole-wheat English muffins, and potatoes are among some of the higher chromium-containing foods. Chromium and picolinic acid are not naturally found together, but studies in animals have found that when supplemental sources of chromium are complexed with picolinic acid, absorption is improved.

How it works: The exact mechanism of chromium is not known, but it is believed to be related to its capacity to increase the effectiveness of insulin's ability to bind to cells and upregulate (or increase) receptors (Lukaski et al., 1996). It is hypothesized that this ability could enhance the anabolic properties of insulin, thus increasing lean body mass. In addition, chromium may stimulate metabolism and suppress appetite.

Performance benefit: If the proposed benefits of chromium are true, it would be of benefit for athletes wanting to gain lean muscle mass, improve body composition, and lose body fat and weight.

>continued

Chromium Picolinate >*continued*

Research: Excitement about the potential fat-burning and muscle-building effects of chromium picolinate began in the late 1980s following a study in which males who were supplemented with 200 mcg/day of chromium picolinate saw greater gains in strength and improvements in body composition verses a placebo (Lukaski et al., 1996). The results of this study were followed by several duplicate research trials that were unable to produce the same positive results. Pittler, Stevinson, and Ernst did a meta-analysis project in 2003 and compared the results of 10 studies related to chromium picolinate. Their results concluded that chromium picolinate provided a relatively small reduction in body weight, roughly 1.1-1.2 kg over 10-13 weeks in overweight and obese individuals. More recently, in 2010, a pilot study was conducted on overweight adults to assess the impact of 1,000 mcg of chromium picolinate over a 24-week supplementation period. The results found no significant benefits from supplementation. The authors of this trial concluded that chromium picolinate does not appear to be beneficial for healthy overweight populations (Yazaki et al.). However, it was noted that more research is needed relative to the use of chromium during intense periods of physical training and in prediabetic or diabetic populations suffering from insulin resistance.

Common usage: Typically, 200-1,000 mcg of chromium picolinate are supplemented daily, in either one or two smaller doses per day.

Health concerns: Few adverse events have been linked to high intakes of chromium; therefore, the Institute of Medicine of the National Academies has not established an upper tolerance limit. Certain medications may interact with chromium, especially when taken on a regular basis. It is advisable to check with a doctor or a qualified healthcare provider before supplementing with chromium.

Chrysin

aka *5,7-dihydroxyflavone*

What is it: Chrysin is a naturally occurring flavonoid present in plants. Significant amounts can be found in honey and honeycomb, and it can be chemically extracted from the blue passionflower or Indian trumpetflower. Flavonoids are natural antioxidants that exhibit a wide range of biological effects. Currently, more than 4,000 types of active flavonoids have been identified. These flavonoids are further subclassified into flavonols, flavones, flavanols, flavanones, anthocyanins, and isoflavonoids. Chrysin is considered a flavone. The effects of flavonoids can include antibacterial, antiinflammatory, antiallergic, antithrombotic, and vasodilatory results (Khoo, Chua, & Balaram, 2010).

How it works: Chrysin is largely promoted as an antiestrogen and testosterone-boosting supplement. It is believed to inhibit aromatase, an important enzyme involved in the production of estrogen. Aromatase enzymes are involved in the conversion of androgens into estrogens (Monterio, Azevedo, & Calhua, 2006). Inhibition of aromatase would increase androgens, such as testosterone, and limit the production of estrogens. Another potential mechanism is chrysin's ability to bind to estrogen receptors, limiting estrogen binding and estrogen's effects in the body.

Performance benefit: Athletes, mostly bodybuilders, have used chrysin supplements to promote anabolic hormones such as testosterone and limit estrogen. Anabolic hormones help build lean body mass and increase strength and power.

Research: Early studies in vitro related to chysin's ability to inhibit aromatase were positive (Campbell & Kurzer, 1993). Unfortunately, studies in animals and humans have not been effective, and while more research is needed, our current understanding is that chrysin does not inhibit aromatase activity (Monteiro, Azevedo, & Calhua, 2006; Saarinen et al., 2001). A group of scientists studied the impact on testosterone in males of 21 days of treatment with proplis and honey containing chrysin. The results showed no changes in levels of testosterone (Gambelunghe et al., 2003). Other studies have also failed to show a positive effect of chrysin on testosterone. Chrysin is often combined with other herbal ingredients to form a natural testosterone-boosting supplement. In a 2001 study, the effects of a natural testosterone-boosting cocktail that included androstenedione, dehydroepiandrosterone, saw palmetto, indole-3-carbinol, chrysin, and *Tribulus terrestris* were evaluated for 28 days. Total testosterone was unchanged, and while free testosterone levels were increased, so too were levels of estradiol, which can increase levels of estrogen and result in the development of female sex characteristics in males (Brown et al.).

Common usage: Chrysin is sold individually as a dietary supplement, often with a recommended daily dose of 1,000-2,000 mg. It is also commonly sold in combination with a variety of other so-called natural testosterone-boosting ingredients.

Health concerns: The use of chrysin appears safe. No known adverse effects have been noted in scientific research studies. However, many natural testosterone boosters often contain impurities such as prohormones, which are known to cause gynecomastia, lower HDL cholesterol, and negatively affect a person's psychological state. Athletes should use extreme caution when considering the use of these types of supplements.

Cinnamon

aka *cinnamomum*

What it is: Cinnamon is a common spice used for cooking. It originates from the bark of two medicinal herbs, *C. zeylanicum* and *C. cassia.* Aside from its use in cooking, cinnamon has been used for many years as a medicinal herb to treat stomach complaints and other ailments. However, scientists recently have discovered that cinnamon has a plethora of other potential benefits most significant of which is its ability to control blood sugar levels and improve insulin sensitivity. In addition, cinnamon is also believed to have antiinflammatory, antimicrobial, antioxidant, and blood pressure–lowering effects (Gruenwald, Freder, & Armbruster, 2010).

How it works: Cinnamon is comprised of a number of components that are speculated to be responsible for its beneficial effects. Volatile oils such as cinnamaldehyde, eugenol, linalool, and camphor are found in different quantities within the bark, leaf, and root bark of *C. zeylanicum and C. cassia* (Gruenwald, Freder, & Armbruster, 2010). These volatile oils are thought to be responsible for the beneficial effects of cinnamon. The quantities of these volatile oils vary within the different species of cinnamon. In addition, cinnamon contains powerful polyphenols that can function as antioxidants and have antiinflammatory effects.

Performance benefit: Cinnamon's ability to increase the effects of insulin could have strong implications for athletes, especially postworkout. Cinnamon could improve glycogen restoration and further stimulate protein synthesis through its insulin-augmenting effects. Improvement of glycogen restoration and protein synthesis could aid and speed muscle recovery. In addition, cinnamon could protect against chronically inflamed muscles and joints, reducing the severity of delayed-onset muscle soreness (DOMS) and tendonitis. Additionally, the antioxidant properties of cinnamon could support the immune system and decrease the immune suppression that often results from heavy exercise and training.

Research: The majority of research has focused on the impact of cinnamon on blood glucose and potential benefits in the treatment of diabetes. A meta-analysis in 2011 concluded that cinnamon intake either as whole cinnamon or as cinnamon extract improves fasting blood glucose in type II diabetics or prediabetics (Davis, 2011). In another study 22 subjects with prediabetes and metabolic syndrome consumed 500 mg daily of cinnamon extract for 12 weeks. Cinnamon extract resulted in significantly lower fasting blood glucose levels and increases in lean mass (Ziegenfuss et al., 2006). Another study using 3 g of cinnamon per day for 8 weeks found no significant reductions in body composition compared to a placebo (Vafa, 2012). Clear conclusions related to cinnamon's impact on body composition are difficult to make at this

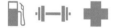

time, and more research is needed. In vitro studies show cinnamon extract increases glucose uptake and glycogen synthesis (Couturier et al., 2010). Unfortunately, no specific studies have involved athletes or investigated cinnamon's impact on glucose uptake and glycogen restoration postexercise or its impact on protein synthesis. In vitro and animal studies also support cinnamon as an antiinflammatory and inhibitor of cyclooxygenase-2 (COX-2) (Gruenwald, 2010). Unfortunately, there is no evidence in humans related to treatment or prevention of arthritic conditions; thus, supplementation for joint or muscle pain is not supported at this time.

Common usage: Supplementation dosages of cinnamon between 3-6 g daily appear to be most effective. In addition the source of cinnamon, either *C. zeylanicum* or *C. cassia,* may have different effects, and further well-designed studies are needed to confirm the most effective sources.

Health concerns: Cinnamon appears to be safe, especially within recommended doses of 3-6 g/day. Preclinical and other human trials have not shown any significant toxic effects (Ranasinghe, 2012).

Citrimax HCA

(see *hydroxycitric acid*)

Citrulline Malate (CM)

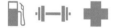

aka *citrullus*

What it is: A nonessential amino acid (L-citrulline) bound to an organic salt compound (malate), citrulline malate (CM) is a special nutrient combo marketed as an ergogenic aid for its purported role in reducing muscle fatigue, enhancing aerobic energy production, and facilitating optimal recovery.

How it works: Individually, citrulline is synthesized from the amino acid glutamine within the intestines and plays a part in a series of biochemical reactions important for the removal of ammonia. Ammonia is a byproduct of both anaerobic and aerobic exercise that at high levels can negatively affect the production of energy, thereby leading to fatigue and reduced performance. Malate, also known as malic acid, is found naturally in fruits such as apples and plays a role in a series of chemical reactions known as the Kreb's cycle that produce energy from carbohydrate, fats, and protein within the mitochondria. Furthermore, malate is able to recycle lactate for energy production, critical in protecting the muscles from fatigue and aiding recovery. Together, CM is thought to enhance aerobic performance by accelerating the clearance of fatigue-inducing ammonia and recycling lactate for improved energy production (Sureda & Pons, 2013).

>*continued*

Citrulline Malate (CM) >*continued*

Performance benefit: Athletes may benefit from increased endurance during aerobic training and competition as well as faster recovery between high-intensity bursts of energy common in interval training as well as stop-and-go sports such as soccer.

Research: While limited in quantity, human studies evaluating the impact of citrulline malate have shown some promise. One well-designed favorable study found a single dose of 8 g of CM to increase the total number of repetitions completed by healthy men during 8 sets of flat barbell bench presses by nearly 53%, a significant improvement from the placebo trial. Furthermore, a 40% reduction in muscle soreness at 24 hours and 48 hours posttraining was reported as compared to the placebo trial. Study investigators concluded that CM demonstrated promise for athletes engaged in high-intensity anaerobic exercises with short rest times as well as for any athlete looking to reduce muscle soreness and improve recovery (Perez-Guisado & Jakeman, 2010). A lower dose of 6 g/day taken over 15 days also yielded positive results with healthy men, demonstrating a significant reduction in the sensation of fatigue, a 34% increase in the rate of ATP energy production during exercise, and a 20% increase in the rate of phosphocreatine recovery after exercise, indicating a reduced energy cost of muscle contraction as compared to presupplementation trials (Bendahan et al., 2002). An animal study essentially replicated this data, demonstrating a significant decrease in both phosphocreatine (28%) and oxidative (32%) costs of contraction with CM supplementation, leading authors to conclude CM has an ergogenic effect associated with an improvement of muscle contraction efficiency (Giannesini et al., 2011).

Common usage: Research-supported dosages for CM range anywhere from 4-8 g/day. For use as a single dose, athletes may consume 8 g 30-40 minutes before competition. For use as a daily supplement taken throughout a competitive season, athletes may consume 4-6 g split into 2 doses so that 2-3 g are taken 30-40 minutes before exercise and another 2-3 g are taken at bedtime, preferably on an empty stomach.

Health concerns: CM appears to be safe for use though there are some reports of stomach upset at doses of 8 g/day.

Additional performance benefits: CM supplementation can improve the use of amino acids, especially branched-chain amino acids, during exercise, which may further improve recovery from exertion (Sureda et al., 2010).

Citrus Aurantium

(see *synephrine*)

Cobalamin

(see *vitamin B12*)

Cochin Ginger

(see *ginger*)

Cocoa

aka *dark chocolate, cacao, theobroma cacao, cocoa flavonals, gallated flavan-3-ols*

What it is: Foods and beverages that contain chocolate or cocoa are made from the beans of the *Theobroma cacao* tree. Cocoa liquor is a paste made from fermented cocoa beans that have been ground, roasted, and shelled (nibs). The percent cocoa referred to on food packaging is the percentage of cocoa liquor within the product. Cocoa powder, used in baking, is made by removing the cocoa butter from the liquor (Katz, Doughty, & Ali, 2011).

How it works: Cocoa contains fatty acids; minerals such as magnesium, copper, potassium, and calcium; and polyphenols. Polyphenols include a variety of compounds, but cocoa is particularly rich in flavonoids, which include epicatechin, catechin, and procyanidins. Flavonoids can have cardioprotective effects through their antioxidant activity. In addition, flavonoids have immunoregulatory properties and beneficial effects on the vascular system. Flavonoids in cocoa can prevent the formation of atherosclerosis and lower blood pressure. Epicatechins appear to affect vascular function the most (Katz, Doughty, & Ali, 2011; Jalil & Ismail, 2008).

Performance benefit: Cocoa could benefit athletes through its impact on vascular function. Improved vascular function would result in increased blood flow and nutrients to muscles during training, resulting in improved performance. Improved blood flow postexercise would provide benefits as well, better enabling nutrients consumed postexercise to be delivered and thereby affect recovery. The antioxidant and immunoregulatory effects of cocoa provide additional benefits to athletes.

Research: Research related to nonathletes is positive. The majority of research trials suggest that cocoa is capable of decreasing blood pressure and cholesterol and improving vascular function. No study to date has looked at the impact of cocoa on immune function in humans although early animal studies are positive. Only recently have trials investigated the impact of cocoa on exercise. A study in 2011 and another in 2012 investigated the impact of 40 g and 100 g of dark chocolate before prolonged cycling. Results found dark chocolate to be beneficial in reducing oxidative stress and increasing mobilization of free fatty acids (Allgrove et al., 2011; Davison et al., 2012); however, dark chocolate had no effect on immune and endocrine response, nor on time trial performance. More research is needed to clarify the impact of cocoa and its polyphenols relative to sports and exercise.

>continued

Common usage: As little as 5 mg of the polyphenol epicatechin has been shown to provide health benefits. Typically, research trials have used 300-800 mg/day of cocoa polyphenols, which is the recommended supplementation level. Roughly 50 mg of polyphenols are present in 1 g of cocoa powder; a 40 g dark chocolate bar contains 300-600 mg, while a 40 g milk chocolate bar averages 100-200 mg.

Health concerns: The biggest concerns related to cocoa and dark chocolate are the high calorie and fat content and the risk of associated weight gain. No other health concerns are known at this time.

Coconut

aka *coconut water, coconut milk, virgin coconut oil, Cocos nucifera*

What it is: Coconut is the fruit harvested from the *Cocos nuciferea* tree. It is a dietary staple in Philippian, Polynesian, and Malaysian cultures. These cultures commonly use coconut as a complementary medicine. Coconut water, milk, and oils (found in the fleshy component of the fruit) are commonly used portions of the fruit and are becoming more popular as dietary supplements.

How it works: Coconut's uses in medicine include its antibacterial, antifungal, and antiviral properties. In addition, coconut contains powerful antioxidants and is an immunostimulant. Coconut is unique in that it contains large amounts (roughly 70%-80%) of medium-chain triglycerides (MCTs). MCTs are smaller and can be absorbed directly into the blood compared with longer chains, which must travel through the lymphatic system and the liver before being oxidized by the muscles as fuel. Recently, coconut water has been touted as a superior fluid replacement compared to Gatorade and other sport drinks.

Performance benefit: Coconut water is speculated to enhance fluid replacement, prevent dehydration, and limit the drops in physical performance that result from dehydration. Coconut milk, oil, and to some extent water provide powerful antioxidants and support healthy immune function. These properties could aid athletes in managing the stresses of training that can suppress the immune system, as well as limit the inflammation produced by muscle damage or injury. MCTs, which are absorbed directly into the blood, can be quickly oxidized as a source of fuel during exercise, enabling endurance athletes to spare muscle glycogen and improve performance. Some evidence exists that MCTs can increase metabolic rate, assist in weight loss, and improve body composition.

Research: Kalman and colleagues conducted a study in 2012 examining coconut's hydrating abilities compared to water and a carbohydrate electrolyte sport drink. No significant differences were noted in performance or markers of rehydration. Other studies have produced similar results. While coconut water is equally effective in promoting rehydration, it is not superior to sport drinks and has also been noted to be less tolerable, causing GI tract distress (Kalman et al., 2012; Saat et al., 2002). Information related to the immune-stimulating and antiinflammatory properties of coconut is limited. Early work in animals is positive, showing coconut's antiinflammatory effect at high doses; however, no studies have evaluated this effect in humans or with specific inflammation-related conditions in athletes (Intahphuak, Khonsung, & Panthong, 2010). In weight loss studies, coconut oil provides small improvements and tends to improve losses in abdominal body fat; however, only two studies related to these effects are known, and more data are needed to confirm these results (Liau et al., 2011; Assuncao et al., 2009).

Common usage: Weight-loss studies have used 30 mL (2 tbsp) of coconut oil per day. Recommendations for coconut water as a fluid replacement are similar to those for other fluids: 4-8 oz (.12-.24 L) every 15 minutes during exercise and 20 oz/lb. (.6 L/.45 kg) lost during exercise.

Health concerns: Although they are high in saturated fats, coconut milk and oils do not negatively affect blood cholesterol levels, and consumption is safe.

Coenzyme Q10 (CoQ10)

aka *ubiquinone, ubidecarenone*

What it is: A vitamin-like, fat-soluble compound of the ubiquinone family, coenzyme Q10 functions in all cells of the body, serving as a coenzyme for several of the key enzymatic steps that facilitate ATP production through aerobic respiration within the mitochondrial electron transport chain. Coenzyme Q10 also doubles as potent antioxidant, helping destroy free radicals before they can cause damage to normal cells within the body. Coenzyme Q10 is found naturally in highest concentration within organs and muscles demanding the most energy, such as the heart. Coenzyme Q10 can also be found in such dietary sources as meat, poultry, and fish.

How it works: The human body is on a continuous mission to generate enough energy to support the performance of every cell. It is thought that increased dietary intake of coenzyme Q10, through whole food or supplementation, may help the body keep up the demand for mitochondrial ATP synthesis, especially when demand exceeds production during times of stress, including the stress of physical exertion on the cardiovascular system as well as the stress of muscle recovery from athletic injury. In addition, as a potent antioxidant in both the mitochondria and lipid membranes, coenzyme Q10 helps to combat the 10- to 20-fold increase in molecules called reactive

>continued

oxygen species (ROS) during physical exercise that can contribute to muscle injury and decreased performance.

Performance benefit: Purported performance-focused benefits of coenzyme Q10 supplementation include improved oxygen usage in the heart and skeletal muscles, leading to increases in maximal aerobic capacity, anaerobic endurance, and overall work capacity. Coenzyme Q10 is also marketed as a recovery agent, helping to reduce exercise-induced muscle injury.

Research: While research has shown intense physical training to lower blood levels of coenzyme Q10, there are mixed results on the validity of daily supplementation to produce enhancements in cardiovascular-focused performance variables. The majority of double-blind and placebo-controlled studies fail to demonstrate any significant enhancement with a daily supplementation protocol of 60-150 mg followed over 4-8 weeks regardless of fitness status (trained vs. untrained) (Zhou et al., 2005; Bloomer et al., 2012; Ostman et al., 2012). Some scientists believe this may be due to inefficient absorption of coenzyme Q10 into the mitochondrial membrane, leaving open the possibility of better results with increased bioavailability (Liao et al., 2007). Nonetheless, while the current consensus remains primarily negative with respect to coenzyme Q10's impact on cardiovascular performance parameters, the studies evaluating its impact on muscle recovery remain positive. A double-blind study on elite martial arts athletes, for example, discovered that a daily supplementation protocol of 300 mg of coenzyme Q10 for 20 days during a period of intense training significantly lowered levels of the lipid peroxide, a free radical that contributes to oxidative stress in the body, and creatine kinase, an enzyme that signals muscle damage and injury, thereby helping protect against exercise-induced muscle injury and improving recovery (Kon et al., 2008).

Common usage: Per study protocols, recommended doses for adult athletes over 18 years range from 60 to 300 mg/day taken continuously for at least 3 weeks. For doses higher than 100 mg/day, it is best to split the does into 2-3 smaller doses and take them with meals containing some fat to facilitate more efficient absorption. While coenzyme Q10 is available in many forms, soft gels tend to be better absorbed than capsules or other preparations.

Health concerns: Coenzyme Q10 is generally safe, with the exception of infrequent reports of nausea, loss of appetite, upset stomach, and diarrhea. Due to several drug-nutrient interactions, however, athletes taking any form of medication are advised to consult a physician before starting a supplementation protocol.

Additional performance benefits: Athletes with muscle wasting diseases, such as muscular dystrophy, as well as diabetic and master's level athletes are thought to carry lower levels of coenzyme Q10 and might benefit the most from supplementation.

Colostrum

aka *mother's milk, bovine colostrum (BC)*

What it is: The milk secreted by a cow during the first few days after giving birth, bovine colostrum (BC), contains a wide array of nutrients essential to the overall health of the athlete as well as growth-promoting and disease-fighting compounds that are thought to facilitate quicker recovery times during intense cycles of training and competition. BC contains 3-4 times more protein than regular cow's milk, an estimated 150 g/L, and is lactose free.

How it works: In 2009 a review of studies exploring the positive, performance-focused attributes of BC and corresponding mechanisms of action concluded that supplementation seems to elicit a favorable impact on the recovery of athletes engaged in high-intensity or high-volume training (Shing, Hunter, & Stevenson). Several reasons were cited. First, BC seems to increase blood levels of a hormone called IGF1, otherwise known as insulin-like growth factor 1, which enhances glucose and amino acid transport to cells; promotes protein synthesis while protecting against protein breakdown, all key factors to recovery; and may also help contribute to lean body mass gains. Second, BC appears to improve intramuscular buffering capacity, helping protect against muscle fatigue during high-intensity training as well as enhance recovery between high-intensity exercise sessions. Finally, BC has been shown to increase levels of an antibody called IgA (immunoglobulin-A) within saliva that may help activate immune defenses, protecting the athlete from various sidelining bugs throughout training and competition.

Performance benefit: Athletes may benefit from quicker recovery times and enhanced immune function, especially when the body is exposed to increased stress levels common at the peak of training and competition.

Research: The bulk of current research evaluating the performance impact of BC has produced mixed results. One double-blind, placebo-controlled study failed to demonstrate an impact on blood or saliva immunoglobulin levels after a 4-week daily supplementation protocol incorporating 25 g of a low-protein colostrum; however, the incidence of upper respiratory symptoms reported by elite swimmers decreased by 36% as compared to a calorie-matched placebo (Crooks et al., 2010). In contrast, an earlier double-blind, placebo-controlled study of adult male and female athletes found a BC dose of 20 g taken during 2 weeks of training produced significant increases in serum IGF1 and saliva IgA (Mero et al., 2002). Additionally, a lower dose (10 g/day) of BC taken over 10 weeks not only reduced the incidence of upper respiratory symptoms but also yielded significant improvements in highly trained cyclists compared to a placebo group in a 40 km time trial performance after completing a high-intensity training session (Shing et al., 2006).

>continued

Researchers attributed these results in part to a significant level of favorable changes in the concentration of several antibodies. It is evident that the performance impact of BC is likely multifaceted, meaning small improvements across several variables versus a single variable contributing to the potential benefits associated with supplementation. Future studies should focus on the impact of a standardized supplement protocol (e.g., dose, length of time) on the proposed mechanisms of actions and the performance of athletes in a variety of exercise protocols.

Common usage: BC is available in a variety of forms, including tablets, powders, bars, and liquids. Research-supported doses are variable but, on average, a dose of 10-50 g/day has been used.

Health concerns: While BC is generally well tolerated, there have been some reports of gastrointestinal distress, including such symptoms as bloating, nausea, vomiting, and diarrhea, as well as diminishing performance returns at high doses (>50 g/day).

Additional performance benefits: BC taken in doses of 20 g/day over 14 days before completing a high-intensity exercise trial may help reduce the exercise-induced increase in gut permeability of athletes by helping to reduce the incidence of gastrointestinal symptoms such as an upset stomach or diarrhea often seen as a result of endurance competition (Marchbank et al., 2011).

Coneflower

(see *echinacea*)

Conjugated Linoleic Acid (CLA)

What it is: Conjugated linoleic acid (CLA) is an isomer of linoleic acid. Linoleic acid is an omega-6 fatty acid, one of two fatty acids considered essential since they cannot be made in the body and must be consumed in the diet. The chemical formula of CLA is the same as linoleic acid; however, its chemical structure is different. CLA is commonly found in two shapes: trans-10, cis-12-CLA (10-CLA) and cis-9, trans-11-CLA (9-CLA). CLA is found in milk, butter, and meat fats. Roughly 75%-90% of the CLA found in milk is of the 9-CLA variety.

How it works: CLA is believed to improve body composition by lowering fat mass and increasing fat-free mass. There are a variety of proposed mechanisms, which include decreased enzyme activity leading to a decreased uptake of triglycerides by fat cells. CLA is also believed to influence transcription factors that regulate production of new fat cells. Lastly, CLA is thought to increase β-oxidation, the metabolic pathway used to burn fat.

Performance benefit: CLA is a popular supplement among bodybuilders, fitness competitors, and other athletes interested is reducing body fat and increasing lean.

Research: A significant amount of research has been done on CLA, producing a wide variety of results. Early studies in animals were positive: CLA use led to losses in body fat and increases in lean body mass, especially in mice. However, studies in humans were not nearly as conclusive or effective. In 2007 scientists conducted a meta-analysis looking at 18 scientific studies related to CLA and its impact on body composition. They concluded that a 50:50 mixture of 10-CLA and 9-CLA did produce a slow decrease in fat mass (.05 kg/week) over the course of 6 months to 2 years. Fat loss peaked between 1 and 2 years (Whigham et al.). A similar meta-analysis was completed in 2009 to determine if fat-free mass or muscle mass was affected. The same 18 studies were used, and it was concluded that CLA was not effective in increasing muscle mass (Schoeller, Watras, and Whigham). More recently, in a 2011 study of the effects of CLA for 8 weeks on body composition in overweight men, CLA did not affect body weight, composition, or beta-oxidation, which is a marker of fat use (Joseph et al.).

Common usage: Research suggests that 10-CLA is most effective in producing changes in body fat; however, when supplemented alone, it produces insulin resistance. This negative affect is counteracted when 10-CLA is supplemented with 9-CLA. A dosage of 3.2 g/day of 50:50 (10-CLA:9-CLA) is suggested, and higher doses are not recommended.

Health concerns: Higher intakes of CLA increase liver and spleen size and can result in insulin resistance. In addition, some studies have found CLA to increase makers of inflammation, such as the C-reactive protein.

Copper (Cu)

What it is: An essential trace mineral that is not synthesized by the body and thus must be consumed in the diet, copper plays a role in a wide range of biochemical processes key to optimal health and performance. It can be obtained naturally from such foods as organ meats, seafood (especially shellfish), nuts, seeds, whole grains, legumes, and chocolate as well as in dietary supplement form.

How it works: Because copper is lost in small amounts via sweat during exercise, athletes may be more vulnerable to deficiencies if intake from whole foods or supplementation does not offset these losses. Deficiencies in copper can lead to a number of symptoms detrimental to the health and performance of an athlete. For one, the body requires copper to produce ATP energy; without it, energy waivers. Copper is also critical for optimal use of iron. If iron is hindered, oxygen delivery to red blood cells becomes impaired,

>continued

Copper (Cu) >*continued*

leading to diminished respiratory function as well as muscle fatigue and weakness. Furthermore, copper is important for the function of a variety of enzymes essential to an athlete's health. One of these enzymes, superoxide dismutase (SOD), is considered one of the most powerful antioxidants, helping to scavenge damaging free radicals and counteract some of the damage to cells the body's own defense mechanisms cannot offset during particularly hard training cycles. Copper's antioxidant defenses may better support an athlete's immunity as well as aid recovery. Another enzyme, lysil oxidase, aids in the formation of collagen and elastin, two proteins necessary for bone and connective tissue health.

Performance benefit: Athletes may benefit from enhanced energy and endurance as well as gain better immune support and quicker recovery times.

Research: Most available research has evaluated the impact of strenuous exercise on copper status and the ramifications for a variety of body functions important to health and performance; however, many studies are animal based and merely draw conclusions based on purported benefits of increased copper intake through diet or supplementation. One study of sorts evaluated the correlation between neutropenia (abnormally low numbers of white blood cells called neutrophils), a marker of immune status, and serum copper levels in an Olympic sailing crew during training for the Beijing Olympic Games. As suspected, the serum copper concentration of sailors with neutropenia was significantly lower than those with normal neutrophil content, leading authors to conclude that low serum copper may be a cause of impaired immune function in elite athletes and that supplementation may be helpful for this population (Lewis et al., 2010). Another study of race dogs determined prolonged run training over 3 days and a 12-15 day sled race depressed the blood activities of three copper enzymes with antioxidant qualities: plasma ceruloplasmin, plasma diamine oxidase, and erythrocyte superoxide dismutase. Study investigators concluded this effect could have been prevented by increased copper intake (DiSilvestro, Hinchcliff, & Blostein-Fujii, 2004). Future research needs to focus on the actual impact of copper supplementation on the variables important to human athletic performance in both deficient and nondeficient populations.

Common usage: The current RDA for copper is 0.9 mg, though up to 3 mg may be consumed through whole food or dietary supplementation, generally in multimineral form, to support health. Copper should be taken separately from vitamin C and zinc for optimal absorption. While the recommended daily intake for copper is met by most North American diets, athletes, especially those who follow a vegetarian diet or who have undergone gastric bypass surgery, are at greater risk for deficiency due to special circumstances that increase daily requirements.

Health concerns: Excessive copper intake, generally defined by levels above the upper safe and adequate daily dietary intake of 1.5-3 mg/day for adults, can trigger severe stomach pain, nausea, vomiting, and diarrhea. Copper can be toxic to the body at levels above 10 mg/day.

Cordyceps Sinensis

aka *Chinese caterpillar fungus, Dong Chong Xia Cao,* medicinal mushroom

What it is: A wild fungus discovered at high altitude in China, *Cordyceps sinensis* (CS) has long been used in Chinese medicine to protect the lungs from a variety of ailments. Nicknamed "summer plant, winter worm" due to its growth on the larvae of a Leipidoptera moth, a cycle that takes approximately 6 years, CS is an extremely rare find in nature and expensive in its wild form. As a result, CS is generally cultivated. The popularity of the supplement in sports boomed in the early 1990s after a series of records set by Chinese elite distance runners were attributed by their coach to a dietary protocol that included CS during training.

How it works: Animal studies have shown CS to increase the ratio of ATP to inorganic phosphate in the liver, allowing for more efficient use of oxygen and a higher tolerance to acidosis, thereby showing potential performance applications for sports that require both aerobic and anaerobic endurance.

Performance benefit: As exertion level increases, so does the demand for oxygen. By improving oxygen usage, CS may help an athlete better respond to these demands, enhancing anaerobic threshold, reducing lactic acid, and extending time to exhaustion.

Research: While animal studies have demonstrated several potential positive applications for athletes, especially those competing in endurance events, the translation to sport performance in human studies have not been consistent. For example, a 2004 double-blind study found no significant differences in $\dot{V}O_2$max, peak power output, blood lactate levels, time to exhaustion, and overall time trial performance between a placebo-fed and a CS-fed group of trained cyclists after 5 weeks of CS supplementation. Similar results were documented just a year later in a smaller double-blind, placebo-treatment study on trained cyclists (Parcell et al.). However, a 2010 double-blind, placebo-controlled, prospective trial yielded significant improvements in the metabolic and ventilatory performance of older (50-75 years) active subjects completing a symptom-limited incremental exercise protocol on a cycle ergometer after a 12-week daily supplemental protocol with 333 mg CS taken 3 times/day (Chen et al.). Such results are consistent with animal studies demonstrating a higher tolerance to acidosis and resistance to fatigue (Kumar et al., 2011).

Common usage: Research-supported doses of CS range from 4.5-10 g/day, often split into 2-3 doses.

Health concerns: While CS is generally considered safe, there is little known about the safety of long-term use. In the short term, reported side effects

>continued

include diarrhea, dry mouth and nausea. Athletes with immune system disorders such as multiple sclerosis, lupus, and rheumatoid arthritis or who are pregnant or breastfeeding are advised against using CS.

Additional performance benefits: Animal studies have shown CS to improve stress-induced physiological changes within the adrenal gland, thymus, and thyroid, thus presenting promise from an immune function, resistance to fatigue, and recovery standpoint. CS may further help enhance the body's defense against infections and inflammation by stimulating the activity and numbers of several immune markers, including T-helper cells and natural killer cells.

Creatine

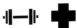

aka *N-(aminoiminomethyl)-N-methylglycine, creatine monohydrate, creatine citrate, creatine ethyl-ester*

What it is: Creatine is a naturally occurring nutrient that can be obtained in the diet from meat and fish. It can also be synthesized in the liver and pancreas from the amino acids arginine, glycine, and methionine. Approximately 95% of the body's creatine is stored in muscle, mostly in the form of phosphocreatine. Phosphocreatine and creatine provide a vital reservoir of energy that is used to replenish ATP during high-intensity exercise. Although the supplementation of creatine did not become popular until the early 1990s, the interest in creatine and its metabolism dates back over 160 years. In 1992 the London *Times* revealed that Linford Christie, a British sprinter and gold medalist in the Barcelona Olympic Games, used creatine (Rawson & Venezia, 2011). Since the 1990s creatine has become increasingly popular and to date is among the best-selling dietary supplements on the market.

How it works: During high-intensity anaerobic exercise lasting 5-15 seconds, muscles rely on stores of phosphocreatine to resynthesize ATP. Once these stores become depleted, the body is forced to rely on other forms of metabolism for ATP, and performance begins to decline. Supplementation with creatine increases stores of phosphocreatine, allowing muscles to work at higher intensities for a longer time. This is extremely beneficial for performance in high-intensity, strength, and power sports that rely heavily on phosphocreatine stores for energy.

Performance benefit: Creatine offers a number of performance benefits. It can produce small but immediate effects on maximum strength and power. This allows athletes to perform more high-intensity work in competition and training, resulting in improved performance and an enhanced training effect.

Research: Scientific research has proven that supplementation with creatine results in 10%-40% increases in phosphocreatine stores within muscles. Athletes who consume diets low in meat and fish or who are vegetarian typically see the highest increases in phosphocreatine stores. Short-term supplementation has been shown to improve maximal strength and power by 5%-15%, single-effort sprint performance 1%-5%, and work performed during multiple sets of maximal strength training or sprinting 5%-15%. In addition, long-term creatine supplementation can improve the training effect by 5%-15%, improving gains in strength, power, and lean body mass (Kreider, 2003). A number of forms of creatine exist, including creatine salts (creatine citrate, maleate, fumarate, tartrate, pyruvate), creatine ethyl ester, and Kre-alkalyn. No forms of creatine are scientifically proven to be more effective than creatine monohydrate. D-pinitol and Russian tarragon (*Artemisia dracunculus*) are commonly added to creatine supplements to improve effectiveness; however, evidence to support this is inconclusive (Jager et al., 2011). One of two research studies on D-pinitol found low doses to be effective and enhance creatine uptake; however, results from another research trial found no benefits (Greenwood et al, 2001; Kerksick et al., 2009).

Common usage: It is advised that athletes use a loading protocol for the most immediate effect on phosphocreatine stores. This involves consuming .3 g/kg of body weight or .25 g/kg of fat-free mass for 3-5 days followed by a dose of 3-5 g/day thereafter. The uptake of creatine within the muscle is best when creatine is consumed in combination with protein and carbohydrate. During the 3- to 5-day loading phase, the total daily dose should be separated into 4-5 smaller servings consumed throughout the day. Following loading, a 3-5 g maintenance dose can be consumed pre- or postworkout. A longer-term strategy that does not involve loading for 3-5 days but rather involves consuming 4-6 g daily can also be used and is effective; however, the effect is not as immediate (Buford et al., 2007). Typically, phosphocreatine stores remain elevated for 4-6 weeks after supplementation stops.

Health concerns: Creatine is considered safe despite speculation that it negatively affects renal function. Creatine has also been scrutinized because of a lack of long-term research; however, long-term use has been studied up to 5 years. Creatine does not increase the risk of cramping nor cause dehydration. Interestingly, recent evidence suggests that creatine might have additional health benefits in the treatment of a broad range of diseases including neurodegenerative disorders, cancer, rheumatic diseases, and type 2 diabetes, in addition to improving cognitive function in the elderly (Buford et al., 2007).

Creatine Pyruvate

(see *pyruvate*)

Curcumin

aka *Curcuma longa, tumeric*

What it is: Curcumin is a constituent of *Curcuma longa,* also known as turmeric. Turmeric is cultivated in India and other parts of Southeast Asia where it is a common spice used in Indian dishes such as curry. Turmeric is what gives these dishes their strong yellow color. In addition to its use as a spice, turmeric has been used in Ayurvedic medicine (traditional system of medicine from India) for a wide variety of conditions most commonly related to inflammation. Curcumin polyphenols are the active constituents in turmeric.

How it works: Curcumins have antiinflammatory and antioxidant effects on the body. The antiinflammatory effects of curcumins have sparked so much interest that between 1999 and 2009 over 2,400 articles were published on curcumins and their role in the treatment of conditions such as cancer, heart disease, rheumatoid arthritis, and even obesity (Kidd 2009). Curcumins inhibit COX-2, as well as transcription factors and down regulate NF-κB, which is involved in the regulation of many different inflammatory proteins. The mechanisms behind curcumins antiinflammatory effects can seem complex and overwhelming (Jurenka, 2009). However, most important to understand is that curcumins act via many mechanisms, and this diversity has a powerful antiinflammatory effect.

Performance benefit: Athletes commonly use antiinflammatories to limit inflammation and pain from muscle injury, arthritic joints, or DOMS (delayed-onset muscle soreness) resulting from heavy, intensified training. Curcumin is a promising supplement for athletes looking for an alternative to nonsteroidal antiinflammatories (NSAIDS) such as ibuprofen. Curcumins could also be used to lessen muscle soreness and speed recovery following training, thus improving and speeding athletic gains from training.

Research: Numerous studies are positive related to the use of curcumins as a therapy for cancer, rheumatoid arthritis, and osteoarthritis (Jurenka, 2009). Animal and human trials are confirming the antiinflammatory and antioxidant effects of curcumins. In addition, these trials are uncovering the various mechanisms by which curcumins work. Davis and colleagues were the first to test the impact of curcumins on DOMS produced in rats via a downhill running protocol. Results found curcumins blunt various inflammatory markers, improve muscle recovery, and improve performance in a time trial 48-72 hours after induction of DOMS (2007). No human trials related to muscle recovery or the prevention of DOMS are known.

Common usage: Supplementation doses of curcumin have ranged from a total of 500 mg-3 g daily. This dosage has been provided once or twice a day in most studies. Unfortunately, the most effective strategy has yet to be determined. The bioavailability of curcumins is poor and variable between subjects. Scientists are working to develop strategies to improve bioavailability. Currently, it is recommended that daily intake not exceed 3 g (1 tsp) per day.

Health concerns: Curcumin appears to be safe; however, there is some concern that turmeric or curcumins can cause urinary oxalate levels to rise resulting in an increased risk of kidney stones. For this reason, keeping turmeric intake below 3 g (1 tsp) daily is advised (Tang, 2008).

Cyanocobalamin

(see *vitamin B12*)

Dark Chocolate

(see *cocoa*)

Deer Velvet

aka *deer velvet antler, deer antler extract, elk velvet antler*

What it is: Deer antler (DA) has been used for over 2,000 years in Chinese medicine. It is purported to provide a range of benefits, including enhancement of musculoskeletal and immune function, rapid healing of tissues and bones, and improved vitality (Allen, 2008). DA received extensive media attention in 2013 when Baltimore Ravens All-Pro linebacker Ray Lewis was accused of using DA spray to speed his recovery of a torn biceps tendon he suffered early in the season. Supplement companies claim that deer antler is a natural source of insulin-like growth factor 1 (IGF-1), which is a substance banned by the NFL.

How it works: DA contains an array of nutritional compounds that could be responsible for its beneficial effects. Proteins, peptides, and minerals as well as omega-3 fatty acids, glycosaminoglycans, and prostaglandins are in DA. More significant are the claims that DA is a natural source of IGF-1, a powerful anabolic hormone that can promote the building and recovery of muscles and connective tissues. Aside from its impact on muscle and connective tissue, DA has been used in clinical studies to improve treatment of arthritic conditions.

Performance benefit: If DA does contain IGF-1 and can increase levels of IGF-1 in the body, it will assist athletes in muscle recovery and regeneration, allowing faster recovery from intense workouts and promoting gains in lean body mass. In addition, DA could benefit athletes with arthritic joints and tendinitis.

Research: In a 2003 study by Sleivert and colleagues, DA was supplemented during 10 weeks of a strength program. No effects on circulating levels of testosterone, IGF-1, or erythropoietin were noted. Furthermore, no differences in strength or $\dot{V}O_2$max were observed. A similar study by Syrotuik and colleagues (2005) that used 10 weeks of DA supplementation also found no significant effects on rowing performance and showed no altered hormonal responses at rest or during exercise. A recent review of the health benefits of DA concluded that claims for DA are not based on research from human trials (Gilbey & Perezgonzalez, 2012). Currently, there is no evidence to suggest that DA can naturally increase levels of IGF-1, nor does it affect muscular strength, recovery, and growth.

Common usage: DA is sold in spray form as well as in capsules and powder. Doses used in clinical trials range from 430 to 1,300 mg in capsule form (Allen, 2002). Similar doses are suggested when used in spray form.

Health concerns: The safety of DA is confirmed by clinical human trials as well as animal studies. However, athletes should use caution because supplements claiming to affect anabolic hormones naturally are often adulterated with pharmaceutical drugs not listed on product labels.

Dehydroepiandrosterone (DHEA)

What it is: Dehydroepiandrosterone (DHEA) is an anabolic prohormone or precursor to testosterone. Prohormones became very popular in 1998 when baseball player Mark McGwire admitted to using a supplement called Andro and claimed it helped him gain muscle mass, strength, power and subsequently improved his home run hitting abilities. Andro was the name for an over-the-counter supplement that contained androstendione.

How it works: DHEA can be converted into androstenediol or androstenedione, both of which can be converted into testosterone. In men after the age of 30, serum-free testosterone concentrations decline 1.2% each year. Oral supplementation with DHEA is believed to increase the availability of precursors to testosterone and prevent this decline. It is also speculated that young athletes would also experience increases in testosterone. There are two significant problems with this thought. First, oral intake and absorption of DHEA must bypass uptake and degradation by the liver. Secondly, DHEA must be converted into either androstenediol or androstenedione, both of which must then be converted into testosterone. Unfortunately, both androstenediol and androstenedione can take a variety of paths that end in the production of female sex hormones like estrogen. In reality, depending on the pathway, DHEA could affect both testosterone and estrogen.

Performance benefit: Athletes may benefit through increased testosterone production; higher testosterone levels will result in increases in lean body mass, strength, and power.

Research: Oral supplementation of 50-100 mg of DHEA raises serum levels of DHEA and DHEA-S 7-fold and increases androstenedione 4-fold. Chronic supplementation of 50-1,600 mg of DHEA appears to affect these weaker androgens with greater than 1,600 mg doses resulting in greater effects. Unfortunately, acute and chronic supplementation have no impact on testosterone (Brown, Vukovich, and King, 2006). While testosterone is not affected, estradiol and female sex hormones do increase. This effect is most clear in young adolescent and adult athletes. Research in older individuals and those with abnormally low testosterone levels is less clear, with some studies showing DHEA capable of increasing testosterone and others showing no effect. Brown Vukovich, and King studied the effects of 50 mg of DHEA taken 3 times daily on young, untrained weight lifters and concluded DHEA did not improve strength or lean muscle mass(2006). A more recent study found similar results in 19- to 22-year-old soccer players

>continued

Dehydroepiandrosterone (DHEA) >continued

consuming 100 mg daily for 28 days; there were no significant changes in body fat or muscle mass (Ostojic, Calleja, and Jourkesh, 2010).

Common usage: Research studies have used a variety of doses ranging from 50-100 mg to 1,600 mg/day.

 Health concerns: Extreme caution should be used when purchasing and using DHEA and other prohormone supplements. The side effects of supplementing with DHEA are less severe than those of other prohormones like androstenedione, which can cause gynecomastia (enlarged breasts in men), lower HDL cholesterol levels, and negatively affect a person's psychological state. Dietary supplements marketed as natural testosterone boosters often contain prohormones, which are not listed on labels, and purity is a concern.

Delta-Tocopherol, Delta-Tocotrienol

(see *vitamin E*)

Devil's Claw

aka *Harpagophyum procumbens, grapple plant, wood spider, harpago*

What it is: Devil's claw is the common name of *Harpagophytum procumbens,* an herb native to regions in South Africa, Botswana, Zambia, and Zimbabwe. The name devil's claw was given to the plant because of its hooked fruit, which can cause pain once inside the claws of animals. The roots of the plant are used for medicinal purposes to treat pain, inflammation, and degenerative disorders. Devil's claw contains a variety of phytochemicals and nutrients. Harpagoside and glycoside β-sitosterol are the major constituents believed to provide the greatest antiinflammatory effects ("Harpagophytum procumbens [Devil's Claw]," 2008).

How it works: Devil's claw inhibits two major inflammatory mechanisms known as lipopolysaccharide-induced nitric oxide and cyclooxygenase-2 (COX-2). Many popular pharmaceutical drugs prescribed as antiinflammatories and pain relievers inhibit COX-2. In addition, devil's claw is chondroprotective, meaning it protects against the degradation of cartilage (Sanders & Grundmann, 2011).

Performance benefit: Devil's claw is a promising supplement for athletes looking for an alternative to nonsteroidal antiinflammatories (NSAIDS) such as ibuprofen in the treatment of pain and loss of function in degenerative and arthritic joints. Devil's claw's chondroprotective effects may also aid in protecting joints from the degenerative stresses of sports and training.

Research: While more research is needed related to devil's claw, early results are promising. Research trials have examined the effectiveness of devil's claw in relieving symptoms of pain and improving joint function in a variety of conditions such as osteoarthritis, fibromyalgia, and rheumatoid and degenerative joint disorders. Many trials are problematic because of smaller sample sizes, short treatment periods, and insufficient quality control. Only two studies to date have looked at long-term supplementation over 1 year, making the safety of long-term use questionable. A 2004 meta-analysis drawing conclusions based on 14 studies involving devil's claw determined there was strong evidence for the use of Harpagophytum extract at a daily dose of 50 mg of harpagoside (the glucoside constituent responsible for the beneficial effects of devil's claw) (Gagnier et al.). This is somewhat in contrast to a 2006 review of the efficacy of devil's claw, which concluded that "the methodological quality of the existing clinical trials is generally poor, and although they provide some support, there is a considerable number of methodologic caveats that make further clinical investigations warranted" (Brien, Lewith, & McGregor, 991). As a result, additional better-controlled, long-term research trials should be undertaken before definitive conclusions are made.

Common usage: The quality of extract found in many dietary supplements can be a concern and affect usage. Typically, 1,000-3,000 mg of devil's claw extract is recommended; however, the harpagoside content is most important, with 50-100 mg of harpagoside recommended. A dose of 1,800-2,400 mg dried devil's claw root powder contains 50-100 mg of harpagoside ("Harpagophytum procumbens [Devil's Claw]," 2008).

Health concerns: Devil's claw should not be used in combination with NSAIDS, anticoagulants such as Coumadin, hypoglycemic medications, antacids, or medications taken to decrease stomach acid. Minor adverse symptoms involve gastrointestinal complaints. Effects on heart rhythm and force of contraction have also been noted (Sanders & Grundmann, 2011).

Dihydrolipoic Acid

(see *alpha-lipoic acid*)

Dimethylamylamine (DMAA)

aka *1,3-dimethylamylamine, geranium stem, geranium oil extract, forthane, methylhexaneamine, geranamine, 1,3 dimethylpentylamine*

What it is: Dimethylamylamine (DMAA) is a pharmaceutical amphetamine derivative. It was originally introduced by Eli Lilly in 1948 as a nasal inhaler; however, it was removed as an approved pharmaceutical in 1970. Today, DMAA is found abundantly in nearly 200 sports supplements, commonly

>*continued*

Dimethylamylamine (DMAA) >continued

recommended as a preworkout enhancer or a so-called fat burner. Its sales topped $100 million in 2010. According to FDA rules and regulations, for DMAA to be sold as a dietary supplement, it must be naturally occurring and have a documented history of use before 1994. Fortunately for many supplement companies, a scientific study found that geranium oil contains a small amount of DMAA (.07%), thereby allowing DMAA to pass both criteria (Cohen, 2012). However, since this study, nearly 6 others have been unsuccessful in confirming this finding. Currently, a significant amount of controversy exists between the FDA and supplement companies producing products containing DMAA. The FDA claims that DMAA is not found naturally in geranium oil, thereby disqualifying it as a natural ingredient.

Popular Supplements Containing DMAA

Jack 3d (USPlabs)

OxyELITE Pro (USPlabs)

Lipo 6 Black (Nutrex Research)

Lipo Black Ultra (Nutrex Research)

Hemo Rage Black (Nutrex Research)

Arson Fat Burner Capsule (Muscle Aslyum Project)

Spirode (Gaspari Nutrition)

Nitric Blast (Sports Nutrition International)

Napalm (Musle Warfare)

Lean EFX (Fahrenheit Nutrition)

HydroxyStim (MuscleTech)

Neurocore Powder (MuscleTech)

How it works: DMAA has strong stimulatory effects on the body. Its exact mechanisms are unknown. Some speculate that DMAA works in a fashion similar to ephedrine and other amphetamines by binding to sympathetic nervous system or adrenal receptors and initiating a strong sympathetic response increasing heart rate, heightening alertness, and increasing force production within the muscles. In addition, increases in resting metabolic rate and lipolysis (fat burning) may also result.

Performance benefit: DMAA is believed to improve exercise performance by delaying fatigue and potentially increasing force production. In addition, it may increase resting metabolic rate and lipolysis at rest and during exercise, resulting in improvements in body composition.

Research: The use of DMAA is contraindicated for athletes as supplementation can result in positive drug tests for amphetamines (Vorce et al., 2011). In addition, use of DMAA can result in serious and life-threatening adverse events (Gee, Jackson, & Easton, 2010). Limited scientific data are available related to its effectiveness. A 2011 study found DMAA increased systolic and diasotolic blood pressure; meanwhile, plasma norepinephrine and epinephrine were relatively unaffected (Bloomer et al., 2011).

Common usage: Most supplements list DMAA as an ingredient included in a proprietary blend; therefore, the amount of DMAA found in most dietary supplements is unknown.

 Health concerns: DMAA has been implicated in a number of serious adverse events, including panic attacks, seizures, and two deaths. It has been described as having toxic effects on animals that were "greater than that of ephedrine and less than that of amphetamine." (Cohen, 2012, E1)

Supplement Warning

 Athletes should avoid using products containing DMAA. It may be listed in the nutrition facts panel of many dietary supplements under a variety of names (see aka names previously listed), making it difficult to identify. Furthermore, the U.S. military has removed DMAA-containing supplements from all its military exchanges worldwide, and Health Canada has banned DMAA from all supplements (Cohen, 2012).

Dimethyl Sulfone

(see *methylsulfonylmethane*)

D-Leucine

(see *leucine*)

Docosahexaenoic Acid

(see *omega-3 fatty acids*)

Dong Chong Xia Cao

(see *Cordyceps sinensis*)

D-Ribose

(see *ribose*)

E

Ecdisten, Ecdysone

(see *ecdysteroids*)

Ecdysteroids

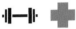

aka *ecdysterone, 20-beta-hydroxyecdysterone, ecdisten, ecdysone, isoinokosterone, 20-hydroxyecdysone, β-ecdysterone*

What it is: There are three classes of steroid hormones. The most familiar are the vertebrate steroid hormones such as androgens, estrogens, progestogens, and others. However, a second class of growth-promoting hormones known as brassinolides can be found in plants, and a third class known as ecdysteroids are found in insects and plants (Bathori et al., 2008). Thus far nearly 300 ecdysteroids have been discovered; 20-hydroxyecdysone (20-HE) is the main biologically significant ecdysteroid found in insects and is also one of the most common plant-derived ecdysteroids (Bathori et al., 2008). Spinach, quinoa, and chestnut are noted to contain considerable amounts of ecdysteroids, such as 20-HE (Bathori et al., 2008; Gorelick-Feldman et al., 2008).

How it works: Ecdysteroids are believed to produce anabolic and cholesterol-lowering effects. In addition, they stimulate and strengthen the immune system and are referred to as being *adaptogenic,* allowing individuals to better adapt to various stresses placed on the body. Ecdysteroids promote vitality and increase resistance to stress. The mechanisms are somewhat unknown. Unlike androgens, which act on androgen receptors and initiate a response, ecdysteroids behave differently because receptors do not exist. However, various nonreceptor-induced signaling pathways have been implicated as potential mechanisms (Bathori et al., 2008).

Performance benefit: If the claims about ecdysteroids are true, athletes would benefit from the anabolic and adaptogenic effects. Similar to anabolic steroids, ecdysteroids could promote gains in lean body mass, increasing muscle size, strength, power, and performance. The adaptogenic effects of ecdysteroids would allow athletes to adapt to the stresses of training and potentially handle higher volumes and intensities, inducing adaptation and improved performance over time.

Research: Research conducted on humans is relatively weak. Wilborn and colleagues conducted a study in 2006 looking into the effects of three supplements often marketed as natural alternatives to steroids. The three supplements included ecdysterone or 20-HE (a common type of ecdysterone), methoxyisoflavone, and sulfo-polysaccharide. Forty-five resistance-trained men were supplemented for 8 weeks while lifting 4 days/week. No beneficial effects on changes in lean body mass, levels of anabolic hormones, or improvements in strength and power were observed. Early studies on mice in the 1960s and 1970s found that ecdysteroids promoted protein synthesis (Otaka, Okui, & Uchiyama, 1976), and more recent studies by have produced similar results (Gorelick-Feldman et al., 2008; Gorelick-Feldman, Cohick, & Raskin, 2010; Toth et al., 2008). A 2009 study found 20-HE capable of improving insulin resistance and decreasing weight and body fat gain in diet-induced obese mice (Kizelsztein et al.). In summary, current research is promising related to ecdysteroids and their impact in promoting protein synthesis and improving gains in lean body mass and body composition in mice. Other proposed benefits of ecdysteroids, such as promoting adaptogenic effects during training, are unstudied and speculative at this time.

Common usage: One of the few human trials used 200 mg of 20-HE daily (Wilborn et al., 2006). Mice models typically use 5-10 mg of ecdysteroids/kg of body weight or 20-HE (Bathori et al., 2008).

Health concerns: Ecdysteroids have low acute toxicity at doses of 6-9 g/kg body weight in mice, and 2 g/kg body weight in rabbits resulted in no toxic symptoms (Kizelsztein, 2009). The common consumption of vegetables with high ecdysteroid content is further proof of safety.

Echinacea

aka *coneflower, Echinacea purpurea, Echinacea angustifolia, Echinacea pallida*

What it is: Also known as coneflower, echinacea is an herbal remedy prepared from both the stems and leaves of the plant that is often used by athletes to ward off the common cold, flu, and other infections. While several species of echinacea exist, the three types commercially available include *Echinacea angustifolia* (narrow-leaved coneflower), *Echinacea pallida* (pale coneflower), and *Echinacea purpurea* (purple flower coneflower).

How it works: The physical stress associated with training and competition can suppress an athlete's immune function, increasing risk for infection. Antibodies known as immunoglobulins within the blood and mucous membranes are critical to an athlete's immune defense against bacterial and viral infection; however, following periods of intense training, decreases in these antibodies have been reported along with increased incidence of upper respiratory infection. Echinacea contains several bioactive compounds, including alkamides, caffeic acid, and polysaccharides, that may help bolster the strength of an athlete's immune function by increasing the number and activity of antibodies as well as several other key immune system cells: white blood cells (macrophages) that destroy bacteria, viruses, and other foreign cells through a process called phagocytosis; and natural killer cells that destroy cells that have become infected with viruses.

>*continued*

Echinacea >*continued*

Performance benefit: Athletes may benefit from less frequent occurrence of sidelining infections throughout their competitive season.

Research: While animal trials have demonstrated favorable immune responses through exposure to echinacea, applications to humans are less conclusive with mixed results being reported in healthy populations. For example, one large study of 755 healthy subjects found supplementation of an alcohol extract from freshly harvested *E. purpurea* (95% herb, 5% root) over a period of 4 months to reduce the total number and duration of cold episodes and protect against viral infections with maximal effects occurring on recurrent infections compared to the placebo (Jawad et al., 2012). Yet, according to a second large-scale study (713 subjects), a placebo effect may contribute to results. Study investigators evaluated whether the severity and duration of illness caused by the common cold are influenced by randomized assignment to open-label echinacea pills (root extracts of *Echinacea purpurea* and *angustifolia*) compared to conventional double-blind allocation to active and placebo pills and compared to no pills at all during a 5-day span. While participants randomized to the no-pill group tended to have longer and more severe illnesses than those who received pills, the differences were not significant. There were also no significant differences between groups in a couple of key markers of immune function. For the subgroup that received pills and believed in the purported role of echinacea in immune function, illnesses were substantively shorter and less severe. This was the case regardless of whether the pills contained echinacea, confirming a placebo effect was indeed present (Barrett et al., 2011).

Common usage: The stems and leaves of the echinacea plant are used fresh or dried to make teas, juices, extracts, tablets, and capsules. Research-supported doses are based on the type of preparation used: capsule 300 mg, dried root (or tea) 1,000-2,000 mg, freeze-dried plant 325-650 mg, juice 2-3 mL, tincture 3-5 mL, fluid extract 1-2 mL. Prescribed doses can be taken 3 times daily over a heavy training block or every 2 hours for 24 hours with the onset of cold-like symptoms.

Supplement Fact

Echinacea loses its effectiveness with long-term use and thus should only be used cyclically throughout a season. For example, an athlete may use echinacea during a particularly hard 3-week training block and then cycle off during a recovery period or merely use echinacea throughout the duration of an infection.

Health concerns: Echinacea seems to be well tolerated by most people though clinical trials have demonstrated gastrointestinal symptoms at doses above 2 g/day. Allergic reactions have been reported in those with allergies to plants within the daisy family, such as ragweed and marigold.

Additional performance benefits: There is preliminary evidence that supplementation with echinacea at doses of 8,000 mg/day for 4 weeks significantly boosts erythropoietin (EPO), a hormone that is naturally produced in the body and primarily functions to stimulate the formation of red blood cells; effects last for 21 days (Whitehead et al., 2005; Whitehead et al., 2012). With increased red blood cell production, the oxygen-carrying capacity of the blood improves, allowing more oxygen to be delivered to muscles for enhanced energy production to fuel performance.

Egg Protein

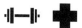

aka *albumin*

What it is: Eggs have long been known as an excellent high-quality source of protein. Eggs are considered a complete protein and contain all of the essential amino acids. As early as 1930, scientists worked to understand and determine protein quality. This led to the development of biological value (BV). BV is a measure of the amount of protein from food that becomes incorporated into the proteins of the body. Early work identified the egg as the gold standard of protein quality with a BV of 100. Protein needs are slightly to moderately higher for athletes verses nonathletes. Some athletes have taken these increased needs to extremes, consuming excessive amounts of protein daily and increasing the demand for protein supplements. Because of its biological value, eggs are commonly used as the source of protein in powders and supplements.

How it works: Egg proteins provide important amino acids that are used by the body as building blocks for the synthesis of new proteins, including muscle. These amino acids can also signal or turn on protein-building pathways in the body. Exercise and training push muscles to their performance limits, inducing damage and the breakdown of proteins within muscle. Supplying dietary protein throughout the day and in relation to workouts and training can help prevent damage during training and spark restoration of muscle. All protein sources are unique in the various combinations and amounts of amino acids they contain. Eggs could contain a superior combination of these amino acids, making them more effective for athletes than other protein sources.

Performance benefit: Eggs provide a valuable, high-quality protein source for athletes that assists in preventing muscle breakdown, maintaining lean body mass, sparking the recovery of damaged muscle, and building new muscle.

Research: Recently, biological value has been scrutinized as a valid measure of protein quality. Typically, BV is measured in fasting states or after

>continued

Egg Protein *>continued*

periods of brief starvation, both of which do not provide real-life scenarios. Also, BV does not take into account proteins that are quickly burned as fuel after consumption, which could be the reason whey protein, a fast-digesting protein, has the highest BV of any protein at 106. Studies comparing the consumption of protein sources before and after exercise tend to conclude that the fast-digesting properties of whey protein make it the best and quickest source of high-quality amino acids before, during, and after exercise. However, egg proteins tend to rank a close second. It should also be noted that while egg protein powders and supplements can provide an excellent source of amino acids, they lack many natural vitamins, minerals, phospholipids, and lipids found in whole eggs.

Common usage: Protein needs are based on body weight. Scientific research studies have found 1.2-2 g of protein/kg of body weight sufficient for nearly all athletes. However, many athletes consume amounts in excess of this. Excessive consumption does not provide additional benefits and only results in increased oxidation or burning of protein as fuel. The consumption of protein before, during, and after exercise is also beneficial. The amount of protein needed for maximal benefits postexercise is roughly 20-30 g. Protein intake before exercise is dependent upon an athlete's ability to tolerate it, but intake should not exceed 10-15 g and 5 g per hour of activity.

Health concerns: High-protein diets do not appear to pose any health concerns; however, athletes must understand that excessive intakes of protein could result in underconsumption of other important nutrients such as carbohydrate, healthy fat, and nutrient-dense fruits and vegetables.

Eicosapentaenoic Acid

(see *omega-3 fatty acids*)

Elderberry

aka *elder, elder flower, Sambucus nigra*

What it is: A large shrub native to Europe, Africa, and parts of Asia, elderberry—and more specifically its bark, leaves, flowers, and berries—has long been used for medicinal purposes in many European and Middle Eastern cultures and has more recently garnered attention in athletics for its immune-strengthening and antioxidant properties. While several species of elder exist, European elder, also known as black elder or *Sambucus nigra*, is the most commonly used.

How it works: The fruit, or more specifically the berry, of the elderberry plant is an excellent source of vitamins A and C as well as several plant compounds, including phenolic acids, flavonoids, catechins, anthocyanins, and proanthocyanidins that are thought to contribute to its therapeutic properties (Barros et al., 2012). Dietary flavonoids, in particular, carry antioxidant properties that may help offset some of the oxidative damage to cells, including those important to immune function, that occur during heavy training cycles. Additionally, animal models have shown elderberry to increase the number and activity of several key immune compounds as well as help initiate phagocytosis, which helps rid the body of harmful foreign particles, bacteria, and dead or dying cells that could otherwise sideline an athlete with a variety of infections including the flu.

Performance benefit: Athletes may benefit from enhanced immune function, allowing them to rebound faster from illness during training and competition.

Research: Few human studies have been conducted to be able to confirm the efficacy of supplemental use in athletes. However, two randomized, double-blind, placebo-controlled studies demonstrate some promise. In the first study, elderberry extract (Sambucol) was given to adult patients in a daily dose of 60 mL (4 tbsp) within the first 48 hours after the onset of flu-like symptoms. These patients were able to recover significantly faster than the control group receiving the placebo. Over 93% of patients receiving the elderberry reported cessation of symptoms after only 2 days of treatment; the placebo group failed to report improvement until day 6. Furthermore, while serum samples analyzing various antibodies did not reveal a significant difference, the trend was in favor of the treatment group. The second study revealed similar results with a treatment protocol that incorporated 15 mL (1 tbsp) of elderberry extract (Sambucol) taken 4 times daily over 5 days; following this protocol essentially cut the duration of flu-like symptoms in half compared to a placebo (Zakay-Rones et al., 1995, 2004). These results suggest elderberry may be helpful in enhancing recovery from the flu, extremely helpful for an athlete who can't afford to be sidelined in the midst of a busy training and competition schedule.

Common usage: Elderberry is available dried (tea) and as a liquid, syrup, wine, extract, and tincture as well as in capsule and lozenge forms. In the limited human research available, elderberry extract at a dose of 15 mL (1 tbsp) taken 4 times daily upon first onset of flu-like symptoms may be effective in reducing the duration of the flu. As an alternative, 3-5 g of dried elder flower, standardized to at least 0.8% flavonoids, can be prepared as a tea and consumed 3 times daily.

Health concerns: While elderberry appears to be safe when used in recommended doses short term (up to 5 days), certain species such as *Sambucus ebulus* consumed uncooked can cause symptoms that resemble cyanide-like poisoning, including diarrhea, vomiting, vertigo, numbness, and stupor.

>*continued*

Elderberry >*continued*

Additional performance benefits: Preliminary evidence suggests that chemicals found in the elder flower and berries may help reduce swelling in mucous membranes, such as the sinuses, and help relieve nasal congestion, of particular benefit to athletes affected by seasonal allergies.

Elemental Iron

(see *iron*)

Elk Velvet Antler

(see *deer velvet*)

Enterococcus

(see *probiotics*)

Epimedium, *Epimedium Grandiflorum*

(see *horny goat weed*)

Escherichia

(see *probiotics*)

Euterpe Olearacea

(see *acacia berry*)

Evening Primrose Oil

(see *gamma-linolenic acid*)

Evodia Fruit, Evodiamine, *Evodia Rutaecarpa*

(see *rutaecarpine*)

F

Fenugreek

aka *Trigonella foenum-graecum, goat's horn*

What it is: A white-flowered herbal plant from the pea family, fenugreek is commonly used for culinary purposes with its dried or fresh leaves and seeds used as an herb, spice, and vegetable to flavor dishes, especially Indian curry dishes. For athletes, fenugreek is recognized for its potential ability to reduce exercise fatigue and promote recovery.

How it works: Evidence from animal studies suggests that fenugreek may lead to a favorable metabolic response during exercise: Reliance on fatty acids, rather than glucose, to fuel activity is enhanced, helping to spare limited muscle glycogen stores and delay the onset of fatigue associated with depletion, or hitting the wall. Additionally, fenugreek seems to help promote glycogen repletion, which is essential for optimal postworkout recovery. Of further ergogenic benefit, fenugreek is rich in antioxidant compounds known as flavonoids and polyphenols, which may boost protection against damaging free radicals that, during heavy training cycles, can accumulate at a rate faster than the body's natural defense can cover and cause a cascade of inflammatory events that can hinder an athlete's recovery.

Performance benefit: Athletes may benefit from delayed onset of fatigue during endurance training and competition as well as enhanced recovery.

Supplement Fact

Fenugreek seeds contain an amino acid called 4-hydroxyisoleucine that is commonly extracted and used to lower blood sugar in diabetics. In addition, some studies suggest it may help lower body fat through its role in insulin promotion and blood sugar regulation.

Research: Studies evaluating the impact of fenugreek on performance parameters in a trained population are limited and equivocal. One animal study, for example, found fenugreek administered at a dose of 300 mg/kg body weight over 4 weeks promoted a favorable metabolic response: Reliance on fatty acids as an energy source increased, thereby sparing limited glycogen stores and significantly increasing swimming time to exhaustion in mice as compared to a control group (Ikeuchi et al., 2006). Another human trial with trained cyclists found administration of 1.8 g/kg body weight of dextrose in combination with 2.0 mg/kg body weight of 4-hydroxyisoleucine from fenugreek seeds immediately and 2 hours after completion of a 90-minute exhaustive cycling exercise protocol enhanced the rate of glycogen repletion by 63% as compared to the placebo group, supporting the potential benefit of

>continued

Fenugreek >*continued*

fenugreek for recovery (Ruby et al., 2005). However, another human study of similar double-blind design failed to replicate these results. In that study, the same dose of dextrose and 4-hydroxyisoleucine was administered immediately and 2 hours after cycling 5 hours at 50% peak cycling power. In addition, a standardized meal with or without fenugreek was consumed 4 hours after and before concluding with a 40 km cycling time trial (Slivka et al., 2008). Contrary to previous studies, there was no difference between groups in muscle glycogen levels at any point during the study, nor was performance gain experienced by the fenugreek group during the 40 km time trial. It is evident more research is needed before conclusions can be drawn on the performance attributes of fenugreek related to fuel usage, endurance capacity, and recovery.

Common usage: Fenugreek is available as seed powder capsules, teas, and pulverized seeds that can be mixed in water. The appropriate dose of fenugreek for athletes is still unclear, although dose recommendations appear to be weight dependent. One favorable study utilized 2 mg/kg of 4-hydroxyisoleucine (an active ingredient isolated from fenugreek seeds) to solicit a performance benefit (Ruby et al., 2005). Fenugreek has also been used for general health purposes as a tincture at a dose of 3-4 mL taken 3-4 times/day, as well as a defatted seed powder at a dose of 5-30 g taken 1-3 times/day.

Health concerns: Fenugreek is considered safe and well tolerated by most, although athletes sensitive to curry should be cautious as allergic symptoms (e.g., bronchospasm, wheezing, and diarrhea) have been reported. Additionally, because the leaves and seeds of fenugreek are rich in dietary fiber, consumption may initiate gastrointestinal disturbances such as diarrhea and gas. Thus, precompetition use is not recommended. Fenugreek may alter the color and smell of urine, a side effect that is not considered harmful to health.

Additional performance benefit: A study of trained men demonstrated that 500 mg of fenugreek taken daily over 8 weeks in conjunction with a resistance training program significantly enhanced strength gains and body fat loss compared to training by itself (Poole et al., 2010).

Ferrous Carbonate Anhydrous, *Ferrous Fumarate*, Ferrous Guconate, Ferrous Pyrophosphate, Ferrous Sulfate

(see *iron*)

Fiber

What it is: Fibers are types of carbohydrate commonly found in plants that resist digestion and absorption in the small intestine. Many types of fibers exist; however, they are most commonly classified into two categories known as soluble and insoluble. Soluble fibers are soluble in water and include pectins, gums, β-glucans, pysllium, inulin, and mucilages. Insoluble fibers are not soluble in water and include cellulose, hemicellulose, and ligin. Fruits, vegetables, and whole grain foods are all excellent natural sources of fiber (Papathanasopoulos & Camilleri, 2010). Fiber supplements have recently become popular as a means for many whose diets are low in fiber to meet recommended amounts. The average American intake for fiber is less than half the recommended amount. Current recommendations suggest 14 g/1,000 kcal be consumed daily. For the average women consuming 2,000 kcal/day, this is equivalent to 28 g of fiber; for the average male consuming 2,600 kcal/day, this is equivalent to 36 g of fiber/day (Anderson, 2009). These recommendations will be even higher for athletes whose caloric demands are much higher, ranging from 2,500-4,500 kcal/day.

Supplement Fact

There are a variety of types of fiber supplements available on the market. Generally, soluble fiber supplements are suggested. Pysllium and β-glucans are the only two types of fiber with FDA approval as cholesterol lowering agents (Anderson et al., 2009). Psyllium is the most common type of fiber used in research trials. Inulin is another fiber found in foods and supplements. Less specific research has been done on inulin relative to blood cholesterol and weight loss effects, but is a better prebiotic fiber for promoting the growth of bacteria in the GI tract. More research is needed on fibers and the advantages of certain fibers specific to specific health benefits.

How it works: Fiber is proven to provide a number of health benefits. Fiber reduces the risk of coronary heart disease, stroke, hypertension, diabetes, obesity, and certain gastrointestinal diseases (Anderson et al., 2009). Increasing fiber intake will lower cholesterol and blood pressure. Soluble fibers have been shown to improve glycemic control and insulin sensitivity in both nondiabetics and diabetics. Fiber supplementation in obese individuals significantly enhances weight loss. The prevention of weight gain and assistance in weight loss is often attributed to fiber's ability to increase satiety and stabilize blood glucose levels. Finally, fiber is a prebiotic and provides nutrients to support the growth of healthy bacteria in the GI tract. Creating a beneficial environment for growth of these bacteria will strengthen and bolster the immune system.

Performance benefit: Athletes might benefit from the potential weight loss and weight management benefits of fiber, especially those needing to maintain a lower body weight and leaner body composition. In addition, athletes could benefit from the immune-enhancing benefits of soluble fibers.

Research: Animal experiments, epidemiological studies (those identifying trends within population groups), and clinical trials provide support for high-

>continued

Fiber >*continued*

fiber diets to prevent weight gain (Papathanasopoulos & Camilleri, 2010). A recent assessment of five clinical research trials found high-fiber diets to improve weight loss by approximately 2.2 lbs (1 kg) over an 8-week period (Anderson et al., 2009). Fiber improves insulin sensitivity and satiety, and supports the growth of healthy bacteria in the GI tract. It is clear that adequate intake of fiber is essential for optimal health of both athletes and nonathletes.

Common usage: The amount of fiber needed is relative to fiber intake from food. Typically, 5-20 g of fiber is supplemented at smaller doses before meals. Again, a total fiber intake of 14 g/1,000 kcal consumed is recommended. For an athlete burning 3,500 kcal/day, this is equivalent to 49 g of fiber/day. Diets high in fruits, vegetables, and whole grains naturally provide sufficient amounts of fiber.

Health concerns: It is recommended that fiber intake not exceed 60-70 g/day.

5-Diamino-5-Oxopentaenoic Acid

(see *glutamine*)

5-Hydroxytryptophan (5-HTP)

What it is: 5-hydroxytryptophan (5-HTP) is an aromatic amino acid naturally produced in the body from tryptophan. It is extracted from the seeds of the African plant *Griffonia simplicifolia*.

How it works: Serotonin is an important neurotransmitter produced in the body that contributes to the regulation of mood, appetite, sleep, memory, and learning. The amino acid tryptophan is converted to 5-HTP before being converted to serotonin. This is why foods such as turkey that contain high amounts of tryptophan get tagged as inducing sleepiness.

Performance benefit: For athletes, supplementation with 5-HTP may increase levels of serotonin, thereby improving sleep and recovery.

Research: There have be no studies that have looked specifically into the effects of 5-HTP on recovery in athletes. Animal studies and human trials do suggest that 5-HTP supplementation can increase serotonin levels (Birdsall, 1998). Most research has focused on the impact that increasing serotonin levels might have on depression. In a 2006 review article by Turner, Loftis, and Black-well, it was noted that of 11 double-blind placebo-controlled studies, 7 showed 5-HTP to be more effective than a placebo in treating depression. Research studies related to sleep have found 5-HTP supplementation to significantly increase the amount of non-REM sleep (Morrow et al., 2008); however, no studies have evaluated whether this impact on sleep improves recovery for athletes.

Common usage: When used for insomnia or to enhance sleep, a dose of 100-300 mg of 5-HTP before bedtime is recommended. When used in treatment of depression, 50 mg of 5-HTP 3 times daily is suggested. If an effective response is not produced after 2 weeks, it is suggested that an increased dosage of 100 mg 3 times daily be taken.

Health concerns: Caution is necessary when taking 5-HTP in combination with selective serotonin reuptake inhibitors (SSRI) or antidepressants such as fluoxetine (Prozac), paroxetine (Paxil), sertraline (Zoloft), fluvoxamine (Luvox), or an MAOI antidepressant such as phenelzine (Nardil) or tranyl-cypromine (Parnate). 5-HTP in combination with these drugs may lead to serotonin syndrome, characterized by agitation, confusion, delirium, and tachycardia. There are no adequate studies related to use of 5-HTP during pregnancy (Birdsall, 1998).

5,7-Dihydroxyflavone

(see *chrysin*)

Flaxseed

aka *Linium usitatissimum, linseed oil, flax oil*

What it is: Consisting of one-third oil and two-thirds fiber, flaxseed, whose scientific name *Linum usitatissimum* appropriately means "most useful," packs quite the nutritional punch. Its oil is a rich source of essential fatty acids (EFAs), especially alpha linolenic (ALA) omega-3 fatty acid, and the fiberous byproduct of the seed is chock-full of vitamins and minerals as well as a group of chemical compounds called lignans, which are thought to have antioxidant qualities. For athletes, flaxseeds are most recognized for their apparent ability to enhance fat metabolism, aid endurance performance, and promote favorable body composition changes.

How it works: EFAs, especially the omega-3s found in the oil of flaxseeds, are needed for the synthesis of powerful hormones called prostaglandins, which help regulate several aspects of metabolism. Of particular interest to athletes, though, is a metabolic phenomenon known as fuel partitioning: Dietary EFAs facilitate the transport of carbohydrate to muscles to enhance glycogen storage while promoting the oxidation of fatty acids for use as energy. The ability to mobilize and use fat as a fuel is especially relevant during long-duration training sessions when glycogen depletion, or hitting the wall, is of greater concern. Additionally, EFAs appear to enhance the burning of excess fat to produce heat, a process known as thermogenesis, which may help produce fat loss and favorable changes in body composition.

>continued

Flaxseed >*continued*

Performance benefit: Athletes may benefit from extended endurance and favorable changes in body composition.

Research: While research supports the beneficial metabolic and health changes seen with increased EFA intake, especially that of omega-3, the translation to athletic performance of humans is primarily anecdotal; there is limited research from which to draw conclusions. A 2011 study of 12 taekwondo athletes, however, did find daily consumption of foods (primarily toast) enhanced with omega-3s at a dose of just over 1.6 g/day for 6 weeks produced significant increases in all physical performance parameters tested, including peak power, relative peak power, anaerobic capacity, anaerobic fatigue, and total leg strike compared to a washout period of the same duration (Rocha et al.). In addition, favorable changes in body composition were also noted, in particular reduced body fat content and maintenance of lean body mass. While the results were promising, the small subject size is a study drawback. Overall, more research is needed before conclusions regarding the performance benefits of omega-3s from plant foods such as flaxseed can be drawn.

Common usage: Because the whole seed cannot be digested, flaxseed should be taken in ground or oil form at a recommended daily dose of 1-2 tbsp and 1 tsp, respectively. Ground flaxseed can be sprinkled on yogurt and cereals and added to baked goods; its oil form can be mixed with vinegar to form a dressing for salads. A capsule form is also available. The essential fatty acids in flaxseed can become rancid with exposure to heat, light, and oxygen, so storage in a cool, dark, dry place is essential. The oil should not be used in cooking.

Health concerns: Because flaxseed, specifically in whole or ground form, is high in dietary fiber, it is best introduced gradually and in small amounts with water to avoid stomach cramping and diarrhea. It is best taken after competition to avoid such digestive issues.

Additional performance benefits: Athletes consuming a diet rich in ALA omega-3 fatty acids, such as found in flaxseed, may benefit from increased protection against loss of bone mass and consequent fracture (Kim & Ilich, 2011).

Folic Acid

aka *folate, folacin, vitamin B9, pteroyl-l-glutamic acid, pteroylmonoglutamic acid, pteroyl-l-gutamate*

What it is: Folic acid, which is a member of the B-vitamin family, is a synthetic and stable form of its naturally occurring sister, folate. It is a water-soluble vitamin and commonly used in vitamin supplements as well as fortified foods such as cereals and grains. Folate (derived from the Latin word folium, meaning "leaf") is found in dietary sources such as dark green leafy vegetables, liver, legumes, wheat germ, egg yolk, yeast, and sunflower seeds. Because only 50% of dietary folate is available for use in the body, deficiencies are common, making intake of fortified foods or vitamin supplements necessary.

How it works: Folic acid plays a key role in several actions in the body that may benefit performance, especially as it relates to oxygen delivery. In conjunction with vitamin B12, folic acid aids the production and maintenance of new cells, including red blood cells (also known as erythrocytes), which are vital to oxygen transport. A boost in red blood cell count may help facilitate more efficient oxygen delivery to muscles during exercise. Furthermore, by decreasing levels of homocysteine (an amino acid that has been shown to contribute to atherosclerosis or thickening of the arteries), folic acid is thought to enhance vascular function by helping to open up blood vessels and keep the arteries clear of plaque, thereby improving the delivery of oxygen and other nutrients essential to cardiovascular health and performance. This is especially relevant in light of the fact that intense, long-duration exercise has been correlated with increases in blood homocysteine levels, possibly heightening risk for heart attack and stroke in athletes, especially when folic acid intake is insufficient.

Supplement Fact

Deficiencies in folate or vitamin B_{12} can lead to megaloblastic anemia, which causes the production of abnormally large red blood cells that cannot effectively transport oxygen or remove carbon dioxide. Symptoms tend to manifest as neurological problems. Athletes who have undergone gastric bypass surgery or who are sensitive to gluten may be at greater risk for developing these symptoms.

Performance benefit: Folic acid may help increase oxygen delivery to and uptake by muscles, thereby enhancing aerobic performance.

Research: When energy intake is sufficient, athletes seem to consume adequate amounts of folic acid. However, calorie-restricted diets, which are common among athletes looking to lose weight, often contain insufficient amounts of folic acid. According to researchers from Marquette University, such dietary patterning can lead to altered sex hormone levels, known as amenorrhea in females, and compromised vascular function (Lanser et al., 2011). Fortunately, some of the same researchers discovered that a supplemental protocol incorporating 10 mg/day of folic acid taken over 4-6 weeks provides a boost in the vascular function of female runners, regardless of baseline hormonal or serum folate status (Hoch et al., 2010). In addition, there is evidence that increased dietary intake and resulting plasma levels of folic acid are correlated with decreased homocysteine levels (Di Santolo

>continued

Folic Acid >*continued*

et al., 2009). It is currently unknown whether this will aid performance, but based on data from clinical trials, it may help reduce risk factors related to cardiovascular disease in athletes (Hankey et al., 2012).

Common usage: The RDA for folate is expressed as a term called the dietary folate equivalent (DFE) to account for the differences in absorption between naturally occurring folate (1 mcg folate = 1 DFE) and synthetic folic acid (0.6 mcg folic acid = 1 DFE). The current RDA stands at 400 mcg for adult men and women, and recommendations increase to 600 and 500 mcg accordingly for pregnant and lactating women, respectively. Research-supported doses for improvements in vascular function are 10 mg of folic acid taken daily over 4-6 weeks, while reductions in homocysteine concentrations can be achieved at a daily dose of 0.2 mg/day.

Health concerns: As a water-soluble vitamin that is regularly removed from the body through urine, toxicity symptoms are rare, even with doses of 10 mg/day. Some reports of stomach upset, sleep disturbances, and skin problems have been reported with doses above 15 mg/day. The current tolerable upper intake (UL) for folic acid is 1,000 mcg/day for adult men and women.

Forthane

(see *dimethylamylamine*)

Frankincense

(see *Boswellia serrata*)

G

GABA

aka γ-*aminobutyric acid*

What it is: GABA (gamma-aminobutyric acid) is an amino acid neurotransmitter found in the brain. The body synthesizes GABA from glutamic acid. GABA acts as a major inhibitor of the central nervous system (Abdou, 2006). As a neural inhibitor, GABA is believed to have a beneficial role as an antistress agent. It is this ability that is commonly marketed to dietary supplement consumers.

How it works: GABA can bind to GABA receptors in the brain and induce neural inhibition, which has the potential to alleviate stress, induce relaxation, and improve the quality of sleep, concentration, and cognitive performance. In addition, GABA is believed to improve the ability to handle acute stress and reduce cortisol response. Interestingly, as we age, the levels of GABA synthesized in the brain decrease.

Performance benefit: If the speculative benefits are real, GABA could assist athletes in handling the daily physical and emotional stresses of training, improving an athlete's mood and lowering the cortisol response to training. GABA could also benefit athletes by improving the quality of sleep and muscle recovery during sleep.

Research: One problem associated with GABA is that oral supplementation does not cross the blood-brain barrier and reach the brain. A significant number of GABA receptors are located in the brain, and GABA's inability to reach these receptors makes it less likely GABA will have any significant physiological effects on the body. Most research has focused on drugs and other GABAergic substances. These are drugs and substances that can reach GABA receptors in the brain and induce the central nervous system inhibitory effects described previously (Goldberg, 2010). Few well-controlled scientific studies have been carried out on oral GABA supplementation. Those studies that have been done are not considered of high quality, use small numbers of subjects, and commonly come from the same group of researchers. These studies have found GABA to be beneficial in reducing nerve strain and psychological fatigue, but only in chronically fatigued populations (Kanehira et al., 2011, Nakamura et al., 2009). Other trials have looked at the impact of GABA on brain waves and found GABA capable of increasing alpha brain waves, which are associated with relaxation and reduced stress (Abdou, 2006). Unfortunately, only 13 subjects were used for this trial. It is unlikely that GABA supplementation is of any benefit; however, more research is needed before definitive conclusions can be made.

Common usage: Research trials have varied in the amount of GABA provided, but typically 50-100 mg is recommended.

>continued

Health concerns: The use of GABA in 50-100 mg doses appears safe; however, no long-term studies are known at this time. In addition, little is known relative to drug-supplement interactions.

Gallated Flavan-3-Ols

(see *cocoa*)

γ-Aminobutyric Acid

(see *GABA*)

Gamma-Glutamylcysteinylglycine, Gamma-L-Glutamyl-L-Cysteinylglycine

(see g*lutathione*)

G Gamma-Linolenic Acid (GLA)

aka *borage oil, evening primrose oil, blackcurrant seed oil*

What it is: Gamma-linolenic acid (GLA) can be found in a variety of oils in nature and is also produced in the body from the omega-6 fatty acid linolenic acid. Linolenic acid can be found in vegetable oils such as soybean, safflower, corn, and rapeseed, all of which can be converted into GLA. Unfortunately, the rate of conversion of linolenic acid to GLA is very low, below 5% (Czernichow, 2010). GLA is commonly found in a variety of oils sold as supplements, including borage, evening primrose, blackurrant, and fungal oils. It can also be found in organ meats such as eggs and liver, as well as in human milk.

GLA Content in Dietary Supplements Sold as Oils

Evening primrose: 7-10 g/100 g

Blackcurrant: 15-20 g/100 g

Borage: 18-26 g/100 g

Fungal: 23-26 g/100 g

How it works: In the body, the omega-6 fatty acid, linolenic acid is converted into GLA. GLA is then converted into dihomo-GLA, which is finally converted into arachidonic acid (Wang, Lin, Gu, 2012). Arachidonic acid is capable of exerting a variety of physiological effects on the body. In recent years, much attention has been given to omega-3 fatty acids and their important role in health. Omega-3s, like omega-6 fatty acids, are eventually converted into EPA (eicosapentaenoic acid) and DHA (docosahexaenoic acid), which like arachidonic acid exert physiological effects. Omega-3s have been labeled as antiinflammatory in nature, and omega-6 fatty acids as proinflammatory. This, however, is not the entire story. Some actions of arachidonic acid are antiinflammatory, such as its ability to increase prostaglandin (PGE1), which inhibits proinflammatory cytokines as well as inflammatory leukotrienes. The conversion of linolenic acid to GLA is the rate-limiting step in the production of arachidonic acid. As a result, supplementation with GLA is believed to improve production of arachidonic acid and positively affect health.

Performance benefit: GLA is most commonly used in the treatment of chronic inflammation for conditions such as dermatitis, eczema, and rheumatoid arthritis. It is also believed to help alleviate symptoms of menopause and premenstrual syndrome. The exact benefits of GLA supplementation for athletes are speculative; however, it is sometimes added to weight-loss supplements as a source of fatty acids believed to improve weight loss and body composition.

Research: Research to date is not promising since GLA is ineffective as an agent in the treatment of dermatitis and eczema (Bayles & Usatine, 2009). Insufficient evidence exists related to its effects on rheumatoid arthritis (Bayles & Usatine, 2009). One research trial has investigated potential benefits related to weight loss. The study examined the effects of GLA on weight regain. Formerly obese subjects consumed 5 g of borage oil or 5 g of olive oil for 1 year following initial weight loss. The results found the amount of weight regain to be significantly less for the GLA/borage oil group; however, only 13 of 17 subjects completed the trial (Schirmer & Phinney, 2007). More research is required before clear conclusions can be made relative to weight loss. Currently, there is little evidence to support the use of GLA.

Common usage: A range of .16 g to .64 g of GLA is commonly used in research trials. A standard 1 g capsule of evening primrose oil contains roughly .08 g of GLA. A 5 g dose would contain roughly .45 g of GLA.

Health concerns: Minor side effects have been reported, including abdominal pain, nausea, increased bowel movements, diarrhea, and headaches. GLA is safe when used in recommended doses (Bayles & Usatine, 2009). Insufficient research is available to know if any drug-supplement interactions exist.

Gamma-Tocopherol, Gamma-Tocotrienol

(see *vitamin E*)

Ganoderma Lucidum

(see *medicinal mushrooms*)

Garcinia Cambogia

(see *hydroxycitric acid*)

Garden Beet

(see *beetroot*)

Garlic

aka *Allium sativum*

What it is: Also known as the stinking rose plant due to its strong odor, garlic has been cultivated and used for over 6,000 years and is considered one of the first recorded performance-enhancing agents: It was used by the Olympic athletes of ancient Greece to increase strength and endurance during sporting competition and war. Though garlic is currently more widely used for its pungent flavor as a seasoning, scientists have started to evaluate whether the performance-enhancing claims made by early Olympians hold any merit. In particular, research has focused on the 30+ sulfur-based compounds within the plant that may provide immune-boosting and antiinflammatory benefits for athletes.

How it works: The inflammatory process is an important component of the body's immune defense system. When kept temporary and local, it helps protect tissues and organs from damage; however, when inflammation spreads and becomes chronic, common among athletes walking the training tightrope or overtraining, an array of problems from muscle damage and injury to illness can hinder performance. Laboratory studies have demonstrated that sulfur compounds within garlic help regulate inflammation by inhibiting the activity of inflammatory enzymes. Preliminary evidence, primarily from animal studies using aged garlic extract (AGE), suggests that this may benefit the health of the musculoskeletal system during training. Furthermore, the sulfur compounds in the garlic seem to provide immune support to help fight off the common cold and other infections.

Performance benefit: Athletes may benefit from strengthened immune support and enhanced recovery.

Research: While the early Olympians may have believed garlic consumption enhanced strength and endurance during competition, there is no scientific evidence to support such claims, and thus a placebo effect was likely operating. A 2011 animal study discovered no benefit from sulfur-containing compounds found within garlic on exercise time to fatigue (Ferreira et al.). On a more favorable note, especially as it relates to recovery, a small double-blind, placebo-controlled study on well-trained athletes found that a daily supplementation protocol with 80 mg of the sulfur compound allicin, an active ingredient in garlic, over 2 weeks significantly reduced several blood markers of inflammation as well as perceptions of muscle soreness associated with downhill running compared to a placebo (Su et al., 2008). Unfortunately, since this was a stand-alone study with only 16 subjects, conclusions of any merit cannot be made until large-group studies replicate these results. A larger double-blind study found that daily intake of a 180 mg garlic capsule containing allicin over 12 weeks significantly reduced both incidence and duration of the common cold in healthy adults compared to a placebo (Josling, 2001).

Common usage: Garlic can be consumed in whole or supplement form. The amount of active ingredients (sulfur compounds) in each supplement will vary based on how the supplement was processed. Further studies on the effectiveness of garlic from a performance standpoint need to be conducted before conclusive dosing recommendations are appropriate for an athletic population. For general purposes, consuming 1 chopped clove daily or using a standardized extract at a dose of 600-1,200 mg split into 3 doses daily is currently recommended.

Homemade Remedy

A compound in garlic called ajoene has been shown to carry strong antimicrobial properties, and topical application seems to be effective in fighting the fungus that causes athlete's foot. An at-home remedy can be made by mixing a few finely crushed garlic cloves with olive oil and rubbing small amounts on the affected area 2-3 times daily.

Health concerns: The most common adverse effects reported with oral ingestion of garlic and garlic supplements include bad breath and body odor although such gastrointestinal issues as heartburn, abdominal pain, gas, nausea, and diarrhea have been reported. Rare occurrences include allergic reaction and uncontrolled bleeding. Topical application may cause skin irritation and blisters in a small number of users and are considered grounds for discontinuing use.

Geranamine, Geranium Oil Extract, Geranium Stem

(see *dimethylamylamine*)

Ginger

aka *African ginger, black ginger, cochin ginger, ginger essential oil, ginger root, Indian ginger, Jamaica ginger*

What it is: Derived from the horizontal stem of the plant *Zingiber officinale,* ginger is an herb commonly eaten raw or cooked. It is used to add spice to a wide spectrum of cultural cuisines, including such Western favorites as ginger ale and ginger snaps. Containing more than 50 types of antioxidants, ginger has been used in Chinese medicine for several thousand years and is recognized in athletics as a natural alternative to nonsteroidal antiinflammatory drugs (NSAIDs).

How it works: Ginger contains antioxidant compounds called gingerols that, like NSAIDs, block the enzymatic action of cyclooxygenase-1 (COX-1) and cyclooxygenase-2 (COX-2) responsible for the production of inflammation-inducing prostaglandins. Ginger also reduces the body's production of pro-inflammatory chemicals called cytokines while desensitizing a type of pain receptor found in peripheral nerves known as TRPV1.

Performance benefit: Athletes may benefit from reduced levels of inflammation and muscle pain postworkout, thereby facilitating faster recovery from intense training. Supplementation with a 255 mg dose of ginger taken twice daily over a 6-week span has been shown to reduce pain and swelling as well as improve mobility in those suffering from osteoarthritis, a condition common among athletes, especially at the master's level (Altman & Marcussen, 2001).

Research: A pair of placebo-controlled, double-blind studies conducted by researchers from the University of Georgia determined that a 2 g/day dose of ginger, taken either in raw or in heat-treated form, over 11 days reduced exercise-induced muscle pain associated with weightlifting exercise by 25% compared to a placebo (Black et al., 2010). Furthermore, a 2011 systematic review of clinical trials concluded that there is preliminary support for the anti-inflammatory benefits of ginger or specific constituents found within ginger, thereby presenting promising application for pain associated with arthritic conditions, especially osteoarthritis common among athletes (Terry et al.).

Common usage: Prepared from fresh and dried ginger root or from steam distillation of the oil in the root, ginger supplements are available as extracts, tinctures, capsules, and oils. In addition, ginger can be consumed in raw form or added as a spice in cooking. For treatment of muscle pain and inflammation, the research-supported dose ranges from .5 to 2 g/day preferably split into two doses (e.g., pre- and postworkout). If ginger is consumed in capsule form, the recommended approach is a standardized extract with a gingerol content of 5%.

Supplement Fact

A 2 g dose of raw ginger in capsule form is roughly equivalent to 1 tsp of powdered ginger, .5 tsp of ginger extract, or 1 tbsp finely chopped fresh ginger.

Recipe tip: A blend of 1 tbsp grated fresh ginger, 2 tsp olive oil, 1 tbsp honey, and 1 tbsp Dijon mustard can be used as a tangy topping for meat or fish.

Health concerns: While ill effects associated with use of ginger supplements are rare, there have been some reported cases of mild heartburn, stomach upset, and diarrhea with larger doses. Furthermore, because the Food and Drug Administration (FDA) does not currently evaluate the safety, effectiveness, or purity of herbal supplements, extra precaution should be taken if consuming ginger in other than raw form.

Ginkgo Biloba

aka *ginkgo leaf extract, ginkgo seed, Japanese silver apricot*

What it is: *Ginkgo biloba* is an herbal supplement prescribed to preserve memory, improve brain function, and prevent the decline in cognitive function associated with aging. Sales of ginkgo exceed $249 million annually in the United States, making it a popular nutritional supplement.

How it works: A number of mechanisms are hypothesized to be responsible for ginkgo's cognitive benefits. First, ginkgo acts as an antioxidant preventing free radical damage. Secondly, ginkgo may have a neural protective effect on the central nervous system. Third, ginkgo potentially modulates neurotransmitter systems and improves blood circulation. Finally, it has a beneficial effect on mood, resulting from its antidepressant attributes and its ability to improve the handling of stress.

Performance benefit: Ginkgo may be beneficial for athletes involved in sports that require fast decision making and cognitive performance. In addition, ginkgo could reduce the stress of training and improve an athlete's mood.

>continued

Gingko Biloba *>continued*

Research: Most research has focused on short-term cognitive effects following a single dose; longer-term studies have looked at ginkgo's impact on cognitive decline and the prevention of dementia. While some studies show a positive effect, the majority do not (Canter, 2007). A 2009 review of ginkgo studies found only one had significant positive results (Birks, Grimley, & Van Dongen, 2009). Reviews of research related to ginkgo in 2009 and 2007 concluded no convincing evidence existed for the use of ginkgo either as a single dose or long-term for improved cognitive performance, and that benefits for people with dementia or cognitive impairment were inconsistent and unreliable (Canter & Ernst, 2007; Birks, Grimley, & Van Dongen,, 2009). Ginkgo's antidepressant attributes and its ability to help people cope with stress are less researched. In 2002 a group of scientists from the Institute of Experimental Endocrinology found 120 mg/day of ginkgo reduced the rise in blood pressure and cortisol during experimentally induced stress (Jezova et al.). However, these results have not been confirmed by additional research. It is unlikely that ginkgo provides any performance-enhancing benefits for athletes.

Common usage: Most research trials assessing the effects of a single dose of ginkgo on cognitive performance have used 120 mg, 240 mg, or 360 mg doses of ginkgo before performing cognitive tasks. Long-term studies typically have used 120-240 mg of ginkgo/day in either 1 dose or 2 smaller doses.

Health concerns: Ginkgo can interfere with a number of medications such as antidepressants, Warfarin, antiepileptics, antidiabetics, diuretics, and nonsteroidal antiinflammatories (NSAIDs). Those taking any medications for these conditions should check with a doctor before beginning supplementation.

Ginseng

aka *American ginseng, Panax ginseng, Siberian ginseng*

What it is: A slow-growing herb native to East Asia with a light-colored root, single stalk, and long oval green leaves, ginsing is often called "man root" due to its resemblance to a human body. Ginsing is thought to have adaptogenic qualities that may help an athlete better cope with the mental and physical stresses associated with sporting competition, thereby providing a boost to performance. While several types of ginseng exist, the three that make this plant one of the top-selling herbal supplements in the United States include American, Panax, and Siberian ginseng.

How it works: Ginseng is widely used in the United States with the belief that the active compounds found within the root of the plant will improve overall energy and immune functionality, particularly during times of fatigue or stress such as those experienced by athletes in the midst of a busy training and competition schedule.

Types of Ginseng

American: Also known as *Panax quinquefolius* and belonging to the Araliacea family of plants, American ginseng contains active compounds called ginsenosides and saponins that are thought to help fight fatigue and stress by supporting the adrenal glands and the use of oxygen by exercising muscles.

Panax: Derived from the Greek word *panacea* meaning "cure all," Panax ginseng, also known as Korean, Chinese, or Asian Ginseng, also contains active compounds called ginsenosides and saponins as well as B vitamins and dietary flavonoids. These are thought to strengthen the immune system by enhancing the number of immune cells in the blood, helping protect an athlete from a wide variety of ailments that can hinder performance.

Siberian: Also known as eleuthero, ci wu jia, or Russian ginseng, Siberian ginseng contains active compounds called eleutherosides that are thought to help enhance mental acuity and improve the use of oxygen by the muscles, thereby aiding endurance as well as enhancing recovery.

Performance benefit: Athletes may benefit from increased ability to counter the potential detriments of physical and mental stress, including immune breakdown and compromised performance, thereby promoting recovery and allowing more training to be absorbed for increased performance.

Research: Most of the available studies evaluating an athlete's ability to cope with stress have focused on ginseng's impact on exercise-induced changes in immune function and oxidative stress, both components important to recovery. For instance, a small, well-designed study from the National Taiwan Sport University demonstrated that a 4-week daily supplemental protocol with 400 mg American ginseng significantly decreased blood markers of oxidative stress and muscle soreness in active men both immediately and 72 hours after a 60-minute downhill treadmill run compared to a placebo (Hsu, 2010). A second study showed that following a supplementation protocol of 20 grams of Panax ginseng extract consumed in water 3 times a day over 7 days offset a portion of the exercise-induced muscle damage and inflammation associated with an intense uphill treadmill test; it also significantly improved insulin sensitivity of college-aged males, which theoretically should help facilitate quicker restoration of muscle glycogen stores and enhance recovery (Jung et al., 2011). A 2011 animal study found an orally administered extract of Siberian ginseng to significantly extend swimming time of mice to exhaustion (Huang et al.). A further evaluation by the researchers confirmed the isolated eleutherosides (active compounds found in Siberian ginseng) produced several positive effects, including enhanced fat usage and reduced accumulation of lactic acid in the muscles. Immune response to exercise also seems to be enhanced with ginseng; during a

>continued

Ginseng >*continued*

small, randomized, controlled trial, a standardized ginsenoside containing American ginseng extract at a dose of 1,125 mg/day over 4 weeks was shown to significantly improve the immune response in healthy women after undergoing moderate exercise stress on a stationary bike compared to a placebo (Biondo et al., 2010). Because other studies have yielded mixed results, more human trials of a larger nature are warranted before absolute conclusions can be drawn.

Common usage: Ginseng can be made into a powder, capsule, or liquid tincture with important data on supplement labels including the type of ginseng, the plant part used (root), the amount and form of ginseng (powder or extract), and the concentration of ginsenosides or eleutherosides. While a wide range of doses have been used in clinical trials, a low dose is a recommended starting point to avoid side effects: 100 mg of a standardized extract or 1-2 g in powder form taken twice daily..

Health concerns: Reported side effects include heart palpitations, high blood pressure, dizziness, nausea, vomiting, diarrhea, and flushing of the face. Additionally, consuming ginseng with caffeine can cause overstimulation and insomnia in some people.

Glucosamine

aka *glucosamine sulfate, glucosamine HCL*

What it is: Glucosamine is a naturally occurring amino sugar that is a building block for proteins of the connective tissue known as glycosaminoglycans. Roughly 50% of hyaline cartilage, which covers the bones of synovial joints such as the knee, hip, and shoulder, is composed of glycosaminoglycans. Cartilage functions to absorb shock and reduce friction during movement. Two supplemental forms of glucosamine exist: glucosamine sulfate and glucosamine hydrochloride.

How it works: The availability of glucosamine is believed to be a limiting factor in the synthesis of glycosaminoglycan. Therefore, supplementation can prevent the degeneration and loss of cartilage in joints such as the knee, hip, ankle, shoulder, and spine. Glucosamine might also act by suppressing the expression of several mediators of cartilage degradation.

Performance benefit: Many athletes experience chronic joint pain as a result of training. The physical demands of sport and daily training place a significant amount of stress on joints. In addition, many athletes must overcome common injuries to joints resulting in surgery or joint reconstruction. Recovery from these types of surgeries can result in changes to the joint, and glucosamine could have a positive effect on recovery.

Research: A significant amount of research has been conducted related to glucosamine with mixed results, making it difficult to come to clear conclusions. However, a majority of scientists agree that glucosamine can improve symptoms of pain associated with osteoarthritis and delay its progression. It appears that long-term supplementation over at least 1 year may be required before significant improvements take place. In 2005 Poolsup and colleagues reviewed a variety of research studies and concluded there was evidence to support improvement of symptoms with glucosamine sulphate; however, another group of researchers was more cautious, stating that overall, glucosamine was shown to have a moderate clinically significant effect (Black et al., 2009). Early research work suggested that glucosamine sulfate was superior to glucosamine HCL in providing benefit, but some experts believe both are equally effective. Only one known research study has used glucosamine postinjury (Ostojic, 2007). This trial involving athletes who had just suffered knee injuries supplemented glucosamine for 4 weeks. No differences in pain, swelling, or passive knee flexion and extension were noted at 7, 14, or 21 days. However, after 28 days of supplementation, the glucosamine group demonstrated significant improvement in passive knee flexion and extension.

Common usage: It is recommended that 1,500 mg of glucosamine sulfate or glucosamine HCL be supplemented daily in 3 doses of 500 mg each. Recently, scientists have suggested that a 1,500 mg dose is relatively small compared to higher relative amounts used in successful animal studies (Aghazadeh-Habashi & Jamali, 2011). Some believe this is one of the reasons for mixed results in previous research trials. In some European countries and the United Kingdom, glucosamine is prescribed as a pharmaceutical drug to treat osteoarthritis. However, not all countries are as convinced of its effectiveness.

Health concerns: Glucosamine is safe. Recently concerns have been raised related to glucosamine's impact on blood glucose levels, glucose metabolism, and insulin sensitivity. However, this concern is unwarranted (Simon et al., 2011).

Glutamine

aka aminoglutaramic acid, *L-glutamine, 2-aminoglutaramicacid, levoglutamide, (S)-2, 5-diamino-5-oxopentaenoic acid, glutamic acid 5-amide, Q, gln*

What it is: The most abundant amino acid found in the body, predominantly synthesized and stored in the muscles, glutamine participates in a number of reactions important to athletes' health and recovery. Glutamine is classified as semiessential, meaning that under normal circumstances the body can synthesize adequate amounts to support physiological demands.

>*continued*

Glutamine >*continued*

However, while the average Western diet has been reported to supply 5-10 g of glutamine, generally in the form of both animal- and plant-based protein sources, it is thought that athletes may require additional amounts to offset the heightened stress associated with heavy physical training.

How it works: Prolonged periods of heavy training as well as ultraendurance competition, including adventure racing, long-course triathlon, and marathon running, are associated with significant drops in plasma (blood) glutamine levels, which is a postulated cause of exercise-induced immune impairment and increased susceptibility to infection (especially upper respiratory infections). Supplementation with glutamine is thought to help offset these drops, thereby providing athletes with immune support. Glutamine also promotes protein synthesis and thus may help protect athletes against muscle breakdown.

Performance benefit: Athletes may benefit from improved immune response and recovery times during heavy training cycles as well as enhanced ability to rebound from sport-oriented trauma or injury. Glutamine may be of particular benefit to athletes experiencing symptoms of burnout or overtraining, such as fatigue, frequent illness, and poor performance.

Research: A 2012 study of ultraendurance athletes confirmed that heavy training and competition can affect plasma glutamine levels. The study reported a 19% drop in these levels in trained men completing a 24-hour endurance trial consisting of kayaking, running, and cycling (Borgenvik et al.). Even so, intramuscular glutamine levels remained unchanged up to and during the immediate posttraining recovery period. Furthermore, several studies have found no effect of supplementation with glutamine on postexercise alterations in several aspects of immune function (Gleeson, 2008). It is thought that the drop in glutamine levels during exercise by itself may not be significant enough to compromise the immune function of healthy, well-nourished athletes. Even so, during extreme catabolic stress, as that seen with traumatic injury, intracellular glutamine levels can drop by more than 50%, and plasma concentration can drop by 30%. At that point, supplemental glutamine certainly becomes an integral nutritional component to all aspects of recovery, including immune functionality and tissue repair (Askanazi et al., 1980).

Common usage: Glutamine is available in tablet, capsule, and powder form and is often added to recovery-focused sport drinks as well as infused into energy chews and gels. Research-supported doses for added immune and recovery support during intense training cycles range from 1.5 to 4.5 g, generally split into doses taken pre-, during, and postworkout or between meals. In addition, similar doses have been taken 30 minutes preexercise to enhance endurance performance.

Health concerns: Acute intake of glutamine by athletes in daily doses of 20-30 g over 2 weeks seems to be well tolerated though a small number have reported symptoms such as constipation and bloating.

Additional performance benefit: As an important intermediate metabolite in the Kreb's metabolic cycle, glutamine is thought to help spare phospho-creatine and glycogen in muscle fibers, particularly Type I (slow-twitch or aerobic fibers), which may extend endurance. A small study of competitive soccer players found that preworkout consumption of a carbohydrate-gluta-mine solution containing 50 g of maltodextrin and 3.5 g of glutamine to be more effective in increasing the athletes' distance and duration of tolerance to intermittent exercise and lowering subjective feelings of fatigue than a calorie-matched carbohydrate-only solution (Favano et al., 2008).

Glutathione (GSH)

aka *gamma-glutamylcysteinylglycine, gamma-L-glutamyl-L-cysteinylglycine, L-glutathione*

What it is: Synthesized primarily in the liver from the amino acids L-cysteine, L-glutamate, and glycine, glutathione is considered nonessential though it is estimated only 100 mg are obtained via the typical diet, generally from protein-containing foods such as meats, with smaller amounts actually absorbed and available to the body for use. Exercise stress has been shown to lower glutathione levels in the body and negatively affect endurance performance, immunity, and recovery, making supplementation to optimize levels of potential benefit to the athlete.

How it works: As an antioxidant, glutathione is purported to aid perfor-mance by protecting against cellular damage incurred from the production of free radicals during exercise, especially when levels exceed the body's own natural defenses. This can occur when an athlete returns to training after a long layoff, enters a particular tough training cycle, or is exposed to other stressors such as altitude, smog, and extreme heat or cold. Research has shown exposure to such stressors can significantly decrease glutathi-one levels in the body (Gomes, Stone, & Florida-James, 2011; Pinho et al., 2010). Added antioxidant protection through supplementation may enhance endurance, help speed recovery, and better maintain the health of an athlete throughout a competitive season. Additionally, maintaining glutathione levels is thought to protect athletes from infection and reoccurring illness that may otherwise sideline them from critical training and competition by enhancing nutrient and amino acid absorption in cells important to immune function, namely lymphocytes and phagocytes.

Performance benefit: Athletes may benefit from enhanced endurance, immune protection, and recovery.

Research: Because glutathione is not well absorbed across the gastro-intestinal tract, it is virtually impossible to raise circulating levels through direct supplementation. Even an acute, high-dose (3 g) oral administration

>continued

of glutathione failed to affect circulating levels in one study (Witschi et al., 1992). Research focusing on supplemental oral intake of glutathione is virtually nonexistent. Instead, the bulk of research has focused on intravenous administration of glutathione or oral intake of glutathione precursors and derivatives such as N-acetylcysteine, L-cysteine, and L-glutamic acid. In a 2003 case study involving a 61-year-old trained endurance athlete, for example, four separate intravenous doses of 1,000 mg of glutathione over 36 days led to progressive and significant time improvements in an established 18.4 mile (29.6 km) time trial; the end result was a more than a 5-minute improvement or 7.2% performance gain (Misner). In the case of oral supplementation, two separate double-blind, placebo-controlled studies found daily intake of cystine (700 mg), a dipeptide of cysteine, and theanine (280 mg), a precursor of glutamate, over 10-14 days provided a significant protective effect on natural killer cell activity, helping reduce incidence of infection in highly trained athletes during high-intensity resistance exercise and run training compared to a placebo (Kawada et al., 2010; Murakami et al., 2009). Both cysteine and glutamate play key roles in the formation of glutathione. While it is evident that maintaining optimal levels of glutathione is important to an athlete's health and performance, there is not adequate evidence for its oral supplementation use, specifically when taken alone.

Common usage: Glutathione is available in capsule, tablet, and powder form. A combined amino acid cocktail that includes glutathione along with L-cysteine, N-acetylcysteine, glutamic acid, or glycine is thought to have a greater impact on body glutathione levels and consequent antioxidant benefit than taking glutathione alone. Doses generally range from 600-1,200 mg split into 2 doses throughout the day. Hemolytic anemia, also known as hemolysis, which often occurs in runners, can lower circulating levels of glutathione; consequently, affected athletes may benefit from intravenous or oral supplement intervention.

Health concerns: Glutathione, taken either orally or by injection into the muscle or veins, appears to be safe; no adverse symptoms have been reported.

Glycine Betaine

(see *betaine*)

Goat's Horn

(see *fenugreek*)

Golden Root

(see *Rhodiola rosea*)

Grape Seed

aka *Vinis vinifera, grape seed oil, grapeseed, muskat*

What it is: Grapes, a member of the berry fruit family, have long been considered a nutrition powerhouse with medicinal use dating back to ancient Greece. Their seeds contain a unique class of plant compounds called oligomeric proanthocyanidin complexes (OPCs) that contain strong antioxidant qualities of potential benefit to a highly trained athlete.

How it works: As an athlete hits the peak of training, where total volume and intensity often reach uncharted levels, the production of free radicals and oxidative stress may exceed the body's natural defenses, causing damage to muscle tissue and inhibiting optimal recovery from training. Grape seed, whose antioxidant abilities have been shown to be 20-50 times more potent than such popular antioxidants as beta-carotene, vitamin C, and vitamin E, helps strengthen and protect cell membranes, including that of muscle tissue, from oxidative damage caused by elevated levels of circulating free radicals during times of exercise stress.

Performance benefit: Athletes may experience less muscle damage and inflammation during heavy training, thereby facilitating faster recovery times.

Supplement Fact

Grape seed is one of only a few antioxidants that can cross the blood-brain barrier and provide protection for the brain. It is hypothesized that this may help enhance mental alertness, focus, and concentration during training and competition, but there is a lack of research evaluating this potential benefit.

Research: A group of elite sportsmen in the midst of training and competition saw nearly a 10% increase in antioxidant capacity, resulting in reduced biomarkers of skeletal muscle damage, when supplementing with 400 mg of grape seed extract versus a placebo over a month as part of a 2009 randomized, double-blind, placebo-controlled study (Lafay et al.). This result equated to significant increases in the performance of handball athletes, including a 6.4% boost in explosive power, during a structured jumping exercise protocol. There is also some evidence that OPC in grape seed offsets some of the swelling triggered by athletic injury and surgery (Teixeira, 2002; Xu et al., 2012; Constatini, De Bernardi, & Gotti, 1999; Fine, 2000).

Common usage: Grape seed is available as a liquid extract or as a capsule. Research-supported treatment doses for antioxidant protection in athletes range from 25 to 50 mg taken up to 3 times/day. The highest quality grape seed products are standardized for purity and control of the substance to 40-80% proanthocyanidins or have an OPC content of at least 95%.

Health concerns: Grape seed seems to be well tolerated although there have been reports of headache; dry, itchy scalp; dizziness; and nausea in a small population. Animal studies have shown doses up to 100 mg/kg/day to be safe for use; however, safety trials on humans are limited, so it is advisable to consult with a physician before supplementation, especially if taking any medications.

Additional performance benefits: Grape seed helps inhibit the release of chemicals called prostaglandins that can generate inflammation during an allergic response or asthma, making supplementation potentially beneficial for athletes who suffer from allergies or asthma.

Grapple Plant

(see *devil's claw*)

Green Pepper

(see *capsicum*)

Grifola Forndosa

(see medicinal mushrooms)

Gymnema Sylvestre

aka *gurmar*

What it is: *Gymnema sylvestre* (GS) is a large woody herb grown in central and southern India as well as tropical regions of Africa and Australia. For centuries it has been used as a medicinal plant in traditional Ayurvedic medicine. Its leaves, which are typically the active part of the plant, are believed to assist in reducing blood sugar, resulting in its use as a treatment for diabetes. In addition, the plant is believed to benefit digestion, promote circulation, protect against viral infection, and prevent obesity. GS is sold by itself as a dietary supplement to promote health or is often added to so-called fat-burning supplements.

How it works: There is a lack of quality research studies on GS; as a result, how it works is relatively unknown. The majority of research has focused on diabetes, and GS's mechanisms are speculated to involve insulin production and sensitivity. GS is thought to enhance the uptake of glucose by adipose and muscle tissue as well as decrease the intestinal absorption of glucose and the production of glucose in the liver. All such actions would have beneficial effects on blood sugar, obesity, and the storage of body fat.

Performance benefit: The potential benefits for athletes are in GS's ability to assist in weight loss and reduction of body fat.

Research: No scientific studies have evaluated the effectiveness of GS in improving weight loss and reducing body fat in humans. Claims of improved body composition and fat burning have not been validated scientifically. A study performed in 2012 on rats found a 100 mg/kg of body weight dose of GS was capable of decreasing body weight, food consumption, triglyceride levels, and total cholesterol in obese rats fed a high-fat diet (Reddy et al.). A 2007 review of GS in the treatment of diabetes concluded that the clinical efficacy of GS is supported only by a small number of nonrandomized, open-label trials, and that further research is urgently needed (Leach, 2007). Currently, GS lacks enough evidence to support any of its claims.

Common usage: Open-trial diabetic studies have used doses ranging from 200 to 800 mg daily. The longest study on GS is 18-20 months in length.

Health concerns: The use of GS appears to be safe; however, one report of toxic hepatitis was noted in a diabetic patient treated with GS.

Harpago, *Harpagophyum Procumbens*

(see *devil's claw*)

Herba Epimedii

(see *horny goat weed*)

Hippophae Rhamnoides L

(see *sea buckthorn*)

Hoodia Gordonii

aka *P57*

What it is: Hoodia is a cactus-like plant grown in South Africa. The plant was first recognized in 1932 where it was recorded as a source of food for the Khoi-San people, who consumed hoodia during long hunting trips when food was scarce to suppress appetite and thirst. In 1963 a compound known as P57 was isolated from hoodia that was believed to be responsible for the plant's appetite-suppressing affects. In 1998 a patent was granted for different pharmaceutical compositions of hoodia. Between 1998 and 2009 large pharmaceutical companies such as Pharmacia, Unilever, and Phytopharm worked to develop products containing hoodia that could be used to treat obesity. Since 2009 all companies except Phytopharm have terminated their efforts because of safety and efficacy concerns (Vermaak et al., 2011).

How it works: Hoodia is believed to work by affecting the central nervous system and hypothalamus. A 2004 study showed that P57, the active constituent of hoodia, increased ATP content in the hypothalamus of rats. The elevated ATP content countered decreases in ATP content that would be expected from a reduced-calorie diet (MacLean and Duo).

Performance benefit: Athletes such as wrestlers needing to restrict calorie intake for weight loss might benefit from the appetite-suppressing affects of hoodia.

Research: To date, no clinical studies in humans have been reported in peer-reviewed scientific journals. Private companies wanting to produce a profitable, functional food have conducted the majority of the research. The results of this research are often protected and unpublished. The only other published data are on animal models. These studies often compare the effects of hoodia on food intake in obese and nonobese mice and report substantial reductions in food intake when rats are fed ad lib diets. Although data on animals are positive, much more evidence is needed before hoodia is recommended as a weight-loss supplement. Consumers should be leery, considering the termination of research efforts by many pharmaceutical companies (Vermaak et al., 2011).

Common usage: Studies in rats have determined 1.8-2.7 g/kg of body weight to be the optimal effective dose. Human trials have typically provided 400-500 mg daily. It is difficult to determine a recommendation for safe and effective use without further research.

Health concerns: No adverse effects have been reported, and a history of safe use within the indigenous Khoi-San people of South Africa is known. Those considering supplementing with Hoodia should be cautious about the quality of the product they purchase. Studies on quality control have found fake products claiming to contain *Hoodia gordonii* (Vermaak et al., 2011).

Horny Goat Weed

aka *Herba epimedii, epimedium, icariin, Epimedium grandiflorum*

What it is: Horny goat weed is a more common name used to refer to *Herba epimedii,* a plant used in traditional Chinese medicine. The plant has been sold as a dietary supplement for many years and claims a range of benefits, including an ability to increase sex drive and treat sexual dysfunction. Legend claims that a Chinese goat herder who noticed increased sexual activity in his flock after consuming the plant discovered these abilities. In addition, horny goat weed claims to increase testosterone and improve vitality.

How it works: Horny goat weed is thought to act as a natural testosterone booster. As men age, the levels of testosterone they produce begin to decline. This drop in testosterone limits their ability to build muscle and maintain strength. It also decreases sex drive, lowers vitality, and can leave many men feeling depressed. Horny goat weed contains the flavonoid icariin, which is believed to be the active flavonoid responsible for beneficial effects.

Performance benefit: Supplementation is most common among male athletes looking for a natural alternative to anabolic steroids to increase testosterone levels. Testosterone, a powerful anabolic hormone, increases muscle mass and improves strength and power.

Research: Most research trials on horny goat weed, icariin, and *Herba epimedii* have used mouse and rat models. There are no clinical trials on humans related to its effects on testosterone. More research has focused on its use in treating and preventing osteoporosis and erectile dysfunction. Only animal models have been used to test these benefits. Presently, there is no scientific research backing any claims for horny goat weed as a natural testosterone booster.

>continued

Horny Goat Weed >*continued*

Common usage: Typically, dietary supplements sold as horny goat weed contain roughly 500 mg and recommend using 60-90 mg before physical exertion. These recommendations have no scientific data to validate them.

Health concerns: The safety is unknown at this time. Few human research trials exist, making it difficult to determine any potential health concerns related to use.

Supplement Warning

 Horny goat weed is often marketed as a natural supplement for the enhancement of sexual performance. Consumers should proceed with caution when purchasing natural products making these claims. A recent analysis of nine dietary supplements intended to improve sexual performance found four of the nine to be adulterated with analogues of Viagra. Others were adulterated with drugs not approved for use (Balayssac et al., 2012).

Hot Pepper

(see *capsicum*)

Huang Qi

(see *astragalus*)

Hydroxy-Beta-Methylbutyrate (HMB)

What it is: Hydroxy-beta-methylbutyrate (HMB) is a metabolite of the amino acid leucine. When leucine is metabolized, it is converted into α-ketoisocaproate (KIC), which is further converted into HMB. Roughly 5% of leucine is converted into HMB. HMB became popular in the 1990s when Ross Pharmaceuticals developed a product known as Juven. Juven, which is a combination of HMB, arginine, and glutamine, was developed to help prevent losses in lean body mass in cancer and AIDS patients.

How it works: The exact mechanisms of HMB are unknown; however, a couple of theories exist. HMB is believed to upregulate (increase) the gene expression of the anabolic hormone IGF1 (insulin-like growth factor 1) in skeletal muscles. Increased levels of IGF1 would assist in building muscle as well as preventing muscle breakdown. Additionally, HMB might stimulate muscle building or protein synthesis directly by affecting the mTOR pathway which is a key regulator of protein synthesis. The last theory seems to hold the most promise. It involves an ability of HMB to prevent protein breakdown by inhibiting the ubiquitin-proteasome pathway, which is involved in the breakdown of proteins in the body, including in muscle (Zanchi et al., 2011).

Performance benefit: HMB has a number of upsides for athletes. It has been labeled as anticatabolic because of its ability to prevent protein breakdown. Supplementation would lessen the catabolic effects of exercise and training on muscle. This should assist athletes in maintaining and building muscle mass through training, thereby increasing gains in strength. HMB should limit extreme muscle soreness experienced from heavy training and competition. HMB can assist injured athletes by preventing some of the losses in muscle mass experienced during immobilization or limited activity.

Research: Unfortunately, research studies to date have produced mixed results. A meta-analysis conducted in 2003 concluded that HMB did produce statistically significant effects on both strength and lean body mass; however, this review was criticized for including only 9 studies (Nissen & Sharp, 2003). More recent research continues to produce mixed results—some studies demonstrate benefit and others do not. More research is needed to provide a better understanding of these differences. It appears that the benefits of HMB are most significant in untrained populations who experience more significant muscle damage as a result of training. In addition, HMB might benefit athletes during times of heightened training volume and intensity or when exposed to different types of physical stress or training their bodies have not adapted to (Wilson, G., Wilson, J., & Manninen, 2008). Although no studies to date have been done related to injured athletes, this is a potential area of benefit. One recent study found HMB capable of preventing muscle loss in rats during immobilization (Hao, 2011). HMB is most promising for athletes suffering from injury or during heavy, intensified periods of training and competition.

Common usage: A 1 g dose of HMB provided 3 times/day is recommended for a total of 3 g. This recommendation is based on research showing that 3 g daily produces better results than 1.5 g and is equivalent to the results from using 6 g; however, more research is needed to validate these recommendations (Gallagher et al., 2000).

Health concerns: HMB is safe for use by athletes and has been shown to decrease risk factors related to cardiovascular disease. Research found HMB to lower LDL cholesterol and blood pressure and to have no effect on HDL cholesterol (Nissen et al., 2000).

Hydroxocobalamin

(see *vitamin B12*)

Hydroxycitric Acid (HCA)

aka *citrimax HCA, hydroxicitrate, Garcinia cambogia*

What it is: Hydroxycitric acid (HCA) is found in plants such as *Garcinia cambogia, Garcinia Indice,* and *Garcinia atrovirdis.* These plants are typically native to South Asia and India. HCA is commonly found in weight-loss supplements.

How it works: The mechanisms of HCA are speculative. Some scientists believe that HCA causes weight loss by inhibiting adenosine triphosphatase-citrate-lyase, an enzyme involved in the synthesis of adiose tissue; others believe HCA increases the release of serotonin, leading to appetite suppression. HCA may inhibit the carbohydrate digestive enzyme alpha amylase, thereby reducing carbohydrate absorption and metabolism. None of these mechanisms is currently proven. Most scientific studies note the ability of HCA to reduce food intake or produce an anorectic effect.

Performance benefit: If the proposed benefits of HCA are true, it would be of benefit for athletes wanting to improve body composition and lose weight. Athletes should also be aware that the mechanisms of HCA are related to suppressing appetite and reducing food intake. Athletes must be wise when reducing calorie or food intake to lose weight, and severe calorie restriction can negatively affect performance.

Research: Research studies in animals are positive (Saito et al., 2005). HCA was shown to suppress food intake and prevent weight gain in rats fed high-carbohydrate diets. Human trials have also been investigated, including a recent systemic review and meta-analysis of randomized clinical trials (RCTs) related to HCA (Onakpoya et al., 2011). It was concluded that HCA can generate short-term weight loss; however, the magnitude of loss was small and only observed in less-rigorous RCTs. When more rigorous trials are considered, HCA does not produce a statistically significant amount of weight loss. Therefore HCA's relevance as a weight-loss supplement is questionable. These scientists recommend that more rigorous, longer-duration, and better-reported studies be completed. Finally, a review of herbal weight-loss supplements concluded that "while HCA appears to be well tolerated, there is limited data with regards to its efficacy" (Egras et al., 2011, 5). It is unknown if the source of HCA has an impact on results, and current trials have only ranged from 2 to 12 weeks in duration, highlighting the need for longer-term studies.

Common usage: The dosage of HCA typically ranges from 1 g to 2.8 g/day. This dosage is commonly distributed into 2-3 smaller doses of 300-1,000 mg consumed before meals.

Health concerns: The use of HCA appears to be safe, although some studies report subjects experienced headache, nausea, upper respiratory, and gastrointestinal tract symptoms.

Hypoxanthine Riboside, Hypoxanthosine

(see *inosine*)

Icariin

(see *horny goat weed*)

Indian Ginger

(see *ginger*)

Indian Ginseng

(see *Withania somnifera*)

Indian Pennywort

(see *gotu kola*)

Inosine (I)

aka *hypoxanthine riboside, 9-beta-D-ribofuranosylhypoxanthine, hypoxanthosine*

What it is: A member of a chemical family called purine nucleotides, inosine is a molecule that serves as one of the basic structural compounds comprising cells. It can be found dispersed in all tissues within the human body, in particular cardiac and skeletal muscle. Inosine can be derived naturally from such dietary sources as organ meats and Brewer's yeast. Supplementation use by athletes became popular in the 1990s when inosine was marketed as enhancing muscle-building capacity as well as increasing energy and endurance during training and competition.

How it works: Involved in the production of 2,3 DPG (a substance that facilitates the transport of oxygen from red blood cells to the muscles and heart), inosine is purported to help promote blood flow, enhance the oxygen-carrying capacity of the blood, and increase endurance performance. In addition, as a precursor to the manufacture of adenosine (a molecule involved in the synthesis of ATP energy), inosine is thought to help optimize energy production and protect against muscle fatigue.

Performance benefit: Athletes may benefit from enhanced energy and endurance during training and competition.

Research: Well-designed studies evaluating the ergogenic benefit of inosine are limited and have not been favorable. In fact, in some cases inosine actually impaired performance. For example, one small double-blind study of highly trained runners failed to demonstrate any performance benefit of a 2-day supplementation protocol that incorporated 6,000 mg of inosine/day leading up to a run workout that included a submaximal warm-up run, a maximal 3 mi (4.8 km) treadmill run, and a competitive 3 mi (4.8) treadmill run (Williams et al., 1990). In fact, the placebo group actually posted significantly faster times, suggestive of actual impairment by oral inosine supplementation. Similarly, a study of 10 highly trained cyclists found that a supplementation protocol incorporating 5,000 mg/day of inosine over 5 days actually impaired the performance (compared to a placebo) of a cycling exercise protocol that incorporated a Wingate 30-second test, 30-minute time trial, and sprint to fatigue (Starling et al., 1996). Increasing the dose to 10,000 mg over 5 or 10 days during an exercise protocol that incorporated a series of bike sprints followed by a 20-minute time trial also failed to yield any performance benefit (McNaughton, Dalton, & Tarr, 1999). Consequently, the current consensus is that inosine does not seem to improve endurance performance and may even have a detrimental impact on it.

Common usage: Available in tablet or capsule form, inosine can be consumed daily 45-60 minutes before training or competition, preferably with food. Because study results have not been favorable related to performance benefits, dosing recommendations cannot be made with confidence though study doses have generally ranged between 5,000 and 10,000 mg/day.

Health concerns: Excessive intake of inosine may increase blood levels of a waste product called uric acid, increasing the risk for painful kidney stones. Thus, supplementation should be avoided by athletes with gout or kidney disorders. Other reported symptoms include stomach upset, nausea, and bloating.

Iron (Fe)

aka *elemental iron, ferrous bisglycinate, ferrous carbonate anhydrous, ferrous fumarate, ferrous gluconate, ferrous sulfate, ferous pyrophosphate*

What it is: Iron, a trace mineral, is a major component of hemoglobin, whose role is to transport oxygen from the lungs to the muscles via the blood. Some research has shown that aerobic exercise creates an added demand for iron. Failure to meet this added demand through dietary intake and proper absorption of such whole food sources as whole grains, leafy greens, dried fruit, red meat, fish, and poultry can compromise blood iron stores and lead to iron-deficiency anemia (IDA). An anemic athlete may experience muscle burning, shortness of breath during exercise, nausea, frequent infections, and respiratory illnesses and have a pale, washed-out appearance.

How it works: Without enough iron in the blood, the body becomes starved for oxygen; ATP cannot be properly synthesized, leading to pronounced

>continued

feelings of fatigue and limiting work capacity. IDA occurs in three stages, with stage 3 having the most detrimental effect on athletic performance. Most athletes with iron depletion have a stage 1 deficiency, also known as nonanemia iron deficiency, which is diagnosed when ferritin, the storage form of iron, falls below normal. If stage 1 iron deficiency is left undetected for several months, an athlete may develop stage 2 deficiency when red blood cells and consequent oxygen transfer decrease, negatively affecting exercise capacity. The final stage of iron deficiency, stage 3, is detected by insufficient hemoglobin and a low concentration of red blood cells; stage 3 leads to feelings of intense fatigue, compromised physical ability, and decreased athletic performance.

Athletes' Tip

Sports anemia is a term applied to endurance athletes who have lower than normal hemoglobin levels but normal levels of other iron status indicators. This situation is a response to the increase in blood volume that accompanies training; therefore, it is not a true anemia, nor should it be treated like one.

Performance benefit: By restoring hemoglobin and the blood iron levels of iron-deficient and anemic athletes, oxygen delivery to working muscles and ATP energy production increase, thereby allowing the athlete to better meet the metabolic demands of aerobic activity.

Research: While scientific evidence has shown a significant drop-off in endurance with iron deficiency, in part due to an adverse effect on aerobic capacity, there remains controversy about when (i.e., at what stage of deficiency) iron supplementation becomes beneficial from a performance standpoint (DellaValle & Hass, 2011; Reinke et al., 2012; Fallon, 2008). According to the most recent research in this regard, there appears to be no performance benefit associated with iron supplementation without iron deficiency or with nonanemia (stage 1) iron deficiency, particularly in those athletes with ferritin levels above 30 mcg/L (Borrione et al., 2011).

Common usage: The RDA for iron is 18 mg/day; athletes at risk for iron deficiency, including female athletes whose menstrual blood loss often affects iron or those athletes with ferritin levels under 30 mcg/L, may increase to 20-30 mg/day from whole food or supplementation doses. Properly diagnosed cases of IDA, especially stage 2 and stage 3, should be treated with therapeutic doses of supplemental iron, preferably in the ferrous sulfate or ferrous bisglycinate form due to enhanced absorption rates and in slow-release form to reduce constipation. The treatment dose will depend on the cause and severity of iron deficiency, and thus it is important to work with a health professional in determining an appropriate supplementation protocol. Therapeutic doses of elemental iron range from 50 to 100 mg taken 3 times daily for adult athletes and 4-6 mg/kg of body weight per day split into 3 doses for youth athletes. Taking 500 mg of vitamin C or drinking a glass of orange juice may help enhance absorption of the iron. Typical correction of anemic conditions takes approximately 8 weeks.

Health concerns: Dietary iron supplementation is not recommended for athletes with normal blood iron levels. Some researchers have linked excess iron to diabetes, cancer, increased risk for infection, exacerbation of arthritis, and heart disease. Large doses, generally indicated at levels of 20 mg/kg of body weight/day, are toxic; levels above 60 mg/kg of body weight/day can be fatal.

Additional performance benefits: Iron may help improve both short- and long-term recovery times by improving immune functionality.

Isoinokosterone

(see *ecdysteroids*)

Isoleucine

(see *branched-chain amino acids*)

Isomaltulose

aka *palatinose, 6-0-a-D-glucopyranosyl-D-fructose*

What it is: A natural constituent of honey and sugar cane as well as commercially manufactured from bacterial fermentation of sucrose, isomaltulose, marketed in the supplement industry as Palatinose, causes a slower rise in blood glucose than other sugars. As a result, it may provide beneficial applications to hypoglycemic and diabetic athletes as well as athletes looking for an easy-to-digest preworkout carbohydrate option that better sustains blood sugar.

How it works: As a carbohydrate with a low glycemic index, isomaltulose helps keep insulin level increases at bay which helps protect against blood sugar crashes that can initiate symptoms of dizziness, fatigue, and diminished performance. This is especially relevant for athletes vulnerable to hypoglycemia (low blood sugar). Furthermore, studies suggest isomaltulose enhances the oxidation of fat for energy, thereby demonstrating potential benefit for glycogen sparing and enhanced endurance as well as benefits for those athletes wanting to shed body fat.

>*continued*

Performance benefit: Athletes, especially those inflicted with diabetes or hypoglycemia, may benefit from better control of blood sugar, improved metabolic risk factors, and favorable body composition changes.

Research: The bulk of research evaluating the benefits of isomaltulose has been conducted with subjects having preexisting health issues such as metabolic syndrome and diabetes; even so, the results have been favorable. For example, one well-designed study of overweight or obese men with metabolic syndrome and insulin resistance found total fat oxidation to be significantly higher and blood glucose and insulin responses considerably lower with a pre- and postworkout meal that included isomaltulose versus a glucose-sucrose combination. Each subject consumed a 250 mL drink and 140 g of cookies containing 50 g of isomaltulose or glucose-sucrose before exercising at a moderate intensity on a treadmill for 30 minutes; each subject then consumed a standardized recovery meal consisting of a 250 mL drink with 10% isomaltulose or glucose-sucrose, mini pizzas, and an apple. The study investigators concluded that the increased fat oxidation at rest and during physical activity seen with isomaltulose might help facilitate weight loss and improvement in metabolic risk factors (König et al., 2012). The applications for athletes with type 1 diabetes are also promising after a study demonstrated consumption of isomaltulose at a dose of 0.6 g/kg of body weight in coordination with a reduction in rapid-acting insulin dose improved blood glucose responses to a high-intensity exercise protocol: Subjects maintained both speed and endurance compared to an isocaloric feeding with dextrose (Bracken et al., 2012). Similarly, West and colleagues (2011) found consumption of 75 g of isomaltulose 2 hours before 45 minutes of treadmill running at 80% $\dot{V}O_2$max improved the blood glucose responses of type 1 diabetics during and after exercise through reduced carbohydrate and improved lipid oxidation during the later stages of exercise (West et al., 2011). Whether these benefits will translate to a healthy, athletic population is currently unknown. Even so, isomaltulose offers an attractive, low-glycemic (solicits steadier blood sugar response), easy-to-digest carbohydrate source for athletes to consume preworkout, during carbo-loading protocols, and postworkout (Achten et al., 2007).

Common usage: Isomaltulose is commonly added as an ingredient in weight-gainer meal replacement powders and shakes; it is also available as a stand-alone carbohydrate powder or liquid carbohydrate source. As a preworkout snack, 50 g or 0.25-0.3 g/lb (0.25-0.3 g/.45 kg) of body weight can be consumed 1 hour before starting. A similar dose can be consumed immediately postworkout to support recovery. Isomaltulose can also be incorporated into carbo-loading routines, which entails an athlete consume 3.6-4.5 g of carbohydrate/pound (.6-4.5 g/.45 kg) of body weight daily for 3 days leading up to an endurance event.

Health concerns: Similar to the use of any highly concentrated source of carbohydrate, risk for gastrointestinal disturbances such as stomach upset and diarrhea increase exponentially with concentrations above 10% (more than 25 g carbohydrate/8 oz [.23 L] of water consumed).

Jamaica Ginger

(see *ginger*)

Japanese Silver Apricot

(see G*inkgo biloba*)

L

Lactobacillus

(see *probiotics*)

L-Amino Succinate, L-Aspartic Acid

(see *aspartates*)

Lauric Acid

(see *medium-chain triglycerides*)

Lentinula Edodes

(see *medicinal mushrooms*)

Leucine

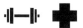

aka *branched-chain amino acids, L-leucine, D-leucine*

What it is: Leucine is considered an essential amino acid that must be obtained from the diet and cannot be synthesized in the body. It is abundantly found in high-protein foods such as lentils, beef, fish, chicken, nuts, pork, eggs, chickpeas, and milk. Leucine is unique in that it is also a branched-chain amino acid, which can be oxidized in skeletal muscle, unlike other essential amino acids, which are mainly catabolized in the liver.

How it works: Amino acids are often viewed as building blocks for the synthesis of proteins in the body. Leucine is much more than a building block and can signal cells to begin protein synthesis or muscle building. A cell-signaling pathway known as mTOR is responsible for initiating protein synthesis. Leucine is thought to act somewhere in this pathway, enhancing the pathway's signals and causing it to increase production of proteins (Pasiakos & McClung, 2011).

Performance benefit: The role of leucine in the stimulation of protein synthesis has a number of applications for athletes. Supplementation with leucine before exercise will prevent the breakdown of proteins and result in less muscle damage as a result of training. Supplementing with leucine during exercise would produce the same benefits. Third, providing leucine postexercise would signal protein synthesis, the recovery and rebuilding of muscles. Finally, as a branched-chain amino acid, leucine could provide a fuel source for muscles during exercise and improve performance.

>continued

Leucine >*continued*

Research: Research studies support the use of leucine to lessen protein breakdown and muscle damage when consumed before exercise and to stimulate and enhance protein synthesis when supplemented after exercise. It is important when evaluating these results to take whole proteins into consideration. It is known that complete proteins found in eggs and whey improve protein balance when consumed before exercise and stimulate protein synthesis after exercise. It is also known that protein synthesis is maximized when a 20 g dose of high-quality complete proteins is consumed, equivalent to roughly 9-10 g of essential amino acids and roughly 1.8 g of leucine (Moore 2009; Kerksick 2008). Recent studies have shown that additional leucine above 1.8 g does not further enhance protein synthesis (Pasiakos & McClung, 2011). There is no benefit to leucine supplementation when adequate amounts of complete proteins are consumed either before or after exercise; however, leucine supplementation is advantageous if adequate amounts of complete proteins cannot be consumed at these times. Research related to the performance-enhancing effects of leucine during exercise is less promising, and most studies show no benefit (Negro et al., 2008).

Common usage: A recommendation of .03-.045 g/kg of body weight is recommended. For a 165 lb (74.8 km) athlete, this would be equivalent to 2.25-3.4 g of leucine before and after exercise.

Health concerns: Leucine supplementation within recommendations is safe and does not produce adverse effects.

Leuzea Carthamoides

(see *maral root*)

Levoglutamide, L-Glutamine

(see *glutamine*)

L-Glutathione

(see *glutathione*)

Linium Usitatissimum, Linseed Oil

(see *flax seed*)

Lipoic Acid, Lipolate

(see *alpha-lipoic acid*)

L-Selenomethionine

(see *selenium*)

L-Tyrosine

(see *tyrosine*)

M

Magnesium (Mg)

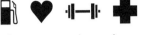

aka *magnesium gluconate, magnesium citrate, magnesium oxide, magnesium chloride, magnesium aspartate, magnesium sulfate*

What it is: As an essential mineral, magnesium is the fourth most abundant element (behind sodium, potassium, and calcium) found in the body, with a total of 50%-60% being stored in the skeletal system and the remainder being stored in muscles and soft tissues. Magnesium can be found naturally in such dietary sources as pumpkin seeds, nuts, whole grains, and legumes. The current RDA is 400-420 mg for adult males and 310-320 mg for adult females. It is thought that athletes may require additional magnesium above the current RDA to accommodate the increased metabolic demands of exercise and offset losses from sweating.

How it works: Magnesium plays an instrumental role in maintaining both structural (bone) and biochemical (muscle contraction, nerve transmission, enzyme production) homeostasis in the human body. Magnesium is responsible for 80% of all enzymatic reactions in the body; it regulates virtually every activity, making attainment and maintenance of magnesium balance crucial to an athlete's overall health. Of particular importance from a performance standpoint is the fact that magnesium is required for both aerobic and anaerobic energy production. Animal data have indicated increased glucose concentrations, lower blood lactate accumulation, and a reduced energy cost of exercise with supplementation (Cheng et al., 2007). Magnesium is also involved in reactions necessary for electrolyte balance. Because prolonged exercise increases magnesium loss via sweat, it is thought that supplementation during exercise, generally in the form of a sport drink or electrolyte capsules, is important for protection against muscle weakness and cramping.

Performance benefit: Athletes, particularly those with poor dietary intake of magnesium, may benefit from enhanced metabolic efficiency during exercise, helping to improve strength, power, and endurance performance. Magnesium also aids bone health by protecting against bone loss and consequent risk of fracture.

Research: A small, well-designed study of women found a month-long period of magnesium restriction (112 mg/day or 36% of the RDA), an intake not uncommon among athletes eating primarily refined, processed foods, to significantly increase the peak oxygen uptake, total and cumulative net oxygen usage, and heart rate for a given training workload in comparison to a period when sufficient magnesium (based on the RDA) was provided through whole foods and supplementation. Furthermore, as the level of magnesium deficiency intensified, so did the metabolic cost of exercise, an established detriment to performance (Lukaski & Nielson, 2002). Another study revealed that the dietary magnesium intake of elite basketball, handball, and volleyball players fell significantly below the current RDA; a regression analysis indicated a direct correlation with performance during several isometric strength and plyometric drills independent of energy intake (Santos et al., 2011). The metabolic benefits for a nondeficient population, however, have not been supported in human research, nor has there been support for supplementation as protection against muscle cramping (Finstad et al., 2001; Soria et al., 2011; Schwellnus et al., 2004). A 2012 study confirmed dietary magnesium intake to be a significant predictor of bone mineral density in elite athletes, which has important applications for the bone health of young, growing athletes and athletes engaged in low-impact (nonweight-bearing) activities such as cycling and swimming, where bone mass tends to be lower (Matias et al.).

Are You at Risk for Magnesium Deficiency?

- I am following a high-protein diet (excessive intake increases urinary loss of magnesium).
- I eat primarily packaged foods and fast food (processed foods are generally lacking in magnesium).
- The fat content in my diet is greater than 30% of my daily calorie intake (high-fat diets reduce absorption of magnesium).
- I drink a lot of carbonated beverages such as soda (phosphoric acid in carbonated drinks prevents absorption of magnesium within the GI tract).
- I'm a heavy sweater and train 3+ hours daily (sweat losses may be great enough to warrant increased intake).
- I regularly consume alcoholic beverages (increases excretion of magnesium).
- I'm taking medication (some antibiotics, diuretics, birth control pills, and steroids can increase excretion of magnesium).

Common usage: Magnesium is generally bound with salts such as gluconate, citrate, and aspartate for supplement use and is available in tablet, capsule, powder, and liquid form. Magnesium is also commonly added as an electrolyte to sport drinks and products. As a daily supplement, typical doses range from 100 to 350 mg. Magnesium is best taken with food to minimize adverse side effects. To offset sweat losses, athletes training or racing longer than 3 hours should replace 20-30 mg of magnesium per 8-12 oz (.24-.35 L) of fluid ingested.

Health concerns: The most common side effect associated with magnesium supplementation, generally at single doses of greater than 350 mg (the current upper tolerable limit for supplement use in adults and adolescents) is diarrhea. Abdominal pain and nausea have also been reported at high doses.

Magnesium Pyruvate

(see *pyruvate*)

Mandukparni

(see *gotu kola*)

Maral Root

aka *Rhaponticum carthamoides, Leuzea carthamoides, Russian leuzeau*

What it is: Maral root, a perennial herb originating in the mountains of southern Siberia, was first observed as a medicinal plant when native hunters noticed that maral deer appeared to renew their strength after eating its roots. This observation gave the plant its more traditional name, maral root. The plant is now grown in central and eastern Europe. In traditional Siberian medicine it is used to restore strength after illness and prevent overtraining. Soviet and Russian athletes were the first to use maral root as an ergogenic aid to assist in handling the physical and psychological stress of intense training (Kokoska & Janovska, 2009).

How it works: Maral roots contain a variety of potentially beneficial compounds. Ecdysteroids such as 20-hydroxyecdysone (20-HE) are believed to have anabolic properties. In addition to ecdysteroids, various sterols such as β-sitosterol, flavonoids or anthocyanins, and triterpenoid glycosides can provide potential health benefits. These compounds are believed to stimulate and support the immune system, prevent free radical damage, increase protein synthesis, improve work capacity, and support cognitive function.

Performance benefit: Athletes may benefit from the anabolic growth-promoting effects. Maral root is also believed to enhance performance during aerobic endurance events and prolonged, intermittent, high-intensity team sports. Lastly, maral root has the potential to boost immune function and prevent free radical damage by functioning as an antioxidant.

Research: Ecdysteroids are believed to be the primary active components responsible for the beneficial effects of maral root, and research has focused on them. Animal studies have found ecdysteroids derived from maral root can promote growth, increase fat-free mass, and in some cases decrease fat mass (Stopka Stancl, & Slama, 1999; Slama et al., 1996). Other animal trials have shown an increase in work capacity in mice running on treadmills and in swimming endurance protocols (Azizov & Seifulla, 1998). Scientists note that in these animal studies significant differences are small, and small sample sizes limit the quality of results. (Kokoska & Janovska, 2009). In 1995 scientists found that ecdysteroid supplementation with track and field athletes improved body composition after 20 days (Gadzhieva et al., 1995). Similar effects on work capacity were found in a study done on Russian athletes in 1997 (Azizov et al., 1997). In addition to improving work capacity, the immunosuppressive effects of training were blunted as lowered levels of immunoglobulin A and G (IgA and IgG) were restored. A reduction in free radicals was also observed. Wilborn and colleagues conducted a study in 2006 examining the effects of ecdysterone on resistance-trained men and found no beneficial effects or changes in lean body mass, levels of anabolic hormones, or changes in strength and power. While some early studies are promising, there is a lack of current scientific evidence to conclude that maral root or its ecdysteroid components are beneficial for athletic performance.

Common usage: The Wilborn study, which is one of the few human trials, used 200 mg of 20- HE daily. Mice models typically use 5-10 mg of ecdysteroids or 20-HE/kg of body weight.

Health concerns: Maral root has been shown to be safe even at high doses. Toxicology studies in mice have found doses up to 40,000 mg/kg did not cause death (Kokoska & Janovska, 2009).

Medicinal Mushrooms

aka *Agaricus blazei murill, Cordyceps sinensis, Ganoderma lucidum (reishi), Grifola forndosa (maitake), Lentinula edodes (shiitake)*

What it is: Typically produced above ground on soil or on top of a food source, medicinal mushrooms are fungi that contain a wide spectrum of nutritional attributes that may enhance health and performance through cardiovascular, antiviral, antibacterial, and antiinflammatory properties. There are over 14,000 species of mushrooms; the following five types commonly appear in supplements used by athletes: *Agaricus blazei murill, Cordyceps sinensis, Ganoderma lucidum* (reishi), *Grifola forndosa* (maitake), and *Lentinula edodes* (shiitake).

How they work: Medicinal mushrooms contain several active ingredients that are thought to contribute to their proposed cardiovascular, antiviral, antibacterial, and antiinflammatory benefits. L-egothioneine and polyphenols, for example, are antioxidants found in abundance in mushrooms. These antioxidants play a key role in protecting an athlete's cells from oxidative damage that can occur during periods of heavy stress, common at the peak of training and competition, ultimately helping to reduce inflammation and pain, optimize joint health, and enhance recovery. Several enzymes within mushrooms also provide added protection against oxidative damage. Beta glucan, a polysaccharide or complex chain of glucose molecules found on the fruiting body of the mushroom, supports immune function by activating macrophage immune cells as well as T cells and B cells, which trap and consume various viral, bacterial, protozoan, and fungal invaders that can cause infection and sideline an athlete from competition.

>*continued*

> ## Supplement Fact
>
> **Agaricus blazei murill:** Native to Brazil, this mushroom provides immune support that, based on animal models, may help protect an athlete against infection as well as allergy and asthma-related symptoms. Extracts from the mushroom have also been found to help provide relief from symptoms associated with inflammatory bowel diseases such as Crohn's and ulcerative colitis.
>
> **Cordyceps sinensis:** Animal studies have shown ingestion of this mushroom to increase the ratio of ATP to inorganic phosphate in the liver, allowing for more efficient use of oxygen and a higher tolerance to acidosis. This result shows potential performance applications for sports that require both aerobic and anaerobic endurance.
>
> **Ganoderma lucidum:** Also known as reishi, this mushroom has been used by mountain climbers to prevent altitude sickness. Research shows that extracts from the fungi may help oxygenate the blood and prevent fatigue. It is also one of the most popular mushrooms in the East and West for strengthening immune function.
>
> **Grifola forndosa:** Also known as maitake, this mushroom has been shown to stimulate the production of T cells, which help defend the body against viruses. Additionally, extracts from maitake have been shown to enhance the forced swimming capacity of mice by increasing fat usage and delaying the accumulation of plasma lactate and ammonia.
>
> **Lentinula edodes:** Beta glucans (sugars found in the cell walls) from this mushroom, also known as shiitake, have been shown to help moderate immune response and thus may help reduce the incidence of illness and symptoms associated with chronic fatigue during heavy training.

Furthermore, medicinal mushrooms contain a large number of secondary metabolites, such as terpenoids, that are involved in a variety of biological processes important for immune functionality.

Performance benefit: Athletes may profit from a wide spectrum of performance benefits, including enhanced aerobic capacity, immune function, and recovery.

Research: While animal studies have presented some promising results, the results on a human population have not been consistent, especially when focused on a healthy, fit population (You & Lin, 2002). Furthermore, the bulk of human trials have been small in nature or of poor design. One well-designed but small human study did find that 6 weeks of supplementation with 500 mcg of ergothioneine, an antioxidant found in mushrooms, significantly reduced pain and improve range of motion in an impacted population compared to a placebo (Benson et al., 2012). However, given the small number of subjects (12) and the fact the supplement also included other ingredients, valid conclusions cannot be made. Therefore, it is evident that larger, double-blind, controlled human studies, especially on a healthy population, are required before the efficacy of medicinal mushrooms for purported health and performance outcomes can be confirmed.

Common usage: Mushrooms can be consumed fresh, dried, as a tincture or an extract, and in capsule or tablet form. While dosing recommendations are hard to make based on the available human data, dietary use of medicinal mushrooms as whole food or a combined daily supplementation protocol incorporating 40-50 mg of shiitake, 50-60 mg of maitake, 50-60 mg of reishi, and 100 mg of cordyceps is considered safe and may provide benefit to athletes, especially those feeling run down or fatigued at the peak of training.

Health concerns: Though only eight types of mushrooms in North America are considered poisonous, consumption of wild mushrooms is discouraged. A small number of allergic reactions, including anaphylactic shock, have been reported with medicinal mushrooms as have mind-altering symptoms brought on by reactions to secondary metabolites within some mushrooms. There is also concern of exposure to heavy metals due to the sponge-like absorption ability of mushrooms; consumption has led to reports of stomachaches, drowsiness, and confusion, as well as heart, liver, and kidney damage. Even so, the bulk of the data indicate that medicinal mushrooms are safe and well tolerated by most.

Medium-Chain Triglycerides (MCTs)

aka *caproic acid, caprylic acid, capric acid, lauric acid*

What it is: Naturally occurring in coconut oil and palm kernel oil, medium-chain triglycerides (MCTs) are a class of fatty acids that, like all triglycerides, consist of a glycerol backbone with three fatty acid molecules; in MTCs, though, the carbon chain is only 6-12 atoms long, far fewer than in its long-chain sibling. Because MCTs require significantly less energy for uptake and storage in the body than long-chain triglycerides yet still provide 8.3 calories/g, they make an appealing choice for athletes looking for an easy-to-digest and energy-dense fuel source.

How it works: Unlike long-chain triglycerides, MCTs do not require the presence of the amino acid carnitine to transport them into the mitochondria, the energy-producing factories that lie within muscle cells. The result is more rapid conversion to a molecule called acetyl-CoA, which is a key intermediate involved in the production of energy. It is thought that these

>continued

Medium-Chain Triglycerides (MCTs) >*continued*

attributes could produce an ergogenic effect by boosting energy output and, by sparing carbohydrate, thereby enhancing endurance.

Performance benefit: Athletes may benefit from increased energy levels and enhanced endurance during moderate- to high-intensity exercise.

Research: Animal data have indicated increased levels of metabolic enzymes along with significant improvements in exercise time to exhaustion with a diet containing 80 g MCT plus 20 g long-chain triglycerides (LCT)/kg over 6 weeks (Fushiki et al., 1995). These results, however, have failed to translate to human subjects, with the bulk of the data failing to show any benefit on glycogen (carbohydrate) sparing and consequent submaximal exercise performance of a prolonged nature at doses of 30-45 g over 2-3 hours (Goedecke et al., 2005; Clegg, 2010; Berning, 1996). Furthermore, doubling this dose over 2 hours has been shown to decrease performance in humans, likely due to increased incidence of gastrointestinal disturbances (Van Zyl et al., 1996; Jeukendrup et al., 1998). Sustained dosing at levels of 60 g/day over 2 weeks has also failed to yield any positive impact on endurance performance in humans (Misell et al., 2001). Thus, while results from animal studies have shown some promise, human subject data have not been supportive of ergogenic purposes in athletes.

Common usage: Commercially available MCT supplements undergo a process called fractionation, which allows the MCT to be separated from other oils and concentrated, making the total content greater than what is naturally found in coconut oil or palm kernel oil. MCTs are also available in several medical food products, generally for use in a clinical setting. Taking 1 tbsp (20 g) of pure MCT, or 5 tsp of coconut oil, 1-3 times daily with food is the current research-supported supplementation protocol.

Health concerns: In one study of endurance-trained cyclists, MCT supplementation produced gastrointestinal distress, primarily intestinal cramping, in half the subjects. Additional reported symptoms include diarrhea, nausea, vomiting, and irritability. Most symptoms occur when 80 or more g (equivalent to 4+ tbsp) of MCT are taken as a single dose. MCTs also contain over 100 calories/tbsp, and thus consuming large amounts without making other dietary adjustments to achieve energy balance can lead to weight gain.

Additional performance benefits: Although completed outside sport research, results from other human studies have demonstrated positive findings on the MCT and body composition front: Supplementation at doses of 18-24 g/day provides a boost to fat oxidation and aids overall weight and body-fat loss (St-Onge & Bosarge, 2008).

Melatonin

aka *N-acetyl-5-methoxytryptamine*

What it is: Melatonin is a hormone produced naturally in the body in response to the normal circadian clock and environmental light. The body develops a 24-hour circadian pattern based on behavior during which important hormones are secreted at various times. Melatonin is released at night during sleep in dark environments and can affect the ability to fall asleep, sleep quality, and sleep duration. The production of melatonin declines with age, which is suspected to play a role in insomnia among elderly adults. Melatonin can also be found in foods and beverages such as cherries and red wine. Melatonin is synthesized from the popular sleep-inducing amino acid tryptophan.

How it works: Typically, melatonin levels peak several hours after the initiation of sleep. This peak is associated with the lowest point of core body temperature, maximum tiredness, and lowest alertness. Melatonin acts on receptors found on various tissues of the body, mostly in the brain and eye but also in peripheral tissues such as the heart, arteries, skin, small intestine, and kidneys. The exact mechanisms are not well understood; however, in theory, supplementing with melatonin either before sleep or during could improve the ability to fall asleep and sleep quality.

Performance benefit: Athletes may benefit from improved quality, length, and quickened onset of sleep. These benefits could produce improved recovery from training and subsequent performance. In addition, melatonin can be used during extensive travel and time-zone changes, thereby assisting jet-lagged athletes in adapting circadian rhythms to new time zones.

Research: Currently, no research is available specific to the effects of melatonin on athletes, their quality of sleep, improved muscle recovery, or performance. Research has focused on the use of melatonin in elderly populations suffering from insomnia, sleep-disordered patients, and in treatment of jet lag. The American Academy of Sleep Medicine has published a positive recommendation for the use of melatonin in treating jet lag and other specific sleep disorders (Zawilska, Skene, and Arendt, 2009). Melatonin supplementation can effectively shift the 24-hour circadian rhythm of those exposed to new time zones, making melatonin a useful supplement for athletes forced to undergo extensive travel and time-zone changes for competition. However, more research is needed before recommendations beyond the use in treatment for jet lag can be made.

Common usage: Smaller doses of melatonin (0.1-0.25 mg) appear to be more effective than higher doses (0.3-10 mg) (Shimazaki, 2007). Most dietary

>continued

supplements contain a 3 mg dose. Melatonin can be taken immediately before or up to 4 hours before bedtime. Melatonin levels typically peak several hours after the onset of sleep. Newer melatonin formulations are experimenting with a time-release melatonin that would minimic the natural rise in melatonin occurring after the onset of sleep (Wade et al., 2010).

Health concerns: No known major health concerns exist related to melatonin, and chronic use for up to 6 months appears safe. Common side effects include daytime sleepiness, dizziness, and headaches. Melatonin can interact with blood-thinning medications, immunosuppressants, diabetes medications, and birth control methods.

Meletin

(see *quercetin*)

Methylcobalamin

(see *vitamin B12*)

Methylhexaneamine

(see *dimethylamylamine*)

Methylsulfonylmethane (MSM)

aka *dimethyl sulfone (DMSO), methyl sulfone*

What it is: Methylsulfonylmethane (MSM) is an organic compound that can be found in a variety of fruits, vegetables, grains, and animal foods. It is most abundantly found in milk, coffee, tomatoes, tea, and corn ("Methylsulfonylmethane (MSM)," 2003). MSM is most commonly used as a dietary supplement to treat joint pain and dysfunction.

How it works: MSM has multiple mechanisms by which it can provide benefits for arthritic joints. First, MSM is a strong antioxidant and antiinflammatory agent, allowing it to combat the damage done by free radicals and reduce pain and inflammation. Second, MSM is believed to enhance the activity of cortisol, a strong antiinflammatory hormone. Cortisol injections are commonly used with athletes to treat joint pain and inflammation. Finally, MSM contains sulfur, an important component of connective tissue, which is reduced by one-third in populations suffering from arthritis (Usha & Naidu, 2004).

Performance benefit: Many athletes experience chronic joint pain as a result of training or injury. The physical demands of sport and daily training place a significant amount of stress on joints. In addition, many athletes must overcome common injuries to joints resulting in surgery or joint reconstruction. Recovery from these types of surgeries can result in changes to the joint, and MSM has potential to improve and speed rehabilitation.

Research: Unlike other popular joint supplements such as glucosamine and chondroitin, which have been studied extensively, much less work has been done related to MSM. Animal studies have produced positive results in reducing joint pain and enhancing mobility (Usha & Naidu, 2004). Clinical trials in humans have also produced positive results. A 2011 study found that MSM improved pain and physical function in older men and women suffering from knee osteoarthritis, although the benefits were small (Debbi et al., 2011). Other studies have had similar results, suggesting MSM has moderate efficacy for use in treatment of osteoarthritis. More research is needed to better understand the mechanisms of MSM and confirm positive outcomes of earlier work since the body of scientific research is not substantial.

Common usage: The recommended supplementation dosage of MSM is 500-1,000 mg 3 times daily for a total of 1,500-3,000 mg.

Health concerns: MSM appears safe at recommended doses. Effects of long-term use are relatively unknown. However, a toxicity study done on rats found that a dose of 1.5 g/kg/day for 90 days did not cause any adverse effects or increased risk of mortality ("Methylsulfonylmethane [MSM]," 2003).

Milk Protein

(see *casein*)

Montmorency Cherry

(see *tart cherry*)

Mother's Milk

(see *colostrom*)

Muskat

(see *grape seed*)

NAC, N-Acetylcysteine

(see *acetylcysteine*)

N-Acetyl-5-Metpphoxytryptamine

(see *melatonin*)

Na-Citrate

(see *sodium bicarbonate and sodium citrate*)

N-(Aminoiminomethyl)-N-Methylglycine

(see *creatine*)

Naringin

aka *naringenin*

What it is: Citrus fruits, particularly grapefruit, contain a flavonoid known as naringin. Naringin is the main cause of bitterness in some citrus fruits and is converted into naringenin in the body. For decades grapefruit have been identified as being beneficial for weight loss. The Grapefruit Diet alleges that a component within grapefruit can trigger fat metabolism and induce weight loss. Some believe naringin to be this component. As a result, naringin has become a popular ingredient in weight-loss and fat-burning supplements.

How it works: Naringin is known to affect the cytochrome P450 enzyme complex. This enzyme complex is responsible for the metabolism of many drugs within the liver. It is speculated that naringin can act synergistically with other dietary supplement ingredients such as caffeine that are known to affect resting metabolic rate and metabolism. Through its impact on cytochrome P450, naringin can slow the metabolism of caffeine and other stimulants, giving them a more potent effect and further increasing their impact on resting metabolic rate, weight loss, and fat oxidation.

Performance benefit: Athletes wanting to improve body composition, decrease body fat, or lose body weight may be interested in supplementing with naringin.

Research: Dow and colleagues (2012) have conducted an investigation of grapefruit and weight loss. In their study a grapefruit group consumed one-half of a fresh grapefruit with each meal 3 times daily for 6 weeks. Results found no significant decreases in body weight, blood lipids, or blood pressure compared to the control group. This is in contrast to a 2006 study of obese patients in which the consumption of one-half of a grapefruit before meals resulted in significant weight loss compared to a placebo (Fujioka et al.). Another study in 2006 found that 200 mg of naringin did not alter caffeine metabolism nor affect resting metabolic rate, despite hypothesizing that naringin would act synergistically with caffeine and increase its effects on resting metabolic rate (Ballard et al.). Currently, there are insufficient and inconclusive data related to the effectiveness of naringin. More evidence is needed before naringin supplements are recommended.

Common usage: The amount of naringin found in an average grapefruit can vary depending on where the fruit is grown; however, the average is roughly 16 mg/100 g of grapefruit. An average grapefruit is roughly 250 g and so contains 40 mg of naringin. Most research trials have used a dose of 60-200 mg of naringin. Narinigin is commonly added to weight-loss supplements in pill form, supporting claims to increase fat and weight loss.

Health concerns: Naringin and furanocoumarins found in grapefruit can affect drug metabolism. The list of drugs affected is vast, and athletes should consult a physician before taking supplements containing naringin to ensure safety.

9-Beta-D-Ribofuranosylhypoxanthine

(see *inosine*)

N-3 Fatty Acids

(see *omega-3 fatty acids*)

O

Oat Bran, Oat-Derived Beta Glucan

(see *beta glucan*)

Olibanum

(see *Boswellia serrata*)

Omega-3 Fatty Acids

aka *n-3 fatty acids, omega-3s, eicosapentaenoic acid (EPA), docosahexae-noic acid (DHA), α-linolenic acid (ALA)*

What it is: Omega-3 fatty acids, one of the major classes of polyunsaturated fats, can be found naturally in such foods as nuts and seeds and their accompanying oils as well as fatty fish. While several forms of omega-3s exist, those considered essential to human health include plant-derived α-linolenic acid (ALA) and marine-derived eicosapentaenoic acid (EPA) and docosahexaenoic acid (DHA), both of which are produced in small amounts from ALA. (See tables 3.3 and 3.4.)

TABLE 3.3   Best Food Sources of ALA Omega-3s

	Serving size	ALA (grams)
Canola oil	1 tbsp	1.3
Chia seeds	1 tbsp	2.4
English walnuts	1 oz (28 g)	2.6
Flaxseed, ground	1 tbsp	1.6
Flaxseed, oil	1 tbsp	7.3
Walnut, oil	1 tbsp	1.4

TABLE 3.4   Best Food Sources of EPA/DHA Omega-3s

	Serving size	EPA (grams)	DHA (grams)
Herring, Pacific	3 oz (85 g)	1.06	0.75
Oysters, Pacific	3 oz (85 g)	0.75	0.43
Salmon, Chinook	3 oz (85 g)	0.86	0.62
Salmon, Atlantic	3 oz (85 g)	0.28	0.95
Salmon, sockeye	3 oz (85 g)	0.45	0.60
Sardines, Pacific	3 oz (85 g)	0.45	0.74

How it works: Physical stress triggers the release of harmful compounds known as free radicals that can penetrate the protective membrane of any cell in the body, leading to cell damage and a consequent inflammatory response. While the body has defense mechanisms to deal with acute inflammation, severe injury or extreme exercise stress can lead to chronic inflammation and the activation of nerves responsible for the sensation of pain, thereby compromising recovery. It is currently thought that the benefits of omega-3s originate, in part, from two compounds appropriately named protectins and resolvins that are derived specifically from EPA and DHA; these compounds protect the structural integrity of cell membranes and fight tissue degradation, resolve inflammation, and significantly downgrade pain.

Performance benefit: Omega-3s may help facilitate quicker recovery times as well as serve as a viable treatment option for a wide range of inflammatory-based conditions, including asthma, arthritis, and traumatic brain injury. Research shows promise for several other potential performance benefits, including these:

- Improved cognitive parameters, such as reactivity and focus, important for such sports as baseball and golf
- Increased blood and oxygen flow to working muscles, including the heart, as a result of reduced blood viscosity or thickness of blood, thereby aiding aerobic endurance
- Improved fuel usage with increased ability to burn fat for energy

Research: Results evaluating the impact of omega-3s on inflammation caused by exercise and sport injury are currently limited and generally equivocal, though some animal and human data present promise. For example, a small, randomized, double-blind human study found that a daily supplementation protocol of 324 mg EPA and 216 mg DHA from fish oil (1.8 g total omega-3) over 30 days held some merit in countering chronic inflammation and associated delayed-onset muscle soreness (DOMS) in untrained individuals after a single 40-minute session of eccentric (lowering phase) loading exercise (Tartibian, Maleki, and Abbasi, 2009). The same supplementation protocol was found to ameliorate exercise-induced markers of inflammation associated with eccentric exercise in untrained men (Tartibian, Maleki, and Abbasi, 2011) Whether or not this would hold true for trained athletes is unknown. According to researchers from Indiana University, however, highly trained athletes with exercise-induced asthma (EIA) may benefit from omega-3's antiinflammatory attributes by following a daily supplementation protocol of 3.2 g EPA and 2.0 g DHA from fish oil over 3 weeks. This protocol has been shown to significantly reduce airway inflammation and enhance overall lung function in highly trained subjects affected by EIA (Mickleborough et al., 2003). Finally, of potential relevance to the contact sport athlete or combat soldier, a daily supplementation protocol incorporating 10 or 40 mg/kg body weight of omega-3s over 30 days was shown to be effective in countering the neural inflammation and damage caused by concussive injuries in rats; the

>continued

Omega-3 Fatty Acids >*continued*

higher dose demonstrated an astounding 98% reduction in neural damage tested (Mills et al., 2011). Further research needs to confirm this benefit in human subjects.

Common usage: For antiinflammatory benefit, target daily consumption is 1-2 g of EPA and DHA in an approximate 2:1 ratio, common in fish oil, krill, and algae supplements. ALA omega-3s, present in plant-based supplements such as flaxseed oil, should be taken at a dose 3-5 times higher due to conversion rates to EPA and DHA that are only estimated at 36% for women and 16% for men. Omega-3 supplements are best taken with food.

Health concerns: Use of omega-3s is generally recognized as safe although reported side effects include indigestion and gas, especially at doses above 3 g of EPA and DHA.

1,3-Dimethylamylamine, 1,3 Dimethylpentylamine

(see *dimethylamylamine*)

Ornithine

aka *ornithine alpha-ketoglutarate*

What it is: Ornithine is a nonessential amino acid. It can be found in protein-rich foods such as meats, fish, dairy, and eggs. As a nonessential amino acid, it can also be synthesized in the body from other amino acids. Ornithine alpha-ketoglutarate (OKG) is a salt that is formed from ornithine and alpha ketoglutarate. OKG is more bioavailable than ornithine alone.

How it works: Ornithine and OKG are precursors of the amino acids proline and arginine. It is speculated that ornithine supplementation can increase concentrations of both arginine and proline. Arginine is important in the production of nitric oxide, a powerful vasodilator that can improve blood flow. In addition, arginine is involved in the production of growth hormone. Proline is an important amino acid found in connective tissues such as collagen. Ornithine supplementation could indirectly promote the availability of both arginine and proline. There is also evidence that OKG supplementation has a better effect on both arginine and proline compared to ornithine alone.

Performance benefit: For athletes, supplementation with ornithine or OKG could improve the availability of arginine and proline. Arginine availability could improve nitric oxide production, promoting blood flow and delivery of oxygen and nutrients to muscles, thereby improving performance. Ornithine and OKG may increase levels of growth hormone, a powerful anabolic hormone, increasing gains in lean body mass and strength. Finally, improving proline availability would increase the strength and density of connective tissues.

Research: Studies have looked at ornithine and OKG supplementation in various populations, including bodybuilders, burn patients, and wound-healing patients. Results are positive in clinical settings for burn and wound-healing patients but not for healthy, well-nourished populations (De Bandt et al., 1998; Donati et al., 1999). These trials found OKG to be superior to ornithine in promoting the availability of arginine and proline. However, this improved availability did not prove to be beneficial for the promotion of nitric oxide, growth hormone, or connective tissues in healthy populations.

Common usage: Because the efficacy of ornithine and OKG supplementation is poor, it is difficult to establish recommendations. Successful research studies for burn and wound-healing patients have used a daily intake of 10 g. A range of 40-170 mg/kg of body weight has also been used; however, intakes above 170 mg/kg of body weight are not recommended.

Health concerns: An upper limit of ornithine to avoid toxicity has not been established, and more research in this area is needed. When used within recommended doses, supplementation is safe.

P

Palatinose

(see *isomaltulose*)

Panax Ginseng

(see *ginseng*)

Pantothenic Acid

aka *vitamin B5, calcium pantothenate, sodium D-pantothenate, pantothenol, pantethine*

What it is: Derived from the Greek word *pantos* meaning "everywhere," pantothenic acid, also known as vitamin B5, is an essential nutrient that is naturally found in a wide variety of plant and animal foods such as peanut butter, liver, wheat bran, cheese, lobster, Brewer's yeast, and royal jelly. It is also available in supplement form, often as part of a multivitamin and multi-mineral formula. While deficiencies are rare, it is thought that athletes may benefit from increased intake as a means to better support the metabolic demands of exercise.

How it works: As a participant in a wide array of key biological roles, including the synthesis of coenzyme A, a key compound involved in the production of energy from carbohydrate, fat, and protein, pantothenic acid is considered essential to all forms of life. Animal studies have found deficiencies in pantothenic acid to compromise storage of glucose (in the form of glycogen) in the muscle and liver, causing decreased exercise tolerance and endurance as a result of carbohydrate depletion, otherwise known as bonking or hitting the wall. In addition, decreased synthesis of heme, the component of hemoglobin that carries iron, has been shown to contribute to anemia in deficient monkeys, and low blood sugar, rapid breathing and elevated heart rates have been reported in deficient dogs (Plesofsky-Vig, 1999). It is hypothesized that supplementation with pantothenic acid may help optimize oxygen usage, reduce lactic acid accumulation and consequent muscle fatigue, and promote optimal glycogen storage for enhanced endurance during exercise. The refining, freezing, canning, and cooking of food causes pantothenic content to drop, making dietary deficiencies an increased likelihood in athletes eating primarily processed foods.

Performance benefit: Athletes, especially those with poor dietary intake of pantothenic acid, may experience benefit from supplementation through reduced muscle fatigue and enhanced endurance. Animal evidence suggests supplementation with pantothenic acid, especially when dietary intake is suboptimal, may help enhance the body's adrenal response to stress, which may help protect an athlete against adverse hormonal and blood sugar changes and immune suppression that can cause performance to suffer.

Research: While clinical deficiencies have rarely been reported in humans, suboptimal dietary intake of pantothenic acid is not all that uncommon, especially in light of the highly processed diet consumed by many. For example, a recent nutritional analysis of adolescent highly trained soccer players determined over half failed to meet Dietary Reference Intake (DRI) goals for pantothenic acid (Gibson et al., 2011). Supplementation, especially for athletes eating primarily processed foods, may be helpful; one study of elite distance runners that found a supplementation protocol providing 2 g of pantothenic acid daily over 2 weeks lowered lactic acid buildup by 17% and the oxygen cost of prolonged, strenuous exercise by 7% (Litoff, Scherzer, & Harrison, 1984). However, the bulk of human research has not demonstrated any performance benefit from supplementation, suggesting most athletes are better off merely focusing on improving intake of whole foods rich in pantothenic acid (Nice et al., 1984; Webster, 1998; Wall et al., 2012).

Common usage: Pantothenic acid is available in capsule, liquid, and tablet form as is included in multivitamin and multimineral formulas, generally as the derivative pantothenol. Pantothenic acid is also available as salts (calcium pantothenate and sodium D-pantothenate) to promote better absorption. Doses of pantothenic acid typically range from 10-50 mg/day in multivitamin and multimineral supplements while single-ingredient tablets and capsules generally provide 100-500 mg. The current DRI for adult men and women aged 14 years and older is 5 mg/day.

Health concerns: While pantothenic acid is generally well tolerated by most in doses up to 1,200 mg per day, gastrointestinal side effects such as nausea and heartburn have been reported in a small number of cases.

Piascledine

(see *avocado soybean unsaponifiables*)

Piruvato

(see *pyruvate*)

P57

(see *Hoodia gordonii*)

Phosphate Salts

  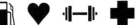

aka *phosphates, sodium phosphate, potassium phosphate*

What it is: Phosphorus, which is found naturally in a wide array of foods such as milk, cheese, grains, beans, peas, soda, and nuts, is an essential mineral. It must be obtained from the diet; after consumption, it is distributed throughout the body's tissues in the form of phosphate, the bulk of which is stored in bone. Phosphate salts, a combination of phosphate and minerals such as calcium and potassium, are commonly included in sport foods, drinks, and supplements, based on the belief that they help protect athletes against premature muscle fatigue during sport competition.

How it works: Phosphates play three key roles that are believed to contribute to their performance-enhancing potential. First, they are relied upon metabolically to generate adenosine triphosphate (ATP), the chemical form of energy within cells, as well as creatine phosphate, an immediate energy source that also can be used to recycle used ATP. Consequently, it is thought that phosphate supplementation may help provide a boost to the energy stores required to propel performance. Second, phosphates serve as an effective buffer against hydrogen ions, lactic acid, and lactate that accumulate within the blood and muscles during exercise, especially high-intensity exercise, helping to protect against a burning sensation symbolic of cellular acidosis that contributes to muscle fatigue and failure. Finally, phosphates increase the concentration of a chemical in red blood cells called 2,3-diphosphoglycerate (2,3-DPG), which helps release oxygen from hemoglobin, promoting quicker delivery of oxygen to muscles for enhanced endurance and recovery.

Supplement Fact

The use of phosphates to improve physical performance dates to World War I when German soldiers reportedly used sodium phosphate to reduce combat fatigue.

Performance benefit: Phosphate loading may help reduce fatigue and the sensation of pain during exercise, extending endurance and enhancing recovery.

Research: Studies investigating the benefit of phosphate loading across the performance spectrum, including anaerobic, power-oriented, and endurance-focused performances, have been equivocal. For example, two double-blind, placebo-controlled studies evaluating the performance benefit of 4 g of sodium phosphate taken in 4 × 1 g doses over 4 days leading to either a 30-second all-out effort or an incremental $\dot{V}O_2$max test using 3-minute stages on a cycle ergometer failed to identify any improvement on such parameters as $\dot{V}O_2$max, blood lactate levels, and overall performance compared to the placebo (Tourville, Brennan, & Connolly, 2001; Brennan & Connoly, 2001). However, a more recent randomized, double-blind study of trained cyclists identified a favorable impact on performance with the same supplementation dose of sodium phosphate taken over 6 days rather than 4 days before completing a more endurance-focused 16.1 km (10 mi) time trial (Folland & Brickley, 2008). The phosphate loading yielded a 10% boost to mean power output, allowing the cyclists to complete the time trial significantly faster than the placebo trial. While not a significant change, the study investigators noted a tendency toward higher maximal oxygen uptake ($\dot{V}O_2$max) after phosphate loading versus the placebo, which was a proposed reason for the improved performance. This evidence suggests that phosphate loading may be of greater benefit to high-intensity activities that are endurance focused rather than sprint focused. Recent evidence also suggests the beneficial effects of sodium phosphate on $\dot{V}O_2$peak (the plateau in oxygen consumption during submaximal exercise),and consequent cycling time trial performance may be cumulative at a supplemental dose of 50 mg/kg of body weight taken daily over 6 days initially and then again 15 or 35 days later (Brewer et al., 2012). These results are especially relevant for athletes engaged in frequent competitions over short time frames.

Common usage: Research-supported doses for phosphate loading are 3-6 g (either sodium or potassium phosphate) split into several 1 g doses throughout the day and taken daily over approximately 5 days leading up to competition.

Health concerns: Because stomach upset, diarrhea, and general GI discomfort have been reported with loading uses of phosphate salts, athletes who choose to supplement should experiment while training before using the salts in competition. It is also important to note that excessive intake of phosphate, especially over the long term, can drive blood levels abnormally high, increasing the risk for electrolyte imbalances.

Phosphatidylserine

What it is: Phosphatidylserine (PS) is a phospholipid nutrient found in the cell membrane of a variety of tissues, including the brain, lungs, heart, liver, and skeletal muscle. The best dietary sources of PS are organ meats such as brain, liver, heart, and kidney. Fatty fish, meats, and white beans can also provide PS in smaller amounts. PS supplements were first derived from the brains of cows; however, concerns related to the transfer of infectious diseases have resulted in soy-derived PS supplements (Starks et al., 2008).

>continued

Phosphatidylserine >*continued*

How it works: Cell membranes contain a variety of receptors, enzymes, and signaling molecules. PS affects the actions of these receptors and signaling molecules in much the same way that diets high in omega-3 fatty acids alter phospholipid membrane composition and create positive physiological changes. Specifically, it is believed that PS can suppress exercise-induced cortisol. Cortisol is a major catabolic hormone that becomes elevated during periods of physical exertion and overtraining. In addition, PS claims to enhance mood, improve memory, and prevent dementia.

Performance benefit: Possible benefits of PS for athletes include the ability to speed recovery, prevent muscle soreness, improve well-being, and enhance performance in endurance and strength sports.

Research: Some but not extensive research has been done on athletes and PS. Scientists completed multiple studies on PS in 2005 and 2006. In both studies PS was ineffective in decreasing markers of muscle damage, oxidative stress, inflammation, cortisol, and creatine kinase in response to exercise (Kingsley et al., 2005; Kingsley et al., 2006). In one of the two studies PS was shown to increase exercise capacity during cycling until exhaustion (Kingsley et al., 2006). Another group of scientists measured the impact of PS on cortisol during a short-duration (15-minute) moderate intensity exercise session. While the number of subjects was small (10), PS did lower cortisol and increase testosterone (Starks et al., 2008). Overall, results are inconclusive, and more research trials are needed to clarify potential benefits for athletes.

Common usage: Typically research studies with athletes have used doses of 300-800 mg of soy-derived PS supplemented 1 time daily; however, these trials were short in duration (10-15 days). A 300 mg/day dose is recommended for treatment of mental stress, and small doses as low as 100 mg/day are common for enhancement of cognitive function (Jager, Purpura, & Kingsley, 2007).

Health concerns: The use of PS appears to be safe: 300-600 mg/day provided for up to 120 days for elderly patients did not result in any adverse effects, and 800 mg doses over 10-12 days have been tolerated without adverse effects in healthy adults.

Pine Bark Extract, *Pinus Pinaster*

(see *Pycnogenol*)

Piperine

aka *black pepper, piperdine, BioPerine*

What it is: Piperine is an alkaloid-amine component of the commonly used spice black pepper. *Piper nigrum* is a flowering vine, and its fruits known as peppercorn are dried and ground to produce black pepper. The vine is native to Southeast Asia, China, and Vietnam, which are the world's largest producers of pepper. As an oriental medicine, black pepper has been used to treat upset stomachs and diarrhea. Recent evidence suggests that black pepper might reduce triglycerides, blood sugar, and cholesterol. Piperine is believed to play an important role in this reduction. Piperine alkaloids are also becoming a common ingredient found in so-called fat-burning and weight-loss supplements.

How it works: Many of the mechanisms behind piperdine are unknown; however, recent studies suggest that it works at the cellular level by influencing gene transcription. Specifically, piperdine influences a number of genes that are downstream targets for PPARγ. PPARγ is involved in the regulation of genes involved in stimulating adipogensis (development of fat cells). Piperdine alkaloids found in black pepper can inhibit PPARγ, decreasing adipogensis and the negative effects of body fat accumulation such as high blood cholesterol and triglycerides.

Performance benefit: Athletes wanting to improve body composition, reduce body weight, and maximize strength-to-mass ratios might supplement with piperine. Piperine can also influence the absorption and bioavailability of other beneficial herbs and spices such as resveratrol and curcumin. A 2011 study of mice found that the addition of piperine significantly increased resveratrol bioavailability (Johnson et al., 2011).

Research: Two animal studies completed in 2011 found piperine to be beneficial in preventing adipogensis and a number of the negative side effects associated with it (Diwan, Poudval, & Brown, 2011). Piperine supplementation at 100 mg/kg, 300 mg/kg, and 375 mg/kg of body weight in mice that were fed an obesity-inducing diet reduced adiposity and weight gain and improved lipid profiles (Jin Kim et al., 2011). Other animal studies have found a beneficial effect of piperdine on antioxidant status suggesting the spice can reduce oxidative stress and increase activity of antioxidant defense enzymes (Srinivasan, 2007). Unfortunately, these benefits have never been studied in humans, and more research is needed before any conclusions can be made. Currently, there is a lack of evidence to recommend piperine supplementation.

Common usage: Not enough research is available to develop an adequate or suggested supplementation dose or usage for humans. Dietary supplements commonly contain 10 mg of piperine.

>continued

Piperine >*continued*

Health concerns: There does not appear to be any risk of toxicity or known adverse effects of piperine.

Potassium (K)

aka *potassium acetate, potassium bicarbonate, potassium chloride, potassium citrate, potassium gluconate, potassium phosphate*

What it is: Found naturally in such dietary sources as bananas, potatoes, tomatoes, prunes, and milk, potassium is an essential mineral stored alongside carbohydrate within the muscles; it is also the primary electrolyte in body cells. Because significant amounts of potassium are lost from muscle and via sweat during exercise, increased dietary or supplementation intake may be warranted in athletes to support optimal muscle function.

How it works: Potassium plays an active role in metabolism, facilitating the synthesis of protein from amino acids in the cell, thereby promoting normal growth and muscle building, and aiding the conversion of glucose to glycogen to enhance the storage of carbohydrate essential for energy production. In addition, as an electrolyte, potassium works with sodium and chloride to control fluid and electrolyte balance and assist in the conduction of nerve impulses critical for optimal muscle contraction and a regular heartbeat. Deficiencies in potassium can trigger nausea, vomiting, slower reflexes, muscle weakness and cramping, and racing heartbeat.

Performance benefit: Athletes will benefit from improved muscle function, including protection against muscle cramps and enhanced muscle endurance.

Research: During exercise, especially at high intensities, potassium is released from the muscles at an accelerated rate, causing potassium concentrations to rise outside the cell as well as in the bloodstream. This activity, according to several studies, is a significant contributing factor to the development of fatigue in human muscle during exercise (Knochel, 1978, 1982; Nielson et al., 2004; McKenna et al., 2008; Juel, 2007). Therefore, scientists agree that maintenance of potassium balance in and outside the cells is a relevant factor in muscle performance. Human sweat data have demonstrated an average potassium loss of 100-200 mg/L of fluid. Most athletes lose .5-1 L of fluid hourly during physical exertion, making replacement of potassium, often via electrolyte replacement beverages such as sport drinks or electrolyte supplements, especially beneficial to performance of activities lasting longer than 1.5 hours.

Common usage: While there is no RDA for potassium, the adequate intake for potassium, outside of replacement needs during physical exertion, has been set at 4.7 g/day for adults. To maintain electrolyte balance and optimize muscle function, athletes should replace 75-150 mg of potassium/L of fluid consumed during physical exertion. Potassium supplements are available as a number of salts, including potassium chloride, potassium citrate, and potassium gluconate; all are available in powder, pill, capsule, and effervescent form. The most common way to replenish electrolytes for most athletes is through use of a sport drink.

Supplement Fact

Use of diuretics, laxatives, alcohol, and large doses of caffeine (>6 mg/kg); prolonged diarrhea or vomiting; and excessive sugar intake can the increase risk for potassium deficiency.

Health concerns: Excessive potassium intake, generally at doses of 18 g or more, alters sodium balance and can lead to gastrointestinal distress, electrical impulse disturbance, irregular heartbeat, and possibly death. Therefore, large doses of potassium or beyond what is commonly found in supplements should never been consumed without the direct supervision and advice of a physician. Athletes engaged in contact sports where blunt-force trauma damages muscle tissue, such as football and hockey, may be at increased risk for abnormally high serum potassium levels due to rapid movement of potassium from the cells into the bloodstream during injury.

Additional performance benefits: Adequate intake of potassium through whole foods or supplements may help improve bone mineral density and lower the risk for osteoporosis and stress-related fractures in athletes (Duke Medical Health News, 2008).

Potassium Phosphate

(see *phoshate salts*)

Potassium Pyruvate, Proacemic Acid

(see *pyruvate*)

Probiotics

aka *bifidobacterium, lactobacillus, escherichia, enterococcus, saccharomyces*

What it is: Probiotics are live microorganisms found naturally within the digestive tract that, when maintained at adequate levels, are thought to support intestinal health and enhance immune function. Most probiotics are of bacterial nature, thus the nickname friendly bacteria, and originate from the Lactobacillus (lactic acid bacteria, LAB, L.) or Bifidobacterium (B.) family. Over 500 types of bacterial species exist with each exerting a unique health benefit by helping fight the growth of harmful bacteria and yeast. Strains of the Bifidobacterium family account for nearly 25% of all probiotics in the body and are found primarily in the large intestine; species of LAB are generally found in the small intestine. Probiotics can be added to the diet from such foods as yogurt, cultured milk products, and beverages as well as taken in capsule, tablet, and powdered form.

Supplement Fact

Probiotics should not be mistaken for prebiotics, which are complex sugars called fructooligosaccharides that serve as fuel for bacteria already present in the digestive tract. Products containing both pre- and probiotics are often labeled as synbiotics.

How it works: Immune functionality after intense exercise has been shown to be suppressed, making the athlete more vulnerable to contraction of upper respiratory tract infections and gastrointestinal illness. Reducing the occurrence of these illnesses is a high priority as full recovery from each bout takes away significant time from training and competition and thus can negatively affect performance. Probiotics may provide added nutritional support in the intestines, where more than 70% of the body's immune defenses work to fight against harmful microbes that can contribute to infection, thereby helping reduce the incidence of illness during heavy training and competition.

Performance benefit: Probiotics may aid the overall health of an athlete, helping to protect against and reduce symptoms of gastrointestinal and upper respiratory tract illnesses.

Research: Results examining the efficacy of probiotic supplementation are promising, though there is a mixed bag of results when focusing on an athletic population. For example, a recent double-blind, placebo-controlled study of competitive cyclists failed to yield any clear trends between patterns of upper respiratory tract infection (URTI) or gastrointestinal illness symptoms and supplement-induced changes in gut bacteria after consuming at least

1 billion colony forming units (CFUs) of the *L. fermentum* strain daily for 11 weeks (West et al., 2011). Gleeson and colleagues (2012) also failed to find any benefit in ingestion of *L. salivarius* over 16 weeks on the frequency of URTI or key immune parameters in endurance-trained athletes during a spring competitive season. On a positive note, Cox and colleagues (2010) found oral administration of *L. fementum* at a daily dose of $1.26 \times 10 (10)$ over 30 days during winter training cut the number of days of respiratory symptoms in elite male distance runners by over half. There was also a substantial downgrade in the severity of respiratory illness compared to the placebo. Gleeson and colleagues (2011) also reported a reduction in the frequency of upper respiratory tract illness in recreational endurance athletes after 8 and 16 weeks of supplementation with *L. casei Shirota*. Additionally, a smaller study determined that daily supplementation with 2 billion CFUs of *L. acidophilus* over 4 weeks produced favorable immune responses in athletes with clinical characteristics of the Epstein Barr virus (EPV), which is well known for symptoms of fatigue, recurrent sore throats, and impaired performance. This finding led the study investigators to conclude that the use of *L. acidophilus* may be effective in ridding the body of viruses and providing a line of support against reinfection (Clancy et al., 2006). Based on these results, it is evident that the probiotic strain and dose used are determining factors in the response yielded.

Common usage: The most potent probiotic supplements will contain more organisms, expressed in terms of billions of organisms or CFUs per serving; products containing a range of 250 million to 20 billion organisms are considered ideal for therapeutic benefit. Each strain of bacteria will elicit a unique health benefit, with bifidobacterium seeming to benefit intestinal health and lactobacillus benefiting both immune functionality and intestinal health. To ensure optimal passage of the bacteria through the stomach, select products with an enteric coating.

Health concerns: Probiotics are considered safe for use, with minimal side effects reported. However, athletes with milk allergies should be aware that some probiotic products, especially those made with lactobacilli or bifidobacterium, may contain trace amount of milk proteins and thus may trigger allergic symptoms.

Additional performance benefits: There is some evidence to suggest that bifidobacterium probiotics can provide some relief for such symptoms as abdominal pain, bloating, and diarrhea, common among athletes affected by irritable bowel syndrome (Ritchie & Romanuk, 2012).

Provitamin A

(see *beta-carotene*)

Prunus Cerasus

(see *tart cherry*)

Pycnogenol

aka *pine bark extract, Pinus pinaster*

What it is: An herbal extract derived from the bark of the French maritime pine tree, Pycnogenol, also known as pine bark, contains plant compounds called oligomeric proanthocyanidin complexes (OPCs) that carry strong antioxidant qualities of potential benefit to human health and physical performance.

How it works: The metabolic demands of sport, reflected by a 10- to 20-fold increase in inhaled oxygen, generate a level of stress that causes the production of detrimental molecules called free radicals. While athletes have natural antioxidant defenses to quench free radicals and protect cells from damage, it is not uncommon to see levels of free radical production exceed natural defenses during high-volume training, leading to problems such as increased muscle damage, inflammation and soreness, and reduced performance. Pycnogenol increases the production of antioxidant enzymes and scavengers, strengthening the body's ability to fight off free radicals and prevent such problems, thereby allowing an athlete to recover more efficiently during cycles of heavy training. Of further benefit to recovery and performance is the apparent ability of Pycnogenol to shut down the production of proinflammatory enzymes such as COX-2 and enhance nitric oxide production, which helps increase blood and oxygen flow to muscles and encourage muscle tissue growth and repair as well as better support aerobic endurance.

Performance benefit: Athletes may benefit from improved recovery times during periods of increased training stress as well as boosts to endurance performance. Pycnogenol also may help inhibit the enzymes responsible for the destruction of lung tissue in chronic bronchitis and decrease the amount of circulating inflammatory substances in the blood stream, thereby helping provide relief to athletes suffering from asthma and chronic bronchitis.

Research: The bulk of current research on Pycnogenol has been focused on preventing muscle pain and inflammation as well as evaluating Pycnogenol's potential ability to enhance aerobic performance. In a 2006 study, a supplementation dose of 200 mg of Pycnogenol taken daily over 4 weeks was shown to significantly reduce subjective ratings of muscle pain as well as the incidence of muscle cramps in athletes compared to a baseline period of 2 weeks when no supplement was provided (Vinciguerra et al.). Another study discovered a daily supplementation dose of 150 mg of Pycnogenol over 5 days significantly reduced the production of enzymes responsible for inflammation in healthy subjects (Canali et al., 2009). An even lower dose may be effective according to German scientists who found a supplemental dose of 100 mg of Pycnogenol/day over 3 months reduced knee pain in subjects inflicted with osteoarthritis by 55% compared to a placebo trial (Becaro et al., 2008). The applications to aerobic performance have also shown some promise, with a 2012 double-blind study demonstrating that a single supplementation dose of 2.4 g of Pycnogenol taken 4 hours before a progressive cycling exercise protocol (5 minutes at 50% peak power output [PPO], 8 minutes at 70% PPO, and 95% PPO to fatigue) extended cycle time to exhaustion by 80 seconds (Bentley et al.). According to Japanese scientists, whose study demonstrated a 42% increase in the blood flow of healthy men after 2 weeks of supplementing with a daily dose of 180 mg of Pycnogenol, aerobic performance boosts are likely related to enhanced healthy nitric oxide production (Nishioka et al., 2007).

Common usage: Pycnogenol is available in tablet and capsule forms in a wide variety of dosing strengths. To help reduce muscle pain and inflammation during heavy training cycles, a range of 100 to 200 mg/day for up to 3 months is recommended. Similar doses seem to be effective for enhancing blood flow. A single dose of 2.4 g taken with water 4 hours before exercise was shown to be effective in extending exercise time to exhaustion.

Health concerns: There have been reports of dizziness, gut problems, headache, and mouth ulcers, especially at doses above 450 mg.

Pyruvate

aka *pyruvic acid, acetylformic acid, alpha-keto acid, alpha-ketopropionic acid, calcium pyruvate, calcium pyruvate monohydrate, creatine pyruvate, magnesium pyruvate, 2-oxopropanoate, 2-oxypropanoic acid, piruvato, potassium pyruvate, proacemic acid, sodium pyruvate*

What it is: Naturally synthesized in the body from glucose (sugar) as well as found naturally in such dietary sources as red wine, dark beer, and red apples, pyruvate, which is the salt derivative of pyruvic acid, is thought to help facilitate body fat loss and enhance endurance performance, making it a popular supplement choice among athletes.

How it works: It is thought that pyruvate increases the uptake of glucose from the blood into working muscles, enhancing the fuel available for immediate use and providing a boost to energy reserves (muscle glycogen) for future use. This helps improve muscle endurance and consequent performance. In addition, as a participant in the Kreb's cycle of metabolism, pyruvate is thought to increase the body's use of fat for energy as well as resting metabolic rate, thereby helping to facilitate body fat loss.

Performance benefit: Pyruvate supplementation may benefit athletes wanting to optimize body composition and boost endurance capacity.

>continued

Pyruvate >*continued*

Research: While early studies showed some promise, the bulk of current data have not been supportive. For example, in a double-blind, placebo-controlled study, a supplementation protocol providing 6 g of pyruvate daily over 6 weeks was shown to significantly decrease body weight, body fat, and percentage body fat in healthy, overweight men and women participating in a fitness program 3 days a week compared to the placebo group (Kalman et al., 1999). A similar supplementation protocol, providing 5 g of calcium pyruvate daily over 30 days, however, failed to demonstrate any significant body composition changes in healthy, untrained women engaged in an exercise program compared to a placebo group (Koh-Banerjee et al., 2005). Furthermore, no significant differences were observed between groups in the metabolic responses to and overall performance during an aerobic exercise routine. Similar void results were identified in an athletic population (soccer players) though the supplementation protocol incorporated only 2 g of pyruvate daily over 4 weeks (Ostojic and Ahmetovic, 2009). The current consensus is that pyruvate appears to be an ineffective strategy for body fat loss in athletes. While there is some evidence to suggest a supplementation protocol containing both pyruvate and the simple carbohydrate dihydroxyacetone may enhance muscle endurance, the applications evaluating pyruvate as a solo ingredient or in combination with creatine have not demonstrated positive results (Van Schuylenbergh et al., 2003; Stanko et al., 1990a; Stanko et al., 1990b; Ivy, 1998; Morrison,Spriet, and Dyck, 2000).

Common usage: Pyruvate supplements are available in capsule, tablet, and bulk powder form; pyruvate is commonly included as an ingredient in so-called fat-burning supplements as well as paired with creatine as a sports supplement. Doses used in research have been highly variable, ranging from 2 to 30 g taken daily either preexercise or with a meal, with conflicting outcomes. It is evident more research is needed before standardized supplementation protocol recommendations are established.

Health concerns: Acute doses of pyruvate above 25 g may trigger gastrointestinal symptoms such as stomach upset, bloating, gas, and diarrhea.

Pyruvate Oxidation Factor

(see *alpha-lipoic acid*)

Pyruvic Acid

(see *pyruvate*)

Q

Quercetin

aka *meletin, sophretin*

What it is: Quercetin is an antioxidant found naturally in the pulp of many citrus fruits and in apple skins, buckwheat, red onions, red grapes, wine, and tea. It is estimated that the average adult diet provides up to 50 mg of quercetin each day; athletes, especially those enjoying healthy amounts of fruits and vegetables, will accumulate significantly more due to higher calorie intakes to support the demands of training and racing.

How it works: Quercetin has recently garnered a lot of attention among athletes for its ability to quench the immense amount of damaging free radicals that accumulates during heavy training and thereby fight the onset of muscle fatigue.

Performance benefit: By delaying the onset of muscle fatigue in endurance athletes, the proposed benefits include an increase in power output and a decrease in time for endurance events.

Research: While much of the research on quercetin is preliminary and primarily in vitro or animal based, the purported health and performance benefits of this flavonoid are nonetheless substantial and touch on multiple variables that may have positive impacts on endurance performance. A 2011 meta-analysis of 11 studies and 254 human subjects, for example, found $\dot{V}O_2$max and endurance performance increased by 2% compared to a placebo with a medium daily quercetin intake of 1,000 mg over 11 days (Kressler, Millard-Stafford, & Warren). The difference reached statistical significance, and a 2% boost in performance can have huge performance implications, especially for the elite or professional athlete. For reference, it would be equivalent to a 40-minute 10K runner dropping his or her time to 39:20. McAnulty and colleagues (2011) found that a combined supplementation protocol with either 1,000 mg of quercetin plus 1,000 mg vitamin C (QC) or 1,000 mg quercetin, 1,000 mg vitamin C, 400 mg isoquercetin, 30 mg epigallocatechin gallate, and 400 mg n-3 fatty acids (QFO) taken each day for 2 weeks before and during 3 days of cycling at 57% maximal watts for 3 hours significantly reduced markers of oxidative stress in trained cyclists compared to a placebo. This result is especially relevant from a recovery perspective. Davis and colleagues (2009) have shown that quercetin increases brain and muscle mitochondria capacity in animals, which is encouraging data considering mitochondria are a key limiting factor for endurance performance. However, whether or not these favorable results apply to a human population has yet to be proven.

Common usage: Quercetin is available in tablet, powder, softgel, or capsule form in a variety of strengths and often combined with other nutrients, such

>continued

Quercetin >*continued*

as vitamin C, to form an antioxidant cocktail. In line with research protocols, the recommended daily adult supplementation dose for quercetin is 200-400 mg taken up to 3 times daily and preferably 20 minutes before meals. There is no RDA for quercetin.

Health concerns: Because quercetin is found naturally in several common foods, it is thought to be generally safe and well tolerated through usual dietary intake. Hypersensitive individuals may experience headaches or tingling. While rare, other reported side effects include gastrointestinal discomfort, hematoma, and kidney toxicity. Children and women who are pregnant or lactating should consult with a healthcare professional before supplementing with quercetin as there currently is insufficient available evidence on safety.

Additional performance benefits: There has been scientific evidence demonstrating improvements in energy output as well as significant immune-enhancing and antiinflammatory benefits that aid recovery and even present promise for athletes with allergies or asthma (Chirumbolo, 2010).

R

Radix Astragali (RA)

(see *astragalus*)

Red Beet

(see *beetroot*)

Red Pepper

(see *capsicum*)

Resveratrol

aka *3,4'5 trihydroxystilbene, 3,4',5-stilbenetriol*

What it is: Found in greatest concentration in the skin of grapes as well as on the vine, root, seed, and stalk of a grapevine (also found naturally in peanuts and mulberries), resveratrol is a naturally occurring molecule called stilbenoid that carries strong antioxidant qualities and is marketed to enhance athletes' health, endurance, and recovery.

How it works: Animal data suggest that resveratrol may help enhance endurance of an athlete by significantly increasing the size and number of mitochondria within muscle. Mitochondria, also known as the power-house of the cell, are responsible for breaking down carbohydrate, fat, and protein in the presence of oxygen to create the ATP energy needed to propel performance. Increasing the number of mitochondria allows more energy to be generated during exercise, thereby enhancing endurance. Furthermore, with its strong antioxidant properties, resveratrol is purported to help offset some of the damage caused by the release of highly reactive oxygen species (ROS) that often are generated at a rate faster than the body's natural defense system can control during heavy training. In combination with its antiinflammatory properties—resveratrol inhibits the activity of the enzyme cyclooxygenase-2 (COX-2) to fight acute inflammation much like nonsteroidal antiinflammatories (NSAIDs) do—resveratrol is thought to enhance recovery and may also serve as a natural treatment option for inflammatory-based conditions such as arthritis that are common among athletes.

Performance benefit: Athletes may benefit from enhanced endurance and recovery.

Research: Several animal studies have demonstrated promise. For example, mice provided resveratrol at a dose of 400 mg/kg/day over 15 weeks

>continued

were shown to benefit from increased aerobic capacity and exercise time to fatigue compared to their unfed counterparts (Lagoug et al., 2006). Another animal study found aging mice fed 0.2% resveratrol in combination with exercise over 12 weeks benefitted from a significant increase in oxygen consumption and enzymes important to mitochondrial function, which helped offset the age-associated decline in endurance capacity seen with the control group that simply followed a matched exercise program without the resveratrol (Murase et al., 2009). An in vitro study of healthy runners determined that administration of 100 μm of resveratrol helped mute some of the inflicted DNA damage associated with oxidative stress common with exercise, a finding of possible benefit to an athlete's recovery (Tomasello et al., 2012). Even so, despite these favorable data, it is evident that human data from a healthy, fit population are needed before practical recommendations can be made.

Common usage: Resveratrol is available in capsule and tablet form containing extracts of red wine and giant knotweed, a plant found in China; it is also commonly seen as an ingredient in a combined antioxidant or phytonutrient blend that often sold in a wine bottle. Several functional food products also advertise various strengths of resveratrol. Supplements vary in purity and can contain anywhere from 50%-99% resveratrol. Animal studies have used a daily dose of 22 mg of resveratrol/kg of body weight or 400 mg, which is much greater than is currently available in supplement form (generally 30-50 mg) and also a dose without a safety record in humans. For reference, fresh grape skin contains about 500-100 mcg of resveratrol/g whereas a glass of wine provides 600-700 mcg per glass.

Health concerns: Use of resveratrol appears to be well tolerated by most, but long-term safety has yet to be established.

Additional performance benefit: Resveratrol, by increasing the number of mitochondria and regulating enzymes and genes that affect their functionality, has shown promise as an antiobesity agent and thus may help facilitate fat reduction in athletes wanting to lower body composition (Baile et al., 2011).

Rhaponticum Carthamoides

(see *maral root*)

Rhodiola Rosea

aka *R. rosea, Sedum rosea, golden root, rose root, Arctic root, Aaron's rod, Rhodiola arctica, Rhodiola iremelica*

What it is: Commonly marketed as an adaptogen that enhances the body's resistance to physiological stress, including exercise, *Rhodiola rosea* (RR) is an herbal plant that grows in the mountainous regions of central and northern Europe, Asia, and North America as well as in the cold climate of the Arctic.

How it works: RR is believed to enhance performance through several mechanisms; the most relevant for the athlete is its apparent impact on energy usage. As demonstrated in animal studies, RR improves energy usage by increasing essential energy metabolites, ATP, and creatine phosphate within muscle and brain mitochondria, thereby stimulating protein and amino acid synthesis and boosting fat metabolism. In addition, RR seems to moderate levels of cortisol, a catabolic hormone, during physical stress, helping to limit muscle damage as well as protecting the immune system, thus optimizing both short- and long-term recovery.

Performance benefit: RR is purported to enhance many areas of athletic performance, including speed, strength, stamina, muscle building, energy reserves, and recovery time.

Research: The ergogenic benefits of acute RR supplementation have not been consistently demonstrated in well-designed human studies although it is suspected that the inconsistency in results may relate to discrepancies in herbal potency. A further evaluation of data, specifically looking at RR dosing patterns, confirms a bell-shaped curve, indicating the bulk of negative results have been seen in subjects taking low or high doses of RR. A daily dose of 170 mg taken over 4 weeks, however, seems to demonstrate favorable changes in exercise-related blood markers that are consistent with results of well-designed animals studies, according to a 2010 double-blind, placebo-controlled study of 14 trained male athletes (Parisi et al.). After the athletes completed an exhaustive cardiopulmonary test at 75% of $\dot{V}O_2$max, significant reductions in plasma free fatty acid (indicating increased fat metabolism), blood lactate levels (key to extending endurance), and plasma creatine kinase (a parameter of skeletal muscle damage) were seen compared to the placebo group. More research, however, needs to confirm how these changes in exercise-related blood markers translate into performance improvements. While modest, yet significant, improvements have been shown with an acute (one-time) dose of 200 mg taken before an endurance exercise test, chronic supplementation at the same dose over 4 weeks has failed to deliver any performance benefits (De Bock et al., 2004).

>*continued*

Rhodiola Rosea >*continued*

Common usage: Most commonly available in tablet or capsule form, RR supplements generally contain 100 mg of a standardized amount of 3% rosavins and 1% salidroside, which matches the natural ratio of the most active compounds found in the root of the plant. The research-supported doses of RR range from 200 to 600 mg/day, often split into 2 doses throughout the day and generally taken in the morning and early afternoon since some reports of sleep disturbances have been reported with evening use.

Health concerns: RR appears to be safe for supplementation use with no severe adverse effects being reported in clinical trials at doses under 680 mg/day. Even so, comprehensive safety studies are lacking; the safety of its use in young children, pregnant or nursing woman, and people inflicted with liver or kidney disease has not been established, making supplementation ill-advised for these populations.

Additional performance benefits: As a central nervous system stimulant, RR increases the activity of the hormones serotonin and dopamine, which may help lift mood, sharpen focus, and increase energy (Ishaque et al., 2012).

Riboflavin

aka *vitamin B2, riboflavin-5-phosphate*

What it is: Playing a key role in the production of energy, riboflavin is an essential nutrient and member of the B vitamin family that must be obtained from such key dietary sources as organ meats, shellfish, dairy foods, eggs, green leafy vegetables, legumes, and almonds. It is thought that exercise increases the requirements for riboflavin, making supplementation of potential benefit to athletes, especially those restricting energy intake or following fad diets where intake often falls short of recommendations.

How it works: Along with its vitamin siblings thiamin and vitamin B6, riboflavin, in the form of two coenzymes—flavin mononucelotide (FMN) and flavin adenine dinucelotide (FAD)—plays a key role in the energy-producing metabolic pathways of the body, helping break down carbohydrate, fat, and protein for conversion into available energy. Physical training puts additional stress on these metabolic pathways, which raises the question of whether athletes might benefit from supplementation to help accommodate these increased demands and protect against deficiency that has been correlated with a lower tolerance to high-intensity exercise and consequent reduced performance output.

Performance benefit: Athletes may benefit from enhanced endurance during high-intensity competition with the greatest results likely to be seen in those whose diets are deficient in riboflavin.

Research: Biochemical evidence of riboflavin deficiencies in an athletic population have been reported, with corresponding diminished performance in high-intensity activities, yet study results have not been consistent. For example, one study failed to discover any change in blood riboflavin in collegiate swimmers despite a dramatic increase in the intensity, volume, and energy expenditure during a heavy training cycle (Sato et al., 2011). Similarly, an evaluation of vitamin B2 blood concentration in a cross section of athletes from all sports found that 90% fell above the normal range with a direct correlation being noted for vitamin B2 intake over 7 days and vitamin B2 blood level (Rokitzki et al., 1994). Intentional depletion of riboflavin through implementation of a deficient diet (55% of the RDA) over 11 weeks, however, has been shown to have a detrimental impact on performance, with healthy men demonstrating a significant decrease in $\dot{V}O_2max$ (–12%) and peak power (–9%) from a baseline nondeficient state (van der Beek et al., 1988; van der Beek et al., 1994). It is evident that supplementation is generally not needed unless the dietary intake of riboflavin falls short of recommendations. Research suggests that female athletes, especially those restricting calories or following fad diets that limit intake of specific food groups or macronutrients, are at particularly high risk for riboflavin deficiency, making supplementation of possible benefit for this population (Woolf & Manore, 2006).

Common usage: Available in capsule and tablet form, riboflavin can be supplemented by itself; however, it is commonly added to multivitamin and multimineral supplements as well as B complex preparations. The RDA for riboflavin is 1.3-1.7 mg/day for men and women 19 years old or older, respectively. Typical supplementation doses range from 1.7 to 10 mg daily. Doses above 30 mg/day should be taken in several smaller amounts throughout the day.

Health concerns: Use of riboflavin supplements appears to be safe though there have been reports of diarrhea and polyuria (yellow-orange coloring to urine that is harmless) in a small number of people with long-term daily use of doses greater than 400 mg. Deficiency symptoms, which generally manifest after several months of failing to consume the RDA, include cracked lips and corners of mouths as well as a sore tongue. Child athletes may also experience stunted growth patterns.

Additional performance benefit: Athletes who suffer from migraine headaches may benefit from some relief with riboflavin supplementation at a dose of 400 mg/day (Boehnke et al., 2004).

Ribose

aka *beta-D-ribofuranose, D-ribosa, D-ribose, ribosa*

What it is: Ribose is considered a sugar or monosaccharide. Its chemical formula is $C_5H_{10}O_5$, which is similar to that of glucose: $C_6H_{12}O_6$. Ribose is not commonly found in food but can be synthesized in the body; phosphorylated ribose can become a subunit of ATP and DNA. It is this relationship with ATP that sparked the interest in ribose as a dietary supplement. Ribose became popular in the 1980s as the popularity of creatine became mainstream, and research supporting the use of creatine more substantiated. Both ribose and creatine are involved in the synthesis of ATP.

How it works: Essentially, ribose works in the synthesis of ATP (adenosine triphosphate), the high-energy molecule used by muscles during contraction. During high-intensity exercise, muscles use ATP at high rates. The breakdown of ATP results in Adenosine diphosphate (ADP) and Adenosine monophosphate (AMP). The muscles can recycle some of these ADP and AMP molecules back into ATP through creatine phosphate stores. Unfortunately, during this process some AMP molecules are removed from the cell. Once removed, these molecules can no longer be recycled back into useful ATP molecules. Ribose prevents AMP molecules from leaving the cell. This keeps more AMP molecules inside the cell and capable of being recycled back into useful ATP molecules.

Performance benefit: Athletes engaged in high-intensity strength and power sports would benefit most from ribose supplementation. Higher levels of ATP in muscles would enable athletes to train for longer periods of time at higher intensities.

Research: Initial research trials with athletes were positive. Most of these studies induced ischemia (reduced blood flow) in certain tissues and then measured the ability of ribose to replenish ATP stores compared with a placebo. In these trials ribose was administered intravenously, and results were positive (Peveler et al., 2006). Other human trials have not been successful. Only one of five studies produced any significant beneficial effects of ribose on performance (Hellsten, Skadhauge, & Bangsbo, 2004; Peveler et al., 2006; Kreider et al., 2003; Berardi & Ziegenfuss, 2003; Kerksick et al., 2005). The majority of studies have used cyclists performing a Wingate protocol on a cycle ergometer to evaluate peak or mean power throughout the 30-second test. Research does not support the use of ribose, and it is becoming less popular as a dietary supplement.

Common usage: A wide variety of supplementation strategies have been employed with ribose ranging from 625 mg to 20 g. The majority of research trials have used 10-20 g/day, although 200 mg/kg of body weight is another protocol that has been used.

Health concerns: Supplementation with ribose appears safe. No known drug-supplement interactions or other health concerns are known at this time.

Rose Root, *R. Rosea*

(see *Rhodiola rosea*)

Russian Leuzeau

(see *maral root*)

Rutaecarpine

aka *Evodia rutaecarpa, wu-chu-yu, evodia fruit, evodiamine*

What it is: A nitrogen-containing compound called an alkaloid, rutaecarpine is derived from the fruit of an *Evodia rutaecarpa,* a small tree native to China and Korea. Rutaecarpine has been widely used in Chinese medicine for over 100 years and more recently has emerged as a dietary supplement marketed to naturally treat inflammatory-based conditions.

Supplement Fact

Evodia rutaecarpa is a natural source of synephrine, a common ingredient found in weight-loss drugs due to its purported ability to boost metabolism, enhance fat burning, and decrease appetite.

How it works: While acute inflammation serves as a normal physiological response, one that is critical to protecting muscle tissue and cells from damage, inflammation that lingers is suggestive of an overactive inflammatory response detrimental to recovery, sport performance, and the overall health of an athlete. Animal data suggest rutaecarpine helps mediate the activity of the proinflammatory enzyme COX-2, helping to protect an athlete against chronic inflammation that can hurt performance and inhibit recovery (Moon et al., 1999). Additional animal studies have shown that rutaecarpine promotes the release of nitric oxide, which opens up the blood vessels for enhanced delivery of nutrients to support muscle performance and recovery (Wang et al., 1999).

Performance benefit: Athletes may benefit from enhanced protection against chronic inflammation that can hurt performance and slow recovery.

Research: Claims marketed to the athlete population have been drawn purely from results of animal-based or in vitro studies, with human data

>continued

Rutaecarpine >*continued*

on healthy, fit subjects currently nonexistent. As a result, applications and recommendations for rutaecarpine use in humans are impossible to make.

Common usage: There are not sufficient data to confirm optimal doses for supplementation use though available doses generally range from 10-100 mg, often in combination with other ingredients. Rutaecarpine can be prepared as an extract by boiling 1.5-12 g of the dried fruit in water for 5-10 minutes and then straining. Athletes can then drink the extract up to 3 times daily, including 1 hour before workouts.

Health concerns: Rutaecarpine appears to be safe when consumed in recommended doses though studies evaluating adverse effects are limited. Because rutaecarpine slows blood clotting, athletes undergoing surgical procedures are advised to avoid its use for at least 2 weeks leading up to a surgery.

Additional performance benefit: Rutaecarpine carries thermogenic properties, meaning it has the ability to increase the production of body heat, which may enhance overall calorie and fat burn (Kim et al., 2009). In addition, rutaecarpine stimulates the production of natural molecules called vanilloids that, in animal studies, have demonstrated the ability to reduce the uptake of fat as well as increase the rate of fat burning (Kobayashi et al., 2001). Thus, it is proposed that rutaecarpine may facilitate favorable body composition changes in athletes, although human studies have not confirmed this theory.

S

Saccharides (Mono-, Di-, Poly-, Oligo-)

(see *carbohydrate*)

Saccharomyces

(see *probiotics*)

S-Adenosyl Methionine (SAMe)

What it is: S-adenosyl methionine (SAMe) is produced naturally in the body from the amino acid methionine. Since its discovery in 1952, it has been known to play an important role in cellular biochemistry and has become a popular supplement used as an alternative medicine for the treatment of depression. Recently, the use of SAMe as a treatment of joint pain and osteoarthritis has become more common.

How it works: SAMe has a role in three biochemical pathways that influence the body at the cellular level. Osteoarthritis is a disease affecting cartilage, which is composed of water, collagen, proteoglycans, and chondrocytes. Chondrocytes are the active cells of cartilage and produce both collagen and proteoglycans. Degeneration of cartilage and joints can result from decreased proteoglycan production, increased activity of degenerative enzymes resulting in the breakdown of connective tissue, or an increase in the death of chondrocytes. The mechanisms of SAMe are not known; however, a number of theories exist. Some speculate SAMe decreases the production of inflammation-promoting cytokines such as TNF-α and alters gene expression of enzymes involved in degenerative pathways. In addition, SAMe may stimulate the production of proteoglycan.

Performance benefit: Many athletes experience chronic joint pain and degeneration as a result of training or injury to cartilage. Nonsteroidal anti-inflammatories (NSAIDs) are commonly used to treat pain and inflammation in these joints. Unfortunately, NSAIDs are also associated with heartburn, ulcers, bleeding, liver and kidney dysfunction, and skin reactions. SAMe could offer a safe alternative to NSAIDs. Psychologically, SAMe may boost moods in athletes feeling overwhelmed and depressed from the constant demands of training.

Research: Short-term studies have found SAMe to be more effective than a placebo and just as effective as many commonly prescribed antiinflammatory drugs such as ibuprofen, naproxen, and Celebrex in the treatment of osteoarthritis. It was noted that while NSAIDs typically offered immediate relief, 2 weeks of supplementation with SAMe were required before beneficial effects were reported (Najm et al., 2004.) A 2002 meta-analysis of 11

>continued

S-Adenosyl Methionine (SAMe) >*continued*

studies concluded that SAMe appeared to be as effective as NSAIDS in reducing pain and improving functional limitation in patients with osteoarthritis without the adverse effects often associated with NSAIDS (Sofken). No studies have specifically measured the psychological impact of SAMe in athletes undergoing heavy training. A 2005 meta-analysis of the use of SAMe in the treatment of depression reviewed five intervention trials and two randomized, controlled studies. All trials reviewed showed positive significant effects (Williams et al.). More research is needed to continue to confirm and identify the exact mechanisms of SAMe in the treatment of osteoarthritis; however, there appears to be enough evidence to suggest a beneficial effect.

Common usage: A recommended daily dose of 400 mg provided 3 times daily for a total of 1,200 mg is most commonly used in research trials for treatment of osteoarthritis.

Health concerns: SAMe offers a safe alternative to NSAIDs with fewer side effects. No serious adverse effects have been noted in research trials; however, minor side effects such as headaches, restlessness, insomnia, and diarrhea have been reported.

Salicin, Salicylates, Salix, Salix Daphnoides Vill., Salix Fragilis, Salix Purpurea L.

(see *willow bark*)

Sallowthorn

(see *sea buckthorn*)

Salt

aka *sodium chloride (NaCl), table salt*

What it is: Comprised of the elements sodium and chloride with sodium making up 40% of its weight, salt is an ingredient commonly included in sport foods and drinks to help offset the losses in human sweat and promote hydration. Also known as electrolytes, sodium and chloride carry and transmit electrical charges important to muscle and nerve function.

How it works: Salt helps maintain optimal fluid levels outside the body's cells with sodium, in particular, being the key determinant in how much water will be retained within the body versus excreted as urine. Failure to replenish at least a portion of salt losses during exercise, which generally range between 2.25 and 2.4 g/L of fluid loss, can lower blood volume and cause the heart to work overtime trying to pump sufficient blood and oxygen to the brain and muscles for peak performance.

Supplement Fact

The concentration of salt within human sweat decreases as fitness levels increase and with heat acclimatization, a process in which an athlete regularly trains and competes in heat.

Performance benefit: Athletes may benefit from enhanced hydration status and consequent muscle and nerve function when supplementing with salt during exercise, especially when exercise is conducted in extreme environmental conditions such as heat and humidity or at altitude over prolonged periods when losses tend to be greater.

Research: The amount of salt needed to support athletic performance is a subject under much dispute, mainly due to the fact that the human body has defense mechanisms intact to protect against a sodium deficiency during exercise, including the release of sodium from internal body stores. There is evidence that supplementation with additional salt during exercise does nothing to affect serum electrolyte and hydration status or affect the incidence of muscle cramping. For example, a randomized prospective study of Ironman athletes found the addition 3.6 g of sodium during the 140.6 mi (226.3 km) race produced no significant difference in finishing time, serum sodium concentration before and after the race, weight change during the race, rectal temperature, or systolic and diastolic blood pressure after the race compared to placebo and nosupplementation groups (Hew-Butler et al., 2006). Similarly, in another study, treatment of cramp-prone football players with additional salt intake during a competitive season failed to affect the incidence of muscle cramps, suggesting salt intake may not play as large a role as believed (Horswill et al., 2009).

Common usage: While the recommended ceiling intake for salt, and more specifically sodium, is 1,500 mg/day for the general public, athletes may need more to offset losses via sweat during training and competition. In addition to a minimal physiological requirement of 500 mg/day, the American College of Sports Medicine (ACSM) recommends replacing 500-700 mg/L of fluid ingested during exercise. Because sweat losses vary from athlete to athlete and also are highly dependent on environmental conditions, this amount may not always be sufficient to fully replace losses. Thus, additional salt may be needed in the recovery period postexercise. Salt is most commonly consumed in the form of sport drinks during exercise though energy gels, energy chews, and salty foods such as pretzels can be used. Athletes who are salty sweaters, especially those who don't eat a lot of processed food (i.e., they have a lower dietary salt intake), may benefit from supplementation

>continued

Salt >*continued*

with electrolyte capsules that contain sodium and chloride as well as other key minerals lost in sweat such as potassium, magnesium, and calcium.

Salt and Muscle Cramping

Sodium losses in athletes vulnerable to muscle cramping can approach rates 2 times those of their noncramping counterparts. These athletes are often labeled salty sweaters and can usually be spotted by the white crusting (salt crystals) on the skin and uniform postexertion. Some research suggests that salt in sweat may merely be a reflection of a high dietary intake of salt, common in the Western world, rather than a need to increase salt intake during exercise. Thus, increasing dietary intake of salt leading up to competition, a practice known as salt loading, as well as upping the intake of both salt and fluids as tolerated during competition, has not been proven to be an effective treatment for all athletes.

Health concerns: To maintain proper functioning of cells, tissues, and organs, sodium levels within extracellular fluid should remain within a range of 130 to 160 mmol/L. Low levels of sodium, also known as hyponatremia, generally are caused by excessive intake of fluids or inadequate replacement of salt. Initial symptoms include confusion, nausea, fatigue, muscle cramps, and weakness. As the condition worsens, the nervous system becomes impacted; seizures, coma, and even death become possibilities. Because nonsteroidal antiinflammatory agents (NSAIDs) such as aspirin, ibuprofen, and acetaminophen (Tylenol) interfere with kidney function and seem to increase risk for hyponatremia, using these in and around competition is discouraged. On the opposite end of the spectrum, bloating and GI discomfort are common symptoms in athletes consuming too much salt (>920 mg of sodium/L of water consumed). Excessive dietary salt intake can contribute to a variety of health problems, including high blood pressure, stroke, heart disease, edema (water retention), and osteoporosis (brittle bones).

Salvia Hispanica

(see *chia seeds*)

Sambucus Nigra

(see *elderberry*)

Sandthorn

(see *sea buckthorn*)

Sea Buckthorn

aka *Hippophae rhamnoides L., sandthorn, sallowthorn, seaberry*

What it is: A plant with distinctive orange berries that grows in mountainous regions of China and Russia as well as coastal regions of Europe, sea buckthorn has long been used as a medicine. It has more recently garnered attention for its purported ability to fight fatigue and reduce inflammation that can hurt performance.

How it works: While every part of the sea buckthorn plant has historically been used for medicinal purposes, it is the nutrient-packed orange berry and its seeds that are thought to provide antiinflammatory and energy-boosting qualities of potential benefit to athletes. The sea buckthorn berry is recognized as a potent dietary source of antioxidants, including vitamins C and E, beta carotene, lycopene, and flavonoids. Animal studies have shown sea buckhorn to limit the production of damaging free radicals and reduce oxidative stress, helping to maintain the integrity of the mitochondria, the cell's energy-producing factory. In addition, sea buckhorn has been shown to provide a boost to the body's natural antioxidant defense system by restoring levels of such key antioxidants as reduced glutathione (GSH) and glutathione peroxidase (GPx), which may help an athlete better withstand heavy cycles of training and competition. Furthermore, sea buckthorn seems to help reduce levels of creatine kinase and C-reactive protein, two markers of inflammation that can negatively affect the overall health and performance of an athlete.

Performance benefit: Athletes may benefit from enhanced endurance during competition as well as quicker recovery times postcompetition.

Research: Data evaluating the potential performance benefits of sea buckthorn are primarily limited to animal studies; however, these studies present some promise. In one study of male rats, sea buckhorn leaf extract (SBT) provided at doses of 200 and 800 mg/kg of body weight/day over 1 week was shown to significantly extend swim time to exhaustion as well as counter the oxidative stress associated with the exercise protocol (Zheng et al., 2012). In addition, markers of inflammation were lowered in the treatment group versus rats just exposed to exhaustive exercise without SBT. Similarly, another study of rats found that administration of sea buckthorn juice, also known as hippophae juice, over 6 weeks of training extended exercise time to exhaustion, significantly enhanced levels of antioxidant enzymes in skeletal muscle, reduced oxidative stress within skeletal muscle, and significantly reduced inflammation as indicated by levels of creatine kinase compared to the nontreatment group (Qiao & Pan, 2010). Investigators from these two studies concluded that SBT, either in extract or juice-concentrate

>*continued*

Sea Buckthorn >*continued*

form, can enhance exercise capacity, boost the antioxidant capacity of skeletal muscle, and protect against oxidative damage and inflammation caused by exhaustive exercise in rats. A double-blind placebo-controlled study of healthy humans confirmed the antiinflammatory benefits of SBT with a daily dose of 28 g of frozen sea buckhorn puree over 90 days, demonstrating significantly lower levels of C-reactive protein compared to the placebo group (Larmo et al., 2008). Even so, more human studies need to be conducted to explore the potential applications of animal data before conclusions can be made.

Common usage: Sea buckthorn can be consumed in whole food form, either frozen or fresh, and is also used in juices, jams, and teas. As a dietary supplement, it is commonly available in capsule, tablet, seed oil, powder, and extract form. While only limited human clinical trials are currently available to draw dosing conclusions from, a daily intake of 28 g of a frozen berry puree or 300 mL of a juice concentrate has shown some benefit.

Health concerns: No adverse effects have been documented, and thus it appears that use of sea buckthorn as a whole food is safe. However, the safety of sea buckthorn oil has yet to be established, so extra caution should be exercised with its use.

Sedum Rosea

(see *Rhodiola rosea*)

Selenium

aka *L-selenomethionine, selenium amino acid chelate, selenium proteinate, selenium yeast, selenomethionine, sodium selenite*

What it is: An essential trace mineral of the sulfur family, selenium is required by the body in small amounts and can be found naturally in variable amounts in plant foods as well as some meats and seafood. The actual content of selenium in food is dependent on the soil the plants were grown in and where the animals were raised. In the United States, for example, soils in the high plains of northern Nebraska and the Dakotas have typically demonstrated high selenium content, but parts of China and Russia fall on the opposite end of the spectrum. In the body, selenium is concentrated in the lining of the GI tract and lungs, liver, and skeletal muscle. As with many minerals, it is thought that physical sport training increases the body's requirement for selenium.

How it works: Through its antioxidant qualities, selenium is believed to help protect an athlete against cellular damage that can negatively affect immune functionality, recovery from sport, and overall performance. In particular, selenium is essential to the production of glutathione peroxidase (SeGPx), an enzyme that is responsible for a portion of the antioxidant actions within the body. Animal research has shown increased levels of muscle damage and fatigue during prolonged exercise are associated with declines in SeGPx production suggesting that supplementation may help augment some or all of this detrimental effect and have a favorable impact on endurance as well as recovery.

Performance benefit: Athletes may benefit from reduced muscle damage, better endurance, and enhanced recovery during heavy cycles of training and competition. Athletes with gastrointestinal disorders such as Crohn's disease or who have undergone gastric bypass surgery are at greater risk for selenium deficiency due to impaired absorption and thus may benefit from increased intake through supplementation.

Research: Studies evaluating the efficacy of selenium supplementation on a healthy, athletic population have brought mixed results. One study of long-distance runners, for example, failed to find a significant or clinically relevant drop in blood selenium levels or activity of SeGPx upon completion of running a marathon (26.2 miles [42.17 km]), suggesting that endurance exercise, in itself, does not warrant supplementation with selenium (Rokitzki, Logemann, & Keul, 1993). Furthermore, a cross-sectional study of 118 athletes discovered that only 2.6% demonstrated low blood selenium levels despite 23% of the males and 63% of the females failing to achieve recommended dietary allowances for selenium (Margaritis et al., 2005). Nonetheless, a recent meta-analysis of randomized, controlled trials published from January 1988 to December 2010 (Jiang et al., 2012) concluded that supplementation with organic selenium does have a significant impact on SeGPx activity in healthy adults, which may be of benefit to athletes. This finding was according to results from a small, double-blind, placebo-controlled study of healthy males that found supplementation with 240 mcg of sodium selenite to offset some of the muscle damage incurred during a cycle-to-exhaustion exercise test compared to a placebo group (Tessier et al., 1995).

Common usage: Selenium supplements are available in capsule and tablet form with selenomethionine being considered the best absorbed and used form of selenium. While the current RDA is 55 mcg/day for both adult men and women aged 19 years and up, research-supported doses for antioxidant protection fall between 100 and 250 mcg per day.

Health concerns: Prolonged intake of selenium at doses above 900 mcg/day increases the risk for toxicity, which is marked by symptoms of hair loss, skin rash, horizontal streaking and loss of nails, bad breath, fatigue, irritability, nausea, and vomiting. To avoid selenium toxicity, the Institute of Medicine of the National Academy of Sciences has established an upper-intake level for selenium at 400 mcg per day.

>continued

Selenium >*continued*

Additional performance benefits: There is some evidence that supplementation with selenium may help alleviate joint stiffness and pain associated with arthritis (Huang, Rose, & Hoffman, 2012).

Siberian Ginseng

(see *ginseng*)

SierraSil

What it is: SierraSil is made from a mineral deposit found in the Sierra Mountains of the United States. It is comprised of a number of macro- and trace minerals believed to be beneficial in the treatment of joint pain (see Supplement Fact). The mineral deposit was the result of thermal forces that occurred in the area, and the compound is said to have been used as a traditional remedy by indigenous Native Americans for healing purposes. The SierraSil deposit was discovered in the early 1970s; in 2001 Peter Bentley acquired the rights to the mineral deposit and formed the company Sierra Mountain Minerals naming the compound SierraSil.

Mineral Content of SierraSil

Calcium = 23 mg	Silicon = 1.0 mg
Potassium = 20 mg	Manganese = 0.15 mg
Sodium = 12 mg	Barium = 0.10 mg
Aluminum = 6 mg	Copper = 0.033 mg
Phosphorus = 3.1 mg	Cobalt = 0.014 mg
Magnesium = 2.2 mg	Zinc = 0.014 mg
Iron = 1.2 mg	

How it works: SierraSil is thought to affect the development of osteoarthritis at the cellular level by decreasing the effects of proinflammatory cytokines such as interleukin-1β. This results in reduced inflammation and degradation of cartilage in joints. The protective effects of SierraSil on cartilage are believed to be responsible for these benefits.

Performance benefit: Many athletes experience chronic joint pain and degeneration as a result of training or injury to cartilage. Nonsteroidal antiinflammatories (NSAIDs) are commonly used to treat pain and inflammation in these joints. Unfortunately, NSAIDs are also associated with heartburn, ulcers, bleeding, liver and kidney dysfunction, and skin reactions. SierraSil could offer a safe alternative to NSAIDs for treatment of joint pain and limited function.

Research: Research related to SierraSil is weak. Miller and colleagues (2005) conducted a study on 107 patients suffering from mild to moderate osteoarthritis of the knee. Patients were randomly assigned to one of four groups: high dose (3 g/day), low dose (2 g/day), low dose (2 g/day plus cat's claw 100 mg/day), or placebo for 8 weeks. Results showed mild improvement in joint pain and function over the placebo for all three groups during the first 2 weeks; however, significant benefits were not maintained over the 8-week study. This is the only known peer-reviewed study, and follow-up studies have not been done, suggesting SierraSil is ineffective in the treatment of osteoarthritis. Until more research is done, SierraSil is not recommended.

Common usage: There is not enough scientific evidence to provide a recommended usage strategy. However, the company's website suggests that a particular number of capsules be consumed per pound of body weight, 1 time/day with water and on an empty stomach. It also suggests a loading dose be used for first-time users. There is no scientific evidence to warrant these recommendations.

Health concerns: SierraSil appears to be safe. A toxicological study on rats is cited on the company's website. The study suggests that an intake of 35 times the recommended intake level for SierraSil is safe. However, there is a lack of peer-reviewed published research concerning safety. Assessment of the mineral composition of SierraSil would suggest that safety would not be a concern.

6-0-a-D-Glucopyranosyl-D-Fructose

(see *isomaltulose*)

Sodium Ascorbate

(see *vitamin C*)

Sodium Bicarbonate (NaHCO₃) and Sodium Citrate (Na₃C₆H₅O₇)

  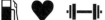

aka baking soda, Na-citrate

What it is: Having been used by athletes for over 70 years, both sodium bicarbonate ($NaHCO_3$) and sodium citrate ($Na_3C_6H_5O_7$) serve as effective buffering agents, offsetting variations in muscle pH triggered by high-intensity exercise. Although stored in limited amounts, sodium bicarbonate is one of the body's most important natural buffering agents; it is commonly known

>continued

Sodium Bicarbonate (NaHCO₃) and Sodium Citrate (Na₃C₆H₅O₇)
>*continued*

as baking soda and is used as a leavening agent in baked goods. Sodium citrate is a byproduct of mixing sodium bicarbonate and citric acid.

How it works: To keep up with the extreme demand for energy to support muscle contraction during sustained high-intensity exercise as well as explosive bursts common in team sports, the body, in the absence of oxygen, breaks down glucose (carbohydrate) to form ATP, a process known as anaerobic glycolysis. The capacity for energy production is limited, however, by the formation of lactic acid and hydrogen ions, two metabolic byproducts that progressively increase muscle acidity (i.e., the burn), which impairs muscle contraction, contributes to fatigue, and diminishes performance. Sodium citrate and sodium bicarbonate enhance the body's natural buffering system by facilitating a faster release of fatigue-inducing hydrogen ions from exercising muscles, thereby reducing acidity as well as aiding the recycling of lactic acid for energy production.

Supplement Fact

Scientific evidence has shown the natural buffering system involved in controlling acidity within muscle cells is about 20% lower in women than in men, making supplementation potentially of greater benefit to female athletes.

Performance benefit: Athletes competing in continuous or repeated periods of explosive, high-intensity activity lasting 1-7 minutes may experience a delay in the onset of muscle fatigue, thereby providing benefit to anaerobic endurance and overall performance.

Research: Numerous studies have explored the supplementation impact of sodium bicarbonate and sodium citrate on human performance, with a 2011 meta-analysis of current data concluding that an acute dose of 0.3-0.5 g/kg of body weight of sodium bicarbonate helped improve 1-minute sprint performance by 1.7%, a margin that often determines whether an athlete earns a spot on the podium (Carr, Hopkins, & Gore, 2011). Adding 5 additional sprinting sessions still translated to improved performance, though the benefit was not as large at 0.6%. By using the current data on sodium citrate, an acute dose of 0.5 g/kg of body weight has been shown to enhance 5 km performance in well-trained college-aged female runners (Oöpik et al., 2003). Interestingly, the same study investigators failed to find the same benefit for trained male runners, a result that falls in line with evidence that the natural buffering system in female athletes is 20% lower than in men (Oöpik et al., 2004). Neither buffering agent appears to have a significant impact on prolonged endurance performance; however, the results of one small study, where 10 trained cyclists completed significantly more work during a 60-minute time trial after ingestion of sodium bicarbonate at a rate of 0.3 g/kg of body weight, suggests additional research may be warranted (McNaughton, Dalton, & Palmer, 1999).

Common usage: Sodium bicarbonate and sodium citrate can be taken as acute doses of 0.3-0.5 g/kg of body weight, split into 5 relatively even amounts and consumed in a staggered fashion starting 3 hours before competition so that loading is complete 1 hour before competition. They can also be taken as a chronic dose with 0.5 g/kg of body weight split into 4 equal doses and consumed every 3-4 hours throughout the day for 5-6 days before competition. While both protocols are effective, the chronic means of loading may help provide an added boost to the body's bicarbonate stores as well as eliminate some of the negative side effects commonly experienced with the acute dosing protocol.

Health concerns: It is not uncommon for athletes to experience nausea, water retention and bloating, vomiting, and diarrhea with sodium bicarbonate loading. Splitting the doses and drinking plenty of fluids seem to help reduce symptoms as does using gelatin capsules. Supplementing with sodium citrate instead of sodium bicarbonate can further reduce adverse GI symptoms.

Sodium Chloride

(see *salt*)

Sodium D-Pantothenate

(see *pantothenic acid*)

Sodium Metavanadate, Sodium Orthovanadate

(see *vanadium*)

Sodium Phosphate

(see *phosphate salts*)

Sodium Pyruvate

(see *pyruvate*)

Sodium Selenite

(see *selenium*)

Sophretin

(see *quercetin*)

Sour Cherries

(see *tart cherry*)

Soy Protein

aka *soy protein isolate, soy protein concentrate*

What it is: The soybean, comprised of 38% protein plus all nine essential amino acids, provides a quality plant-based alternative to animal protein for vegetarian athletes and any athlete looking to enhance cardiovascular health. During soybean processing, the protein is separated from other nutrients, including carbohydrate and fat, and dehydrated to form either a soy protein isolate or concentrate, the dry ingredients commonly used in soy foods and supplements. Soy protein, particularly isolates, contains natural bioactive substances called isoflavones (genistein, daidzein) that may enhance plasma antioxidant activity, thereby minimizing damage to muscle tissue and cells important to immune function and aiding overall recovery and performance in sport.

How it works: With protein contributing up to 10%-15% of the total energy used during strenuous exercise, and muscle tissue constantly being broken down during physical exertion and recovery, an enhanced dietary intake of protein, which may at times be almost 2 times the current recommended dietary allowance (0.8 g/kg of body weight), is of paramount performance to an athlete. The consequences of inadequate intake include inability to repair and rebuild damaged muscle tissue, depressed immune function, poor recovery times, and diminished performance. Beyond helping athletes meet their increased protein demands during training and competition, soy protein, which is absorbed at a slower rate than that of whey protein, may help extend the time at which amino acid acids are delivered to the muscles, thereby maximizing lean body weight gains. Furthermore, of relevance to the endurance athlete, there is some evidence that protein use during ultraendurance competition such as long-distance cycling produces a glycogen-sparing effect, thereby enhancing exercise time to fatigue.

Performance benefit: Athletes may benefit from better endurance, reduced muscle breakdown, and enhanced lean body weight gains.

Research: The bulk of current data evaluating protein and performance has focused on the influence of absorption rates and consequent delivery

TABLE 3.5 Recommended Daily Protein Intake Levels (From All Sources)

	Endurance athletes	Strength athletes
Daily protein goal (g/kg/bw)	1.2-1.4 g	1.2-1.7 g
1-2 hours preexercise	10-20 g	10-20 g
During exercise (hourly)	2-5 g	None needed
Immediately postexercise	10-20 g	10-20 g

of amino acids to muscles on performance and recovery. Double-blind, randomized research presented at the 2012 Experimental Biology Conference in San Diego, for example, determined that postexercise consumption of a protein blend consisting of 25% soy protein isolate (4.5 g), 25% whey protein isolate (4.5 g), and 50% casein (9.5 g) significantly enhanced the body's ability to build muscle (anabolism) compared to whey protein isolate (17.5 g) alone (Reidy et al., 2012). Study investigators attributed this recovery boost to the varying rates at which protein sources are delivered to the muscles. While whey protein is delivered rapidly, soy protein and casein take a little longer for the body to process. Consuming a blend of protein sources postworkout, therefore, extends the time at which essential amino acids are delivered to the muscles, prolonging an anabolic effect for up to 5 hours, helping an athlete maximize lean body weight gains, and supporting recovery.

Common usage: Bars, sport drinks, powders, and meal replacement shakes are all common ways athletes incorporate soy protein into their training menus to help meet daily intake recommendations as well as enhance performance (see table 3.3 for total protein intake recommendations). Because soy isolates carry greater protein potency than soy concentrates, containing 90%-95% versus 65%-70% protein, and are stripped of dietary fiber that can be gas forming, soy isolates are generally the preferred supplementation form for athletes.

Health concerns: Soy protein is well tolerated by most although athletes with allergies to soy should avoid its use. There have also been reports of contamination with potentially dangerous fillers like melamine and lead in some supplement soy protein products. Protein toxicity, which is marked by unexplained vomiting, loss of appetite, and an ammonia-like smell to the breath or sweat, does not seem to be a concern at recommended daily intake levels.

(S)-2

(see *glutamine*)

Sugars

(see *carbohydrate*)

Superoxide Dismutase (SOD)

What it is: As a family of enzymes, superoxide dismutase (SOD) can be found bound to several metals, including copper, zinc, manganese, iron, and nickel. It is consumed naturally in the diet from such green foods as barley grass, broccoli, Brussels sprouts, cabbage, and wheatgrass. In the supplement industry, SOD is marketed as an antioxidant that counters the damaging impact that stress, including exercise stress, can have on the body.

How it works: Exercise triggers the production of chemically reactive molecules known as reactive oxygen species (ROS) that, when produced at a rate that exceeds the body's natural antioxidant defenses, can cause damage to DNA, cell membranes, proteins, and carbohydrates important to the overall health and performance of an athlete. It is thought that supplementation with SOD may decrease the production of ROS, and more specifically superoxide, the most common ROS in the body, helping to mute inflammation triggered by damage to cells that can hurt performance and hinder recovery. While there are several types of SOD, with each type playing a different role in keeping cells healthy, manganese SOD is of particular interest to athletes due to its role in protecting the mitochondria from damage that could negatively affect the production of ATP energy necessary for peak performance.

Performance benefit: Athletes may benefit from enhanced endurance and recovery, especially during periods of heavy training or competition.

Research: It is well established that the physical training common in sport naturally enhances an athlete's antioxidant capacity, allowing the athlete's body to counter the damage associated with exercise stress. However, there is controversy over whether supplementation with antioxidants, such as SOD, can further enhance this activity. In fact, results from some studies suggest antioxidant supplementation, especially in high doses taken long term, may actually hinder this favorable training adaptation, leaving the athlete more vulnerable to the detrimental effects of ROS. Nonetheless, a 2011 small double-blind, randomized study refuted this idea as a supplementation protocol incorporating 500 mg of plant superoxide dismutase extract taken daily during a 6-week training camp was found to significantly enhance SOD antioxidant activity in a group of elite rowers compared to a placebo group (Skarpanska-Stjnborn et al.). In addition, levels of C-reactive protein, a marker of inflammation, were significantly reduced immediately after and

24 hours after completion of a maximal 2,000 m rowing trial, supporting the theory that SOD has strong antiinflammatory properties. Additional research is needed to confirm these results.

Common usage: Available by injection, sublingual administration, topical creams, and in capsule form, dosing recommendations have not been confirmed though limited research suggests a daily dose of 500 mg taken in capsule form during a 6-week competitive or heavy training cycle may be of benefit from an antiinflammatory standpoint. Because SOD is absorbed in the small intestine, enteric-coated pills are essential to avoid destruction by stomach acids before reaching the intestines.

Health concerns: SOD is recognized as a nontoxic substance and presumed safe for supplementation use.

Sweet Pepper

(see *capsicum*)

Synephrine

aka *bitter orange, Citrus aurantium*

What it is: Synephrine is a protoalkaloid found in bitter orange extract, derived from the fruits of *Citrus aurantium* and other citrus species. It can be found in a diverse range of citrus foods such as Seville, mandarin, and Marrs sweet oranges as well as clementines, tangerines, and grapefruits. Synephrine is structurally very similar to ephedrine, a weight-loss supplement banned by the Food and Drug Administration (FDA) in 2003 because of negative health concerns. A variety of synephrine isomers exist as well. Isomers have the same molecular formula; however, they are structurally different and have different physiological effects. P-synephrine is the isomeric derivative found in citrus species, and m-synephrine is not naturally found in plants. It is important to differentiate p-synephrine from m-synephrine and ephedrine when evaluating the health concerns associated with synephrine use (Stohs, Preuss, and Shara, 2011).

How it works: A variety of cells within the body have alpha and beta adrenal receptors. These adrenal receptors are targets for stress hormones and catecholamines released in response to exercise, such as epinephrine and norepinephrine, which initiate the sympathetic fight-or-flight response. This binding induces a strong sympathetic response: increased heart rate, heightened alertness, and increased force production within the muscles, allowing the body to overcome stress. This response increases metabolic

>*continued*

rate and potentially fat oxidation. Alkaloids such as synephrine and ephedrine, like catecholaines, can bind these receptors and induce a sympathetic response potentially increasing resting metabolic rate and fat oxidation. As a result, synephrine and other alkaloids are commonly added to weight-loss supplements.

Performance benefit: Synephrine is most commonly found in weight-loss and so-called fat-burning supplements. It may assist athletes in reducing body fat and weight. In addition, its heightened sympathetic actions could aid in force production, delay fatigue, and enhance performance.

Research: Two groups of scientists in 2004 and 2006 reviewed the scientific evidence of synephrine for weight loss. In 2004 it was concluded that synephrine was ineffective in aiding weight loss and was only lipolytic (fat burning) at high doses (Fugh-Berman and Myers). This was followed by conclusions made by scientists in 2006 stating "while some evidence is promising," more rigorous clinical trials are necessary" (Haaz et al., 2006, 79). More recent studies often use synephrine in combination with caffeine, grean tea extract, and other speculated weight-loss ingredients making it difficult to conclude that synephrine alone promotes body fat and weight loss. These same studies have suggested that synephrine is lipolytic and can induce increases in resting metabolic rate (RMR) of roughly 6.7% without inducing any negative effects on heart rate or blood pressure (Seifert et al., 2011; Stohs et al., 2011). Less is known relative to synephrine's impact on exercise performance. Currently, only one study is known that used a combination of caffeine and synephrine during low- to moderate-intensity exercise. Although the study was not designed to measure exercise performance, it did report an improvement in exercise tolerance among the subjects (Haller, 2008).

Common usage: Research trials have used a range of 13-50 mg.

Health concerns: Scientists have found that p-synephrine does not act on $\alpha 1/2$ and $\beta 1/2$ receptors, unlike ephedrine and m-synephrine. As a result, p-synephrine does not induce the same negative effects on heart rate and blood pressure. In 2004 the FDA concluded that bitter orange extract or p-synephrine was not directly related to adverse events. While p-synephrine appears safe when used within recommended doses, consumers should proceed with caution as weight-loss and fat-burning supplements are often adulterated with additional stimulants and alkaloids that might not be listed on product labels (Stohs, Preuss, & Shara, 2011).

T

Table Beet

(see *beetroot*)

Table Salt

(see *salt*)

Tart Cherry

aka *Prunus cerasus, sour cherries, Montmorency cherry, tart cherry juice, Balatan cherry*

What it is: Containing higher concentrations of naturally occurring plant compounds called phenolics, and in particular anthocyanin, than its sweet sister, tart cherries are the smallest member of the stone fruit family, which also includes plums, apricots, nectarines, and peaches. Tart cherries are grown primarily in Michigan in the United States. There are two varieties of tart cherries, Montmorency and Balaton, both of which are touted as natural alternatives to aspirin and nonsteroidal antiinflammatory drugs (NSAIDs) for the relief of pain.

How it works: Anthocyanins help block two enzymes, COX-1 and COX-2, responsible for the production of inflammatory compounds called prostaglandins. In addition, the antioxidant actions of tart cherries may help ameliorate some of the oxidative tissue damage that can trigger further production of free radicals, inflammation, and muscle soreness.

Performance benefit: Decreasing oxidative stress and inflammation after strenuous exercise facilitates faster recovery times allowing the athlete to accumulate the benefits of more training.

Research: A randomized, double-blind, placebo-controlled study of 54 runners competing in Oregon's 197mi (317 km) Hood to Coast Relay race found that runners consuming 355 ml (~12 oz [.35 L], equivalent to 90-100 cherries) of Montmorency tart cherry juice twice a day for 7 days before the race and twice on race day reported significantly less pain than runners receiving a placebo cherry drink (Kuehl et al., 2010). The same dose of tart cherry juice, taken twice a day for 8 consecutive days before an isometric strength exercise, provided significantly more protection against loss of strength compared to a placebo drink in a well-designed 2006 study of 14 male college-aged subjects (Connoly et al.). The fact that a tapered dose of tart cherries has been clinically shown to reduce circulating concentrations of inflammatory markers in recreational marathoners is a likely reason for reduced pain and enhanced recovery in these subjects (Howatson et al., 2010).

>*continued*

Tart Cherry >*continued*

Common usage: Tart cherries can be consumed fresh, frozen, dried, or as a juice. They are also available in supplement form as an extract, tablet, or capsule. Research-supported dosing with tart cherry is an equivalent of 45-100 cherries or 12 oz (.35 L) of a tart cherry juice concentrate taken 1-2 times daily.

Health concerns: Cherries contain sorbitol, a sugar alcohol that has natural laxative qualities, thereby triggering gastrointestinal distress in some, especially those with irritable bowel syndrome (IBS).

Additional performance benefits: Both Balaton and Montmorency tart cherries contain melatonin, a hormone with antioxidant qualities that may aid sleep, according to a 2011 double-blind, placebo-controlled study of 20 healthy men and women (Howatson et al.). The study found that a 30 ml serving of tart Montmorency cherry juice concentrate (equivalent to 90-100 cherries) taken both in the morning and again before bed significantly increased circulating melatonin while improving sleep efficiency by 5%-6% and overall duration of sleep by 34 minutes per night. The placebo group had no change or a negative change in sleep patterns. It is well known that sleep is an essential component of overall health and necessary for efficient recovery from exercise.

Taurine

aka *2-ethanesuflonic acid*

What it is: Taurine is a sulfur-containing nonessential amino acid. It is one of the most abundant amino acids in the body and is found in muscle and organ tissues such as the heart and liver. Taurine is found naturally in fish, beef, poultry, and lamb. Taurine has become a popular ingredient in many energy drinks, such as Red Bull, which contains roughly 1,000 mg of taurine per 8 oz (.24 L) serving.

How it works: Taurine has a number of mechanisms that may aid in athletic performance. Most significant, taurine is believed to affect cellular excitability by increasing the release of calcium from the sarcoplasmic reticulum (SR). Increases in calcium release from the SR will allow greater actin and myosin interaction improving muscle contractility and force production. Secondly, taurine is a powerful antioxidant capable of combating oxidative free radicals produced during exercise.

Performance benefit: Supplementation with taurine before and during exercise could be advantageous in delaying fatigue and improving performance in endurance athletes and those engaged in high-intensity, prolonged-duration team sports. In addition, taurine may improve strength and power production during muscle contraction.

Research: Exercise has been shown to significantly deplete muscle taurine concentrations, which could precipitate muscle fatigue and reduced performance according to animal data (Hamilton et al., 2006). However, additional animal data have shown administration of taurine to reduce muscle fatigue, improve force production, enhance muscle endurance, and decrease the muscle damage associated with exercise (Yatabe et al., 2009; Goodman et al., 2009). Unfortunately, the number of human trials is small; thus, it is currently unknown if these benefits will apply to humans. One study failed to find any performance benefit with administration of 1.66 g of taurine 1 hour before endurance-trained cyclists completed a 90-minute endurance ride followed by an all-out time trial. However, a significant increase in fat oxidation was noted (Rutherford et al., 2010). Other human trials have used a combination of taurine and caffeine, including two popular sports supplements, Advocare's Spark and Red Bull Energy Drink. Both supplements contain a combination of caffeine and taurine. One study showed no benefit from consuming Red Bull on repeated sprint performance in women (Astorino et al., 2012), while another study found no improvement in sprint performance or anaerobic power in football players consuming Spark (Gwacham & Wagner, 2012). More human trials are needed, but the current consensus is that despite positive research in animal models, taurine does not appear to be beneficial to performance in the human population.

Common usage: Research studies in humans have used 200 mg-1.66 g doses of taurine before exercise. More research is needed to determine if these levels are inadequate and if higher amounts are needed to produce positive performance effects.

Health concerns: The use of taurine appears to be safe. The only noted side effect is diarrhea. The highest dose used in research trials is 12 g.

Theine

(see *caffeine*)

Theobroma Cacao

(see *cocoa*)

Thiamine

aka *vitamin B1, antiberiberi vitamin, B-complex vitamin*

What it is: A member of the B vitamin family, thiamine, otherwise known as vitamin B1, aids the breakdown of carbohydrate for conversion into energy and

>*continued*

can be found naturally in such foods as cereal grains, beans, nuts, meats, and yeast. As a sports supplement, thiamine is proposed to help combat the stress of physical training and increase energy, thereby improving performance.

How it works: Thiamine plays a key role in several reactions important to the metabolism of carbohydrate, including the activation of pyruvate dehy-drogenase (PDH), a mitochondrial enzyme that serves as the gateway for the production of ATP energy. A deficiency in thiamine has been shown to reduce the activity of PDH and consequent energy production as well as increase the production of fatigue-inducing lactate, thereby compromising performance.

Supplement Fact

Are you a coffee or tea drinker? Frequent consumers may be at greater risk for thiamine deficiency as chemicals called tannins found in both beverages trigger a reaction that converts thiamine to a form difficult for the body to process.

Performance benefit: Athletes may benefit from enhanced energy levels and endurance during training and competition.

Research: While most studies have shown the thiamine intake of athletes is sufficient to meet the RDA, athletes may benefit from increased dietary intake or supplementation to offset the heightened level of stress that exercise places on thiamine-driven metabolic pathways. A 2011 study found that the blood thiamine concentration of collegiate swimmers dropped significantly during a heavy training cycle as compared to a preparatory low-volume period; this was in spite of an increased energy intake and sufficient thiamine intake, suggesting a cycle of thiamine supplementation may be beneficial at a certain point during a competitive season (Sato et al.). A well-designed study of nondeficient male athletes, for example, found administration of 1 mg/kg of thiamine pyrophosphate (TPP) enhanced aerobic capacity during exercise while lowering heart rate as well as postexercise levels of blood lactate in comparison to a placebo (Bautista-Hernández et al., 2008). Similarly, an animal study found supplementation with thiamine tetrahydrofurfuryl disul-fide (TTFD) over 5 days to attenuate (reduce) the decrease in ATP content within skeletal muscle caused by a weighted swimming exercise protocol, which helped to significantly delay the onset of fatigue and enhance exer-cise time to exhaustion compared to a placebo group (Nozaki et al., 2009). It is clear that thiamine is an essential component of an athlete's diet, and supplementation may be of benefit, particularly during heavy training cycles and for athletes who struggle to meet the heightened caloric and nutritional demands of competition.

Common usage: The RDA for thiamine in men and women aged 18+ years are 1.2 and 1.1 mg/day, respectively. Supplemental doses generally fall between 100% and 200% of the RDA and are commonly included in B-complex and multivitamin-multimineral supplement blends as well as sold individually in tablet, softgel, and lozenge form. Athletes engaged in heavy training cycles or with mild dietary deficiencies may benefit from elevated doses up to 100 mg taken daily for up to 1 month, preferably split into 2-3 doses throughout the day.

Health concerns: Severe deficiency, also known as beriberi, is rare in developed countries, but mild deficiencies have been reported in those who exercise intensely, are affected by Crohn's disease, follow poor dietary habits (high intake of refined carbohydrate and sugar), and drink a lot of alcohol, coffee, or tea. Symptoms of deficiency include fatigue, irritability, and muscle cramps. Supplementation with thiamine appears to be safe, even at high levels, although rare reports of allergic reactions and skin irritations have been reported.

Additional performance benefits: Through synthesis of key chemical messengers within the nervous system, thiamine, at a dose of 50 mg/day, may help improve reaction time and mental focus (Benton et al., 1997).

Thiotic Acid

(see *alpha-lipoic acid*)

3-Aminopropanoic Acid

(see *beta-alanine*)

3,4',5-Stilbenetriol, 3,4'5 Trihydroxystilbene

(see *resveratrol*)

TMG

(see *betaine*)

Tribulus

aka *Tribulus terrestris*

What it is: *Tribulus terrestris* is an herb native to temperate and tropical climates in Africa, Australia, southern Europe, and Asia. There have been claims that as an herbal supplement, it has provided performance enhancement for many top Bulgarian weightlifters.

>continued

How it works: Tribulus supplementation is believed to increase levels of testosterone in athletes. The anabolic properties of testosterone would equate to gains in muscle mass and improvements in strength and power. There are claims that tribulus increases circulating levels of luteinizing hormone (LH) and testosterone, and that tribulus is a natural testosterone booster. Tribulus contains steroidal saponins, which supposedly block central testosterone receptors, thereby increasing levels of LH and testosterone.

Supplement Fact

The NCAA or World Anti-Doping Agency does not consider tribulus a banned substance. Most banned substance drug testing uses a testosterone/epitestosterone (T/E) ratio as a means of detecting banned supplement use. While tribulus does not affect the T/E ratio, supplements containing impurities and ingredients not listed on product labels may affect this ratio and result in a failed test. Athletes should be extremely cautious if considering taking a tribulus supplement.

Performance benefit: If claims are true, tribulus would benefit strength and power athletes by aiding in the development of lean body mass, strength, and power through increased levels of anabolic hormones.

Research: In 2007 a group of scientists studied the effects of tribulus supplementation on strength and body composition in rugby players. The 5-week study found tribulus to be ineffective in increasing strength or improving body composition, and it did not affect any levels of anabolic hormones (Rogerson et al.). Similar results were found in a 2000 study involving 8 weeks of supplementation in resistance-trained men (Antonio et al.). Additionally, a 2001 study evaluated the effectiveness of a supplement containing a cocktail of tribulus as well as androstenedione, dehydroepiandrosterone, saw palmetto, chrysin, and indole-3-carbinol. The supplement cocktail was concluded to be ineffective in promoting levels of testosterone (Brown). No evidence currently exists to support the use of tribulus as a testosterone-boosting ergogenic aid for strength and power athletes.

Common usage: The three research studies previously mentioned used a range of 450-750 mg or 3.21 mg/kg of body weight (equivalent to 240 mg for a 165 lb [75 kg] athlete). Most supplement labels recommend 750-800 mg of tribulus be consumed 3 times daily in the morning, about noon, and before bed.

Supplement Warning

 In a recent study of nine dietary supplements, four were found to contain sildenafil (Viagra) analogs. These types of supplements often contain impurities, such as prohormones, which are known to cause gynecomastia, lower HDL cholesterol, and negatively affect psychological state.

Health concerns: Tribulus is also marketed for sexual enhancement. Many supplements sold for sexual enhancement contain ingredients not listed on the labels and other impurities.

Trigonella Foenum-Graecum

(see *fenugreek*)

Trimethylglycine

(see *betaine*)

Tumeric

(see *curcumin*)

20-Beta-Hydroxyecdysterone, 20-Hydroxyecdysone

(see *ecdysteroids*)

25(OH)D

(see *vitamin D*)

2-Aminoglutaramicacid

(see *glutamine*)

2-Ethanesuflonic Acid

(see *taurine*)

2-Oxopropanoate, 2-Oxypropanoic Acid

(see *pyruvate*)

Tyrosine

aka *L-tyrosine*

What it is: Tyrosine is a nonessential amino acid; therefore, it can be synthesized within the body and is not required from dietary sources. However, it can be easily obtained from high-protein foods such as, soy, chicken, turkey,

>*continued*

Tyrosine >*continued*

fish, peanuts, almonds, and dairy foods. Tyrosine is used in the production of proteins; it also has an important function as a precursor of neurotransmitters such as dopamine and epinephrine.

How it works: Tyrosine is an important precursor of the neurotransmitter dopamine. Dopamine and another neurotransmitter, serotonin (5-hydroxytryptophan), function antagonistically. When levels of serotonin are high in relation to dopamine, feelings of fatigue, tiredness, and reduced motivation result. In contrast, when dopamine levels increase, feelings of fatigue are reduced and increased motivation ensues. It is speculated that supplementation of tyrosine during prolonged exercise will help improve the dopamine:serotonin ratio, thereby reducing fatigue and improving performance.

Performance benefit: Supplementation with tyrosine during exercise could improve performance for endurance athletes and for strength and power athletes engaged in long-duration, high-intensity sports.

Research: In 2002 Chinevere and colleagues studied the effect of tyrosine supplementation in cyclists during a 90-minute steady-state ride followed by a time trial. The athletes were provided with 25 mg of tyrosine/kg of body weight, and the exercise was performed in temperate conditions. Tyrosine had no significant effects on performance. Other studies have used a pharmaceutical drug known as bupropion to increase dopamine levels during exercise and produced similar results. Interestingly, when bupropion was provided in warm environments (30°C [86°F]), a significant improvement in exercise performance was found in comparison to results in temperate environments (18°C [64°F]) (Watson et al., 2005). In 2011 a group of scientists found tyrosine improved cycling time to exhaustion by 11% under warm (30°C [86°F]) conditions (Tumility). While performance was improved, no differences in core temperature, heart rate, or rating of perceived exertion were noted. More research is needed to confirm these results; however, it appears that tyrosine supplementation is capable of improving performance during prolonged exercise in warm conditions.

Common usage: Tyrosine can be found in a variety of forms, pill and powder being most common. It's difficult to recommend an optimal usage strategy as more research is needed to confirm best-use procedures. A 2011 study of cyclists used a 150 mg/kg of body weight dose provided 1 hour before exercise. This would be equivalent to a 9.5 g for a 140 lb (64 kg) athlete and up to 15 g for a 220 lb (100 kg) athlete (Tumilty et al.). Tyrosine is sometimes recommended for treatment of depression, in which case 500-1,000 mg doses consumed 3 times daily is recommended.

Health concerns: The use of tyrosine is safe when consumed within recommended levels. The toxic dose is roughly 5,000 mg/kg of body weight, which is equivalent to 375 g for a 165 lb (75 kg) athlete.

U

Ubidecarenone, Ubiquinone

(see *coenzyme Q10*)

Uncaria Guianensis, Uncaria Tomentosa

(see *cat's claw*)

Undenatured Type II Collagen (UC-II)

What it is: Glycosylated undenatured type II collagen (UC-II) is a dietary supplement that is produced from the sternum of chickens and is speculated to benefit arthritic joints and conditions such as osteoarthritis and rheumatoid arthritis. It is produced using a low-temperature procedure that prevents the proteins from being broken down, which is important for its effectiveness (Gupta, 2010).

How it works: The exact mechanisms of UC-II are unknown; however, initial research suggests that stomach acids partially digest UC-II upon consumption leaving chains of soluble collagen that can actively induce an immune response within the small intestine. In the case of rheumatoid arthritis, these proteins can downregulate autoimmune inflammatory responses that result in arthritic conditions. Essentially, UC-II stops the immune system from attacking its own joint cartilage. In addition, UC-II has been shown to deactivate killer T-cells, which also can induce an inflammatory response (Crowley et al., 2009).

Performance benefit: Many athletes experience chronic joint pain as a result of training. The physical demands of sport and daily training place a significant amount of stress on joints, often resulting in pain, reduced mobility, and decreased function. In addition, many athletes must overcome injuries to joints resulting in surgery or joint reconstruction. UC-II may provide relief for athletes suffering from chronic joint pain or aid in recovery from injury.

Research: Animal studies in dogs and horses have been positive, showing treatment with UC-II beneficial in decreasing overall joint pain (Deparle et al., 2005; Gupta et al., 2010). Crowley and colleagues (2009) examined the effects of 40 mg of UC-II containing 10 mg of bioactive undenatured type II collagen on subjects with osteoarthritis of the knee. UC-II was found to be twice as effective as 1,500 mg of glucosamine and 1,200 mg of chondroitin in promoting joint health after 90 days. Improvements in physical function, stiffness, and pain were observed. Unfortunately, aside from this study, few recent trials on humans exist. More research is needed before clear conclusions can be made relative to the effectiveness and mechanisms

>*continued*

Undenatured Type II Collagen (UC-II) >continued

involved in the use of UC-II for treatment of joint pain and dysfunction in athletes. However, early findings are positive.

Common usage: A supplementation protocol of 40 mg containing 10 mg of bioactive undenatured type II collagen provided in the evening was used by Crowley. Based on recent research trials, this protocol is recommended.

Health concerns: The use of UC-II appears to be safe. A 2010 toxicological study concluded a broad spectrum of safety existed related to its use (Marone et al., 2010).

V

Valerian

aka *Valeriana officinalis*

What it is: *Valeriana officinalis* is a perennial herb found in North America, Europe, and Asia. More than 2,000 years ago Greeks used the herb as a treatment for anxiety, stress, insomnia, and other sleep disorders. It was used to relieve the stress of air raids in England during World War II. The use of valerian for treatment of anxiety, stress, and sleep disorders is still common today. Supplements are made from the roots, rhizomes, and stems of the plant, and extracts are often put into capsules of tablets.

How it works: The exact mechanisms of valerian are unknown; however, it is composed of a variety of constituents believed to be responsible for its biological effects. These include volatile oils, such as valeric acid, iridoids, alkaloids, and amino acids, including γ-aminobutyric acid (GABA), tyrosine, arginine, and glutamine (Hadley & Petry, 2003).

Performance benefit: Athletes may benefit from improved quality, length, and quickened onset of sleep. These benefits could produce improved recovery from training and subsequent performance. In addition, valerian can be used during extensive travel and time zone changes, assisting jet-lagged athletes in adapting circadian rhythms to new time zones.

Research: In the most recent meta-analysis related to valerian, a total of 29 controlled studies were included; most found no significant differences between valerian and a placebo in healthy individuals suffering from general sleep disturbances or insomnia. As a result, it was concluded that while the use if valerian is safe, it is not effective (Taibi et al., 2007). This review was in contrast to another review in 2006, which concluded that valerian might improve sleep quality; however, more research was recommended. It was noted that many studies included in the 2006 review had methodological flaws (Bent et al.). A 2011 study conducted with oncology patients found valerian ineffective in relieving sleep disturbance in cancer patients (Barton et al.). These results are similar to other recent studies, which were better controlled and less methodologically flawed. In conclusion, while early research suggested a potential benefit, more recent scientific studies have failed to show benefits. No studies have been conducted with athlete-specific populations and the impact of improved sleep through valerian supplementation on recovery and performance.

Common usage: The effective dosage of valerian used in scientific trials ranges from 300-600 mg and should be ingested between 30 minutes and 2 hours before bedtime.

Health concerns: No adverse side effects of valerian are known nor are there contraindications to its use. Unlike some sleep aids, valerian use does not result in dependence.

Valine

(see *branched-chain amino acids*)

Vanadium

aka *vanadyl sulfate, Amanita muscaria, amavadine, sodium metavanadate, sodium orthovanadate*

What it is: Vanadium is considered a trace element. Its discovery is credited to the Swedish chemist Nils Gabriel Sefstrom, who named it vanadium after the Nordic goddess of beauty, Vanadis. Vanadium is found in foods such as mushrooms, shellfish, black pepper, parsley, dill seed, and grains. *Amanita muscaria,* a species of mushrooms, contains amavadine, which is a natural vanadium-containing compound ("Vanadium/Vanadyl Sulfate," 2009).

How it works: Vanadium is not considered an essential nutrient in the diets of humans; however, there is much controversy related to this among experts. Vanadium is an essential nutrient for some animals, for example chickens that develop adverse effects in bones, feathers, and blood as a result of deficiency. Vanadium plays a role as a cofactor in a variety of enzymes, and some studies have shown it to mimic the actions of insulin. This effect is believed to produce a variety of beneficial effects on blood glucose control and possibly body composition. Various forms of vanadium are commonly added to dietary supplements marketed for weight loss and improvement of body composition.

Performance benefit: Athletes wanting to improve body composition may use vanadyl sulfate or vanadium.

Research: A 12-week study completed in 1996 is the only known study related to vanadyl sulfate supplementation and athletes. The study on 31 weight-training athletes found no significant effects of supplementation on body composition (Fawcett et al.). No other more current trials are known. Another study in 2002 found that vanadyl sulfate supplementation did not affect insulin sensitivity in healthy active individuals (Jentijens & Jeukendrup). While vanadium appears to have a role in insulin sensitivity, it does not improve body composition and is not recommended for use in athletes.

Common usage: There is no RDA for vanadium; however, a daily intake of 10-100 mcg is considered adequate. The average diet contains 6-18 mcg of vanadium/day. In scientific trials related to diabetes, a therapeutic dose of 100-300 mcg is often used. Another supplemental strategy often used in clinical trials is 50 mcg consumed twice daily.

Health concerns: Vanadium does not appear to be toxic; however, some mild affects such as abdominal cramps and diarrhea have been reported with higher doses (50-100 mcg). The vanadate form of vanadium can increase the effects of anticoagulants such as heparin ("Vanadium/Vanadyl Sulfate," 2009).

Vanadyl Sulfate

(see *vanadium*)

Vincaria, Vinicol

(see *cat's claw*)

Vinis Vinifera

(see *grape seed*)

Virgin Coconut Oil

(see *coconut*)

Vitamin B1

(see *thiamine*)

Vitamin B2

(see *riboflavin*)

Vitamin B5

(see *pantothenic acid*)

Vitamin B12

aka *cobalamin, cyanocobalamin, hydroxocobalamin, methylcobalamin*

What it is: Often considered nature's most beautiful vitamin due to the striking red color of its crystals, vitamin B12 is a water-soluble vitamin that belongs to a family of chemically complex compounds containing the mineral cobalt—thus its secondary name, cobalamin. Naturally found in foods of animal origin such as organ meats, egg yolks, clams, crab, and salmon, vitamin B12 plays an integral role in the formation of red blood cells, energy metabolism, normal nerve cell activity, and proper brain function.

>continued

Vitamin B12 >*continued*

How it works: Because of its role alongside folic acid in the creation of red blood cells important for oxygen transport throughout the body as well as DNA synthesis, a deficiency in vitamin B12 can result in such anemia-based symptoms as fatigue, poor energy levels, nausea and diarrhea, decreased appetite, weakening of the muscles, headaches, and tingling sensations. Vitamin B12 also protects the outer covering of nerves, called the myelin sheath, which helps facilitate optimal conduction of energy throughout the nervous system. Suboptimal vitamin B12 levels thus may compromise an athlete's ability to see, hear, think and move. While deficiencies are rare thanks to the body's ability to maintain stores for several years, the added stress of intense exercise on the body's energy-producing pathways and tissues may leave an athlete at elevated risk for diminished stores.

Performance benefit: Deficient athletes may benefit from enhanced energy levels and better endurance through reversal of anemia symptoms.

Research: Limited research has been conducted to examine whether exercise increases the need for vitamin B12. It has been confirmed that severe deficiency of B12, especially in combination with folate, results in anemia and reduced endurance performance (Lukaski, 2004). However, there have not been any studies demonstrating a performance-enhancing benefit from use of vitamin B12 supplements in nondeficient athletes.

Common usage: The most common and recommended supplement form of vitamin B12 is cyanocobalamin. Delivery can be sublingual (under the tongue), in pill form, as part of a beverage, or by injection. According to the current Dietary Reference Intake (DRI), those 14 years and older should aim for 2.4 mcg daily; pregnancy and lactation warrant increased daily intake of 2.4 and 2.6 mcg, respectively. For reference, 1 oz (28 g) of salmon meets the 2 mcg/day recommendation. Supplementation of 25-100 mcg daily has been used to maintain vitamin B12 levels in at-risk populations while therapeutic doses to correct deficiencies are often prescribed at doses of 125-2,000 mcg daily under the supervision of a doctor. Vitamin B12 shots (injectable B12) are often marketed to boost metabolism, enhance energy, and speed weight loss. Unless a deficiency is present, however, none of these claims carry any scientific merit.

Health concerns: Athletes competing at the master's level, following strict vegetarian or restrictive diets, or who have undergone gastric bypass surgery are at greatest risk for deficiencies due to poor dietary intake or absorption. Severe deficiency cases, which are extremely rare even within an at-risk athletic population, can lead to anemia, gastrointestinal lesions, and neurological damage. Due to the body's ability to store vitamin B12, it is generally considered nontoxic even in large doses. However, there have been a small number of anaphylactic reactions reported.

Vitamin C

aka *ascorbate, ascorbic acid, antiscorbutic vitamin, calcium ascorbate, cevitamic acid, sodium ascorbate*

What it is: A water-soluble vitamin with powerful antioxidant qualities, vitamin C is an essential vitamin (not produced by the body) found naturally in abundance within fresh fruits and vegetables such as broccoli, peppers, Brussels sprouts, strawberries, and kiwifruit.

How it works: Vitamin C aids the growth and repair of injured tissue by facilitating the production of collagen, the glue that strengthens many parts of the body, including muscles and blood vessels, and enhances wound healing. It also raises concentrations of key antibodies (IgA, IgM, IgG), helping to strengthen immune function. As an antioxidant, it hinders lipid peroxidation and reduces oxidative DNA and protein damage. Additionally, vitamin C serves as an enzyme cofactor for carnitine, important for the transport of fat into mitochondria for energy production, and aids the synthesis of peptide hormones, which are key factors for enhancing muscle size and strength.

Performance benefit: Playing a key role in the growth and repair of many tissues and supporting immune function, vitamin C may help enhance both short- and long-term recovery from intense exercise.

Research: Major reviews of vitamin C confirm that supplementation with the vitamin only aids physical performance in times of deficiency. In fact, a 2008 double-blind, randomized study of 14 nondeficient trained men and 24 rats actually demonstrated a decline in physical performance with an oral dose of 1 g of vitamin C (dose altered in accordance to body mass in rats) taken over 6 weeks (Gomez-Cabrera et al.). Specifically, vitamin C supplementation hindered important training adaptations such as increases in cytochrome C (a marker of mitochondrial content) and the powerful antioxidants superoxide desmutase and glutathione peroxidase, which limited improvements in aerobic capacity and time to exhaustion in supplemented subjects. Exposure to long-term physical stress, often seen in endurance-training programs, however, can rapidly deplete vitamin C stores in an athlete, and increased intake via whole food or supplementation may be needed to offset the losses. Vitamin C at daily doses of 1,500 mg over a 10-day period was found to be effective in staving off the increases in circulating cortisol, adrenaline, and antiinflammatory polypeptides seen after completion of a 90 km ultramarathon in a 2001 study of 29 runners; therefore, it may be beneficial for protecting immune function and aiding recovery after intense, prolonged activity (Peters et al.).

Common usage: Available in capsule, tablet, and powder form as well as in multivitamin and antioxidant formulations, vitamin C is one of the most

Vitamin C >*continued*

commonly supplemented vitamins. The RDA for vitamin C is 90 mg for adult males and 75 mg for adult females. Research-supported doses for vitamin C range from 500-1,500 mg/day, generally split into 2-3 doses and taken with meals.

Health concerns: Severe vitamin C deficiency can lead to the onset of scurvy, a potentially fatal disease marked by fatigue, bleeding gums, joint pain and swelling, and hair and tooth loss. While rare in developed countries, it has been reported in children and the elderly on highly restricted diets. On the other hand, intake of vitamin C at levels well above the RDA and upward of 3 g/day are generally well tolerated although some experience stomach distress and diarrhea with high doses. Chronic supplementation at or above the threshold dose of 3 g/day also increases the risk for kidney stones.

Additional performance benefit: Athletes requiring surgery may benefit from enhanced wound healing with a vitamin C supplementation protocol that incorporates 500-1,000 mg for 3-7 days before a procedure (Fukushima and Yamazaki, 2010).

Vitamin D

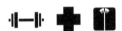

aka *vitamin D2, vitamin D3, 25(OH)D, calcidiol (25-hydroxy-vitamin D), calcifidiol (25-hydroxy-vitamin D), calcitriol (1,25 dihydroxy-vitamin D)*

What it is: Vitamin D is produced in the skin from exposure to ultraviolet B (UVB) radiation and is thus commonly referred to as the sunshine vitamin. Vitamin D is classified as a fat-soluble vitamin even though technically speaking it is a prohormone (any substance that can be converted to a hormone) with its hormonally active form, calcitriol, playing a key role in calcium metabolism and bone health.

How it works: The active form of vitamin D, derived from sunlight and dietary sources, works in conjunction with the parathyroid hormone and the hormone calcitonin to regulate serum calcium and phosphorus concentrations, generally by enhancing intestinal absorption of these minerals, facilitating normal bone mineralization, and protecting against debilitating osteoporotic and stress-related fractures. Vitamin D, which is obtained from sun exposure, food, and supplements, must undergo two chemical reactions within the body before it's available for use. Initially, vitamin D is converted to 25-hydroxyvitamin D [25(OH)D], also known as calcidiol, within the liver and then forms physiologically active 1,25-dihydroxyvitamin D [1,25(OH)$_2$D], also known as calcitriol. As a steroid hormone, calcitriol also regulates more than 50 genes in tissues throughout the body, including muscle and nerve tissue, a mechanism of action thought to have a positive impact on athletic performance especially as it relates to the neuromuscular system.

Vitamin D Deficiency

In recent years scientists have debated what constitutes adequate vitamin D levels. While still being debated by experts, the following ranges can be considered:

<15 ng/mL = severe deficiency
15-30 ng/mL = moderate deficiency
30-40 ng/mL = mild deficiency
40 ng/mL+ = optimal

Also note that ranges are often reported in nmol/L (1 ng/mL = 2.5 nmol/L).

Performance benefit: Vitamin D–deficient athletes may benefit from stronger bones and increases in muscle strength and speed by increasing vitamin D stores through whole food intake, supplementation, and sun exposure.

Research: Despite exposure to sunlight, traditionally thought of as an acceptable means to achieve optimal serum 25(OH)D concentrations (for athletes 30-50 ng/mL), several sun-kissed populations, including elite gymnasts in Australia (Lovell, 2008) and young skateboarders and surfers in Hawaii (Binkley et al., 2007) have been shown to carry suboptimal levels, with some falling under 20 ng/mL. Another study discovered an astonishing 73% of athletes to be vitamin D insufficient with dancers (94%), basketball players (94%), and taekwondo fighters (67%) leading the way (Constatini et al., 2010). A 2011 study of female Navy recruits discovered serum 25(OH)D concentrations less than 20 ng/mL to double the risk for stress fractures of the tibia and fibula as compared to concentrations of greater than 40 ng/mL (Burgi et al.). A threshold level of 30 ng/dL has been indicated for optimal muscle function, including overall strength and mass, according to a study of senior-age men and women (Kenny et al., 2003). Indeed, as serum 25(OH)D concentrations rise, numerous studies have demonstrated increases in intracellular levels of calcitriol within muscle and nerve tissue and consequent improvements in the size and number of Type II (fast-twitch) muscle fibers (Larson-Meyer & Willis, 2010). Although the translation as it relates to performance in a young athletic population is limited, there is some promise. For example, a 2012 study found a supplementation protocol incorporating 5,000 IU of vitamin D3 over 8 weeks to significantly increase serum 25(OH)D concentrations in athletes and consequent performance in 10 m sprint time and in a vertical jump test (Close et al.).

Common usage: Vitamin D is found naturally in such food sources as cod liver oil (1 tbsp =1,360 IU), salmon (3.5 oz [99 g] = 360 IU), and egg yolk (1 = 20 IU); fortified in several products such as milk (1 c = 98 IU); and as a supplement. The Institute of Medicine currently recommends an adequate intake, rather than a specific daily amount of vitamin D, ranging from 600 IU for adults under age 70 to 800 IU for age 71+. Athletes with serum 25(OH)D levels below 30 ng/dL, as revealed by a simple blood test, are encouraged to discuss ways to increase vitamin D via whole food intake, sun exposure, or supplementation

>continued

Vitamin D >*continued*

with a doctor or a registered dietitian. A serum 25(OH)D concentration of 40 ng/mL or greater has been shown to be achievable with a daily supplementation protocol that incorporates 4,000 IU of vitamin D3.

Health concerns: Chronically low serum 25(OH)D concentrations (<10 ng/dL) can lead to rickets in children and osteomalacia in adults, both characterized by soft bones and increased susceptibility to fracture. At the other end of the spectrum, toxicity symptoms, indicated at serum 25(OH)D levels ranging from 200-240 ng/mL or supplementation doses of 10,000-40,000 IU/day, include weakness, muscle pain, bone pain, loss of appetite, nausea, intestinal cramps, headache, metallic taste, and in most severe cases renal impairment. Athletic performance has shown to decline with a supplementation protocol of 5,000 IU or more.

Additional performance benefits: By reducing the production of proinflammatory cytokines and increasing the production of antiinflammatory cytokines, vitamin D may help speed the recovery process between hard workouts.

Vitamin E

aka *alpha-tocopherol, beta-tocopherol, delta-tocopherol, gamma-tocopherol, alpha-tocotrienol, beta-tocotrienol, delta-tocotrienol, gamma-tocotrienol*

What it is: Found naturally in such foods as wheat germ, sunflower seeds, almonds, and vegetable oils, vitamin E, which collectively represents eight fat-soluble compounds, is a powerful and essential antioxidant that protects cell membranes and other fat-soluble parts of the body from free radical damage that can negatively affect both health and performance. Of its eight compounds, alpha-tocopherol is the only form actively maintained within blood and tissues and recognized to meet the human requirements for vitamin E.

How it works: The human body, in response to strenuous or unaccustomed physical activity, produces highly reactive oxygen species (ROS) known as free radicals that oxidize DNA, proteins, and lipids within cells increasing the risk for cellular damage as well as cellular death. Such free radical production has been positively correlated with loss of muscle function, release of muscle enzymes, and histological evidence of damage and muscle soreness. Dietary antioxidants such as vitamin E serve as scavengers, repairing the damage free radicals leave behind and providing added protection against oxidative stress, thereby aiding the integrity of a multitude of physiological functions important to both health and performance.

Performance benefit: Athletes engaged in intense or prolonged endurance training may be able to better adapt to elevated levels of oxidative stress, therefore facilitating quicker recovery times.

Research: In 2001 researchers at Oregon State University determined that extreme endurance activity, in particular a 50 km (31 mi) ultramarathon on rugged terrain, resulted in nearly a 2-fold increase in markers of oxidative stress and a consequent rise in the rate of vitamin E usage compared to rest (Mastaloudis et al.). The same researchers, as part of a 2004 double-blind, placebo-controlled study, discovered a combined antioxidant supplementation protocol of 400 IU of vitamin E and 1,000 mg of vitamin C taken daily over 6 weeks before a 50 km (31 mi) ultramarathon competition offered profound protection to the runners (Mastaloudis et al.). Blood markers of oxidative stress in the supplemented group were significantly lower compared to the placebo group, whose blood markers simulated those of heart attack victims. While these studies demonstrate an attenuation (reduction) of exercise-induced oxidative stress with enhanced vitamin E intake and consequent storage, the translation to the rate of postexercise recovery and other parameters of sport performance has been trending toward negative reviews (Takanami et al., 2000; McGinley, Shafat, & Donnely, 2009).

Common usage: Because vitamin E is found in limited amounts in foods that generally are high in fat, such as vegetable oil, some may find it difficult to consume the Dietary Reference Intake (DRI) of 15 mg (22.4 IU) from food alone without increasing fat intake above recommended levels. Thus, many foods are fortified with a synthetic form of vitamin E, also known as all-rac-alpha tocopherol or dl-alpha-tocopherol, though it is not well absorbed by the body. The highest-quality vitamin E supplements are naturally derived, containing only RRR-alpha-tocopherol, also labeled as d-alpha-tocopherol; a supplementation dose of 200-400 IU/day is indicated to help protect against exercise-induced oxidative damage.

Supplement Fact

To convert from mg to IU:
    Natural: 1 mg of alpha-tocopherol = 1.49 IU
    Synthetic: 1 mg of alpha-tocopherol = 2.22 IU

To convert from IU to mg:
    Natural: 1 IU of alpha-tocopherol = 0.67 mg
    Synthetic: 1 IU of alpha-tocopherol = 0.45 mg

Health concerns: Both deficiency and toxicity have rarely been reported in humans although older athletes as well as those with celiac or muscle-wasting diseases are thought to be at greater risk for deficiency; symptoms include neurological damage, muscle weakness, loss of appetite, and anemia. The Food and Nutrition Board of the Institute of Medicine has established an upper tolerable intake level of 1,500 IU/day (1,000 mg/day) for all forms of alpha-tocopherol. Doses above this may cause bleeding problems.

Additional performance benefits: Athletes training or competing at altitudes above 6,000 feet may benefit from enhanced oxygen usage with increased vitamin E intake.

Whey Protein

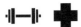

aka *whey protein isolate, whey protein concentrate, whey protein hydrosylate*

What it is: Whey is a type of protein that is found in milk. Milk contains two main proteins: whey and casein. About 20% of total protein in milk is whey. Whey protein concentrate is the most common form used in supplements. Whey can be purchased in powdered forms or is often added to pre- and postworkout supplements.

How it works: Protein is vital for all athletes. Proteins contain amino acids that provide the building blocks for the synthesis or building of muscles, connective tissues, enzymes, and hormones. These amino acids can also act as signalers and initiators of the building pathways in the body. Whey is unique in that it contains higher amounts of specific amino acids known to initiate and signal these pathways. Using whey protein in relation to nutrient timing before and after exercise is believed to enhance muscle recovery and building.

Performance benefit: Because of its role in building new tissues in the body, whey has a variety of benefits. These include gains in lean body mass, which can also lead to improved strength and power; improved recovery from training; and less muscle soreness. Whey can also be used to maintain muscle mass in energy- or calorie-restricted states during weight loss. Finally, the amino acids that are found in whey are also believed to enhance and strengthen the immune system.

Research: Much research has centered on the use of whey protein before and after workouts and shows positive results. Consuming protein before workouts can lessen protein breakdown, improve protein balance, lessen markers of muscle breakdown such as creatine kinase, and spare muscle glycogen. Postworkout, whey protein has also been proven to be successful in stimulating protein synthesis and assisting in restoration of muscle glycogen stores when consumed in combination with carbohydrate (Morifuji et al., 2010). Whey protein's superiority to other proteins at these times is somewhat less understood but appears to be due to whey's characteristic as a fast-digesting protein and its superior composition of amino acids. One study found whey to be superior to casein and soy in stimulating protein synthesis after resistance training (Tang et al., 2009); similar results were found by Pennings and colleagues in 2011. More research is needed to confirm whey's superiority; however, recent research trials suggest this is true. Whey's proposed immunological benefits are less understood.

Common usage: Whey can be incorporated into the diet of an athlete in many ways. Consuming 15-20 g of protein 1 hour before training and within 30 minutes after training are best to ensure benefits; consuming more than

20 g does not appear to provide further benefit (Moore, 2009). Whey also works synergistically in combination with carbohydrate. Various ratios of carbohydrate:protein can be used depending on the workout intensity and duration. Focus on 1:1 or 2:1 ratios for lower-intensity and shorter-duration training sessions and 3:1 or 4:1 ratios for longer-duration, higher-intensity sessions. Data are still limited in terms of which type of whey protein is best; however, there is little current evidence to suggest that any type of whey (WPC, WPI, or WPH) is superior to another (Hulmi et al., 2010).

Health concerns: High-protein diets do not appear to pose any health concerns; however, athletes need to understand that excessive intakes of protein could mean they are underconsuming other important nutrients such as carbohydrate, healthy fats, and nutrient-dense fruits and vegetables.

Willow Bark

aka *salicin, Salix, salicylates, Salix purpurea L., Salix daphnoides Vill., Salix fragilis L*

What it is: Since ancient times the leaves and bark of willow trees have been used to treat pain, fever, and inflammation. *Salix purpurea L., Salix daphnoides ViLL.,* and *Salix Fragilis L.* make up the species of trees used. Willow bark contains compounds known as salicylates, of which salicin is most common and believed to produce beneficial effects. Salicin is a precursor of salicylic acid, which is used to produce acetyl salicylic acid, the chemical name of aspirin. As a result, willow bark is often considered a natural form of aspirin and is used to treat similar conditions for which aspirin is prescribed. Willow bark is often found in dietary supplements used in the treatment of joint pain. In the late 1980s and early 1990s it was often used in combination with ephedrine and caffeine to produce supplements marketed as so-called natural fat burners.

How it works: Although many of the beneficial effects of willow bark are believed to result from salicin, other compounds such as polyphenols and flavonoids are speculated to contribute. This thought is backed by scientific studies, which confirm the benefits of willow bark go beyond its content of salicin. While the exact mechanism is unknown, willow bark's components are believed to inhibit inflammatory cytokines and inflammatory enzymes such as COX-2 (Nahrstedt et al., 2007; Shakibaei et al., 2012). Many experts believe that the additional benefits of polyphenols and flavonoids found within willow bark make it superior to aspirin (Vlachojannis, Cameron, & Chrubasik, 2011).

Performance benefit: Athletes suffering from muscle and joint pain resulting from training, competition, or injury may benefit from the pain-reducing and antiinflammatory effects of willow bark.

>*continued*

Willow Bark >*continued*

Research: Schmidt and colleagues (2001) conducted a study on the use of willow bark in patients with osteoarthritis. A dose equivalent to 240 mg of salicin significantly improved pain experienced by patients in the study. A 2009 meta-analysis of willow bark for musculoskeletal pain concluded that moderate evidence exists for the effectiveness of willow bark extract (Vlachojannis Cameron, & Chrubasik, 2009). No research exists to provide evidence for the use of willow bark as a fat burner. Willow bark is approved by the German Federal Health Agency for use in the treatment of fever, joint pain, and headaches. Willow bark appears to be effective; however, more research is needed to provide insight into the potential mechanisms and confirm optimal doses needed to provide benefit.

Common usage: Currently, a dose of willow bark equivalent to 240 mg of salicin is recommended for treatment of inflammation and pain associated with muscle soreness and joint pain.

 Health concerns: Use of willow bark is contraindicated in individuals with known aspirin allergy. Willow bark can also interact with anticoagulants and blood thinners. Products containing willow bark seldom contain warnings related to aspirin sensitivity and potential drug interactions. Consumers should proceed with caution.

Winter Cherry

(see *Withania somnifera*)

Withania Somnifera

aka *ashwagandha, winter cherry, Indian ginseng*

What it is: *Withania somnifera* (WS) or ashwagandha is a green shrub found in drier parts of the Middle East. WS is commonly used in Ayurvedic medicine, a traditional medical system of India, for treatment of a wide range of ailments.

How it works: WS contains several steroidal alkaloids, withanolides, and sitondosides, which are believed to be the active constituents of the plant. To date 12 alkaloids, 35 withanolides, and several sitondosides are known to exist in various parts of the plant. The diverse number of constituents is believed to be responsible for the multiple medicinal properties of WS (Kulkarni and Dhir, 2008).

Performance benefit: The suggested benefits of WS for athletes include antiinflammatory, adaptogenic (improved ability to adapt to various types of stress), anabolic, antioxidant, and immunomodulatory effects.

Research: Multiple studies on mice have reported WS to have an antistress effect on chronic fatigue induced by forced swimming (Archana & Namasivayam, 1999; Dhuley, 2000). Malondialadehyde (MDA) levels were measured as a marker of stress, and supplementation significantly lowered MDA levels. WS has also been shown to improve enzymatic activity of antioxidant defense enzymes such as superoxide dismutase, catalase, and glutathione peroxidase especially in stress-induced conditions. In another study, WS provided a significant protective effect against footstrike-induced stress in mice (Bhattacharya, 2003). Sumantran and colleagues (2008) found WS to produce antiinflammatory effects in osteoarthritic cartilage. Few studies have evaluated the impact of WS on human performance. Sandhu and colleagues (2010) found that WS at a dose of 500 mg/day for 8 weeks increased velocity, power, and $\dot{V}O_2$max. No training program was implemented during the 8-week period, and sample sizes were relatively low. The only other known study of humans found 5 g/day of WS to improve resting cortisol and enzymatic antioxidant activity in cigarette-smoking men and psychologically stressed men. Unfortunately, no studies to date have specifically evaluated the benefits of WS in athletes or how it might affect an athlete's ability to overcome stress induced by training.

Common usage: The most common method of supplementation used in human trials is 20-50 mg/kg of body weight supplemented once daily. Research studies with mice have used higher dosages of 50-1,000 mg/kg of body weight without any known toxic effects.

Health concerns: Extensive toxicological studies have demonstrated the plant to be nontoxic in a wide range of reasonable doses, and no herb-herb or herb-drug interactions have been reported (Kulkarmi and Dhir, 2008).

Wood Spider

(see *devil's claw*)

Wu-Chu-Yu

(see *rutaecarpine*)

Yeast-Derived Beta Glucan

(see *beta glucan*)

Z

Zinc

♥ ✚

aka *zinc acetate, zinc aspartate, zinc gluconate, zinc methionine, zinc monomethionine, zinc oxide, zinc sulfate*

What it is: An essential mineral derived naturally from such dietary sources as oysters, meat, seafood, and eggs as well as from fortified foods and supplements, zinc plays a key role in several aspects of cellular metabolism, aiding the functioning of over 300 enzymes in the body. While zinc is found in virtually all cells of the body and is especially abundant in muscle tissue, there is no specialized storage system for the mineral, making daily intake necessary to avoid deficiencies. Athletes may need to consume more zinc than the general population to help offset mineral losses via sweat seen during physical training. Zinc is often combined with magnesium and vitamin B6 to form a supplement cocktail known as ZMA, which stands for zinc magnesium aspartate (see the following entry).

How it works: Zinc plays a key role in a wide range of biological functions important to sport performance, including muscle energy production and protein synthesis. Many scientists believe zinc's involvement in energy metabolism to be an important determinant of an athlete's endurance capacity, with suboptimal levels triggering premature fatigue during exercise. Additionally, because blood testosterone levels are in part regulated by zinc, a deficiency may hinder gains in muscle mass and strength. Carrying antioxidant qualities, zinc may also help reduce postexercise free radical activity, thereby promoting recovery. Perhaps zinc's most recognized role, however, is as an immune booster, facilitating the production of immune system cells important to fighting off infection and maintaining the health of an athlete during training and competition.

Performance benefit: Zinc may help enhance recovery by aiding tissue repair postworkout and protecting immune functionality, especially in deficient athletes.

Research: A 2005 double-blind, randomized crossover study on healthy men found poor dietary intake of zinc over 9 weeks at levels of 3.8 mg/day, or less than 50% of the current RDA for adults, to compromise zinc status, impair metabolic responses to exercise, and significantly reduce peak oxygen uptake; this culminated in an 11% decline in total work capacity during submaximal exercise when compared to a supplemental zinc protocol that incorporated 18.8 mg/day over 9 weeks (Lukaski, 2005). The performance effects on a nondeficient population, have not been confirmed although some scientists believe zinc supplementation aids the short- and long-term health of an athlete by enhancing antioxidant activity. A supplementation protocol of 22 mg of zinc/day over 12 weeks in football players

>continued

(de Oliveira et al., 2009) and a shorter protocol of 8 weeks for elite wrestlers (Kara et al., 2010, 2011) have been shown to do just that, decreasing markers of oxidative stress and consequent free radical damage to cells important to immune functionality postworkout.

Common usage: The current RDA for zinc in adult men and women (19+ years) is 11 mg and 8 mg, respectively, with pregnancy and lactation in women increasing needs to 11 mg and 12 mg. Many experts believe intense sport training to warrant an increase in intake to 25-30 mg/day. Deficiencies are generally corrected at doses of 30-40 mg/day. Zinc should not be taken with high-fiber or dairy-containing foods, which can impair absorption. Due to malabsorption and excretion issues, athletes at heightened risk for a zinc deficiency and thus most likely to benefit from supplementation include strict vegetarians, senior athletes (60+ years), those carrying the sickle cell trait, pregnant and lactating women, and those having undergone gastrointestinal surgery (e.g., gastric bypass) or experiencing digestive disorders such as Crohn's disease, ulcerative colitis, and irritable bowel syndrome.

Health concerns: Consuming large doses of zinc, especially above the current upper limit of 40 mg/day, increases risk for copper deficiencies and altered iron status as well as such symptoms as nausea, vomiting, fatigue, neuropathy, and metallic taste.

Additional performance benefits: Female athletes may be treated to reduce symptoms associated with premenstrual syndrome (PMS) by supplementing with zinc, according to preliminary research from Baylor College of Medicine in Houston. The research showed significantly lower levels of zinc among women with PMS during the luteal phase (13 days preceding) of menstruation (Chuong & Dawson, 1994).

Zinc Magnesium Aspartate (ZMA)

What it is: Zinc magnesium aspartate (ZMA) is a nutritional supplement that has been popular for a number of years. Its main ingredients are the minerals zinc and magnesium; however, various proprietary blends can be found that include additional B vitamins, herbs, and plant sterols. ZMA is marketed to athletes wanting to increase lean body mass, improve sleep and recovery, and enhance testosterone levels.

How it works: Research has identified that zinc deficiency results in low testosterone levels. Impaired actions of the gonadotropin-releasing hormone, luteinizing hormone, and follicle-stimulating hormone and alterations in enzyme activity related to testosterone conversion appear to be the main mechanisms responsible. Magnesium intake affects the secretion of insulin-like growth factor 1(IGF1) and increases testosterone bioactivity. However, its relationship with anabolic hormones such as testosterone in men has not been studied. It is known that magnesium has a variety of diverse roles in the body affecting over 300 metabolic reactions, which include hormonal function. A possible relationship between magnesium levels and cortisol may exist.

Performance benefit: Athletes may benefit from the enhanced levels of testosterone promoting gains in muscle strength, size, and power. In addition, athletes may benefit from the immune-enhancing effects of zinc and its role in the function of superoxide dismutase, a powerful cellular antioxidant.

Research: A research study in 2000 created a lot of initial excitement related to ZMA as it was found that supplementation of semiprofessional athletes resulted in an increase in plasma testosterone of approximately 30% and significantly improved muscle strength (Brilla & Conte). However, another study on weightlifters in 2004 found ZMA was not effective and did not produce any significant differences in anabolic or catabolic hormones, body composition, strength or anaerobic capacity (Wilborn et al.), Similar results were found in a 2009 study specifically evaluating the effectiveness of ZMA on increasing testosterone levels. No other studies have found zinc, ZMA, or similar supplements to produce any significant benefits (Koehler et al., 2009). ZMA supplementation shows promise only if zinc and magnesium deficiencies exist.

Common usage: Research studies have evaluated supplements containing approximately 30 mg of zinc and 450 mg of magnesium. The RDA for zinc is roughly 11 mg for men and 8 mg for women. The RDA for magnesium is 420 mg for men and 320 mg for women.

Health concerns: Consuming large doses of zinc, especially above the current upper limit of 40 mg/day, increases risk for copper deficiency and altered iron status as well as symptoms of nausea, vomiting, fatigue, neuropathy, and metallic taste. Side effects associated with magnesium include diarrhea, abdominal pain, and nausea.

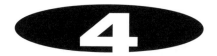

Supplements for Special Groups and Environments

> Unfortunately, everything the experts tell us about diet is aimed at the whole population, and we are not all the same.
>
> *The Scientist* magazine

In a perfect world, there would be a one-size-fits-all strategy for nutrition, but the human body is an intricate machine and dictates otherwise. Every athlete has a different genetic makeup. Some may have food sensitivities and intolerances that create extra performance obstacles unless nutritionally tended to. Others may have metabolic disorders, such as diabetes, that require close monitoring for success in sport. Dramatic differences can exist just based on sex. Furthermore, some athletes make lifestyle choices, such as vegetarianism, that affect nutritional needs. Additionally, every sport has physiological demands that affect an athlete's nutritional requirements. If injury occurs, a specialized nutrition approach may enhance recovery especially if surgery is involved. Even Mother Nature can dictate that a nutrition plan be adjusted for environmental conditions. Thus, a customized approach to nutrition and dietary supplementation recommendation is essential. In this section, we discuss specialized nutrition and dietary supplement recommendations for athletes across the age spectrum and for female athletes, athletes recovering from injury, athletes with diabetes, athletes with food allergies, vegetarian athletes, athletes competing in heat and cold, and athletes competing at altitude.

Athletes With Specialized Concerns

Athletes with specialized concerns are encouraged to work closely with a registered sport dietitian as well as their doctor in developing both a nutritional and supplemental plan best suited towards their needs. A list of qualified dietitians can be found at www.eatright.org.

Master's-Level Athletes

Older athletes must be aware of the physiological changes that result from aging in order to maintain high levels of performance. For the endurance athlete, peak performance is typically maintained until age 35. Performance in strength and power sports peaks and declines slightly sooner, peaking in the mid- to late 20s and beginning to decline in the 30s. Master athletes commonly experience weight gain, slowed recovery time, nagging injuries, and diminished performance. Even so, many master athletes continue to conquer the physiological changes of aging and beat younger competitors: Examples include 42-year-old Yekaterina Podkopayeva, a female Russian distance runner who ran 1,500 meters in under 4 minutes, and marathoner Jack Foster, who conquered 26.2 miles (42.2 km) in 2:19 at the age of 41. As simple as it may sound, peak performance for all ages relies on two factors: smart training and proper nutrition.

Performance Obstacles

A number of physiological changes are responsible for decreases in performance. Impacts on endurance performance have found significant declines in maximal aerobic capacity ($\dot{V}O_2$max), roughly 5%-10% per decade after age 30. $\dot{V}O_2$max is the main contributor to declines as lactate threshold and exercise economy are well maintained. These changes are the result of reduced cardiac output, a product of maximum heart rate and stroke volume. Maximum heart rate declines at a rate of 0.7 beats per year with age starting in early adulthood. Mild decreases in stroke volume are observed in older endurance athletes, who typically have stroke volumes that are roughly 80%-90% of the volume typical for younger trained counterparts. There is still considerable debate whether performance declines are a result of aging or a reduction in the intensity and amount of training typically practiced by older athletes. It has been found that drops in total weekly running distance of approximately 15 miles (24 km) may cause $\dot{V}O_2$max to drop by 2.4%. The loss of muscle mass with aging can also affect $\dot{V}O_2$max. A loss of 3 kg (6.6 lb) of lean body mass can drop $\dot{V}O_2$max 4.5%. Unfortunately, the understanding of the impact of aging on strength and power athletes is less complete. Most significantly for these types of athletes, aging is associated with losses in muscle mass and a decline in the number of fast-twitch muscle fibers. As a result, reductions in speed, strength, and power occur. Metabolic changes within the muscle such as enzyme activity and alterations in the ATP- creatine phosphate energy system can also negatively affect anaerobic exercise. Master's-level athletes should take heart in knowing that although several physiological systems begin to decline with age, these systems are still very adaptable and responsive to training. Both strength and power and endurance master athletes can achieve significant improvements in performance through training. Research related to declines in performance is limited as very few athletes have the time and ability to continue to train at the same intensities and volumes, making it difficult for scientists to conclusively understand the effects of aging on performance.

Other important changes associated with aging include declines in resting metabolic rate (RMR), which can result in increased body fat and weight gain. RMR decreases by about 10% from early childhood to adulthood and another 10% from adulthood to the 60s. Several factors have been shown to directly influence RMR: thyroid hormones, genetics, body or environmental temperature, and stress. Other factors related to RMR are body surface area, total body weight, lean body mass, sex, age, and aerobic fitness. Of these factors, there seems to be the strongest correlation between lean body mass and RMR. When metabolically active muscle tissue is lost and replaced with metabolically inert adipose or fat tissue, RMR inevitably declines. Fortunately, RMR can be kept elevated by master athletes who continue to train at high levels while meeting individual nutritional needs.

More than 25 million people in the United States alone are affected by osteoporosis, leading to as many as 1.5 million bone fractures per year. Bone fractures occur when the calcium stored within the bones is lost, causing the bones to become porous. With aging, there is a progressive decline in calcium content in the bones that begins around age 30, increasing risk for stress fractures and development of osteoporosis. Other risk factors that exacerbate the aging effect on bone include smoking, excessive caffeine or alcohol intake, inactivity, and poor nutrition. Women tend to be more affected by osteoporosis, especially in menopause when levels of estrogen, a bone-protecting hormone, are significantly reduced. In fact, it is estimated that one-third of all women will experience osteoporosis-related fractures in their lifetimes (Riggs and Melton, 1992). Fortunately, bone health can be maintained with a healthy lifestyle, including proper training and a healthy diet.

Aging also affects the immune system. Decreased resistance to infections, increased inflammation, autoimmune activation, lower immune surveillance, and lower vaccination efficiency are all recognized immunological changes. Proper nutrition and certain nutraceuticals (foods that may elicit medical benefits) addressed in this book may assist in preventing some of these changes.

Finally, changes to joint structures and connective tissues can result in pain, dysfunction, and higher rates of inactivity in master's-level athletes. Cartilage, a flexible connective tissue found in many joints, often degenerates over time, a change often responsible for pain and dysfunction. Certain dietary supplements appear to protect against this degeneration.

Nutritional Recommendations

Nutrition can have a significant impact in delaying changes associated with aging. Calorie, or energy, needs of master's-level athletes are often lower due to drops in resting metabolic rate and lower intensities and volumes of training.

The Harris Benedict formula represented in the following equation, which takes into consideration height, weight, age, and sex, is often used to estimate RMR. Consequent daily energy requirements can be estimated by multiplying RMR by an activity factor based on daily physical activity (see table 4.1). Individuals desiring to gain or lose weight should increase or decrease calculated energy needs by 500 calories for a 1 pound (0.45 kg) weight gain or loss per week. Adjustments for weight loss should not exceed 1,000 calories (or 40% of estimated caloric needs) as catabolism of muscle tissue will occur, leading to a compromised metabolic efficiency.

Males: 88.362 + (4.799 × height) + (13.397 × weight) – (5.677 × age)

Females: 447.593 + (3.098 × height) + (9.247 × weight) – (4.330 × age)

Height in centimeters; weight in kilograms; age in years

TABLE 4.1 Activity Factors

Activity factor	Description	Multiply RMR by
Very light	Extremely sedentary; largely bed rest	1.2-1.3
Light	No planned activity; mostly office work	1.5-1.6
Moderate	Walking or stair climbing during the day	1.6-1.7
Heavy	Planned, vigorous activities	1.9-2.1

Protein intake can assist in preventing losses in muscle mass and RMR. The needs for protein are greater for older adults, and intense training can further increase these needs. Fat and carbohydrate intake are also important, however recommendations for older athletic populations do not differ from those for younger athletes. Table 4.2 provides a useful guide for determining macronutrient needs based on time spent training each day. It is difficult to make specific macronutrient recommendations as need varies significantly between individuals and can be manipulated to achieve specific athletic goals. It's best to consult a registered sport dietician to devise a specific macronutrient plan.

Adequate nutrient timing of macronutrients, especially protein and carbohydrate, is essential for older populations. Consuming a small amount of protein (5-15 g) and carbohydrate (15-30 g) before exercise can assist in limiting muscle damage and immune suppression during exercise.

The needs for certain vitamins and minerals also increase with age. Vitamin D is essential for the prevention of many chronic diseases and for immune system and muscle function. It can be produced from exposure to sunlight; however, the body's ability to produce vitamin D from this exposure

TABLE 4.2 Estimated Daily Macronutrient Needs

Daily training schedule			
	1 hour or less	**1-2 hours**	**2-3+ hours**
Carbohydrate (55%-70% of total calorie intake)	3 g/lb (3 g/0.45 kg) body weight	4 g/lb (4 g/0.45 kg) body weight	5 g/lb (5 g/0.45 kg) body weight
Protein (12%-15% of total calorie intake)	0.55 g/lb (0.55 g/0.45 kg) body weight	0.65 g/lb (0.65 g/0.45 kg) body weight	0.75 g/lb (0.75 g/0.45 kg) body weight
Fat (20%-30% of total calorie intake)	0.5 g/lb (0.5 g/0.45 kg) body weight	0.5 g/lb (0.5 g/0.45 kg) body weight	0.5 g/lb (0.5 g/0.45 kg) body weight

decreases with age and makes supplementation essential. Vitamin B12 has a variety of functions, including red blood cell production, DNA synthesis, and nerve function. All are vital for optimal muscle function and performance. B12 requires a special protein produced in the GI tract, known as intrinsic factor, in order to be absorbed. Production of intrinsic factor decreases with age, limiting the ability of the body to absorb B12 and increasing requirements. The need for the antioxidant vitamins C and E can also increase with age; research supports the added supplementation of these vitamins for providing protection against free radicals and preventing some of the declines in immune system function associated with aging. Adequate calcium intake is important in preventing the loss of calcium from bone and the development of osteoporosis. Iron, thiamin, riboflavin, folate, niacin, and vitamin A are also noted as commonly being consumed in inadequate amounts. A daily multivitamin and multimineral supplement with additional antioxidants will serve as a nutrition insurance agent. Research results for any added benefit of nutritional supplementation remain controversial.

Supplement Options

In many cases certain dietary supplements are more or only effective in older populations. Addressing some of the physiological changes associated with aging through nutrition and dietary supplements can assist in preventing declines in function and performance (see table 4.3). Following is a list of physiological changes important for older athletes to consider and potential supplements to address these changes.

- Preservation of lean body mass
- Immune support
- Joint support
- Antioxidant defense
- Skeletal health

TABLE 4.3 Supplement Options for Master's-Level Athletes

Supplement	Potential benefit	Dose recommended
Whey protein	Preserves muscle mass	Can be used as a protein source at meals or snacks to achieve a daily protein intake of 0.55-0.9 g/lb (0.55-0.9 g/0.45 kg) body weight/day; 16-25 g postexercise
Casein protein	Preserves muscle mass	Can be used as a protein source at meals or snacks to achieve a daily protein intake of 0.55-0.9 g/lb (1.2-2 g/kg) body weight/day; 20-30 g supplemented before bed
Egg protein	Preserves muscle mass	Can be used as a protein source at meals or snacks to achieve a daily protein intake of 0.55-0.9 g/lb body weight/day (16-25 g); postworkout
Leucine	Preserves muscle mass	.014-.02 g/lb (0.03-0.045 g/kg) of body weight pre- and postexercise
Branched-chain amino acids	Preserves muscle mass	6-14 g/day; ratio of leucine, valine, isoleucine: 4:1:1
Arginine	Preserves muscle mass	2-9 g/day; multiple doses
HMB	Preserves muscle mass	3 g/day; multiple doses
Glutamine	Supports immune system and preserves muscle mass	5-15 g/day; 1.5-5 g pre-, during, and postexercise or throughout the day
Fish oils	Support immune system and preserve muscle mass	1-3 g EPA and DHA/day
Vitamin D	Supports immune system and preserves muscle mass	2,000-5,000 IU/day
Vitamin B12	Prevents deficiency	25-100 mcg/day
Probiotics	Supports immune system	250 million to 20 billion organisms; 2.5-20 CFU (colony forming units) per day
Curcumin	Provides immune system and joint support	500 mg-3 g/day
Ginger	Provides immune system and joint support	0.5-2 g/day; consumed in 2 doses
Avocado soybean unsaponifiables	Supports joints	300 mg/day
Glucosamine	Supports joints	1,500 mg/day
Chondroitin	Supports joints	800-1,200 mg/day
MSM	Supports joints	1,500-3,000 mg/day (500-1,000 mg 3×/day)
SAMe	Supports joints	1,200 mg (400 mg 3×/day)
Vitamin C	Provides antioxidant defense	100-500 mg/day
Vitamin E	Provides antioxidant defense	200 mg/day
Zinc	Supports immune system	10-20 mg/day
Calcium	Supports skeletal health	1,200 mg/day

Child and Adolescent Athletes

Young athletes must understand that peak speed, strength, power, muscle size, and endurance will take years of well-structured training to achieve. Expectations for these attributes should be realistic. A high school athlete taking a dietary supplement hoping to look like his or her favorite professional body builder will be disappointed with the results unless coaches and parents help athletes understand and have realistic expectations. Young athletes should also be aware that in many cases it is impossible to achieve the same results without illegal performance-enhancing drugs. Adolescence refers to the period of life before the development of secondary sex characteristics. For the preadolescent or adolescent athlete, food is the foundation of fueling. Dietary supplements will not be effective without a proper base of nutrition, hydration, and strategic fueling.

Performance Obstacles

Proper growth and development of the neurological, skeletal, and muscle systems are the primary performance concerns for younger athletes. Peak muscle mass is typically reached between the ages of 16 and 20 in females and 18 and 25 in males. Bone formation is also achieved in the early 20s but can vary significantly between individuals; females typically achieve skeletal maturity 2 to 3 years before males. Young athletes can benefit from resistance training at early ages; however, maximum gains will be developed postadolescence. During adolescence, males experience a 10-fold increase in testosterone, which significantly enhances gains in muscle mass, strength, power, and speed. Child and adolescent athletes should focus on developing proper movement and sport-specific motor skills. As they mature through puberty and adolescence, they can focus on developing the strength and power needed to optimize performance. Focusing on strength and power development before adolescence will not be effective because the athlete will lack the levels of important anabolic hormones needed for optimal development.

Nutritional Recommendations and Supplement Options

It can be difficult for coaches and parents to know when and what types of supplements to recommend for younger athletes. Parents, coaches, and athletes must understand that dietary supplements are only designed to compliment a well-planned diet of whole foods. Food sets the foundation; supplements can then be used to provide additional benefit. This foundation of food for the youth athlete is built on the following five guidelines.

   1. **Meeting calorie or energy needs:** In order to optimize growth and development of the various biological systems during development, nutrition

is of utmost importance. In particular, young athletes must focus on consuming adequate amounts of calories, or energy. This can be difficult because of the busy schedules and significant amount of time that many youth spend practicing, training, and simply being active. Calculating exact caloric needs for youth athletes is difficult as much individual variability exists. However, the Harris Benedict equation provided earlier that is used to determine resting metabolic rate is a good place to start. Macronutrient needs for fats, carbohydrates, and protein in youth are similar to those of adult athletes.

2. **Consume a balanced and varied diet:** All types of food provide a variety of nutrients essential for athletes (see chapter 3 for discussions of many of these nutrients). Fruits and vegetables are rich in many vitamins and minerals; they also contain natural nutrients that function as antioxidants. These foods provide natural sources of quercetin, resveratrol, vitamins, minerals, and more. Dairy foods provide a valuable source of protein, calcium, and vitamin D. Lean meats and proteins are rich in iron, zinc, B12, B6, protein, and amino acids (glutamine, arginine, leucine, branched-chain amino acids). Finally, healthy fats such as olive oil, fish oil, nuts (almonds, walnuts, peanuts), coconut milk, flaxseed, and borage oil contain fatty acids that can benefit health and function of cells within the body. It is evident that athletes and especially young athletes must develop a solid food foundation before considering dietary supplements. By consuming a balanced and varied diet, athletes will ensure they are consuming adequate amounts of vitamins and minerals. Iron, vitamin D, and calcium are the most common nutritional deficiencies reported in children and adolescents; however, deficiencies in magnesium, phosphorus, and vitamins A, C, and E have also been noted.

3. **Nutrient timing:** All athletes regardless of age will optimize training and performance through proper fueling before, during, and after exercise. Recommendations for young athletes are similar to those for adults. Specific guidelines can be found in table 4.4.

4. **Hydration:** Consuming adequate amounts of fluids throughout the day and during exercise is important. Sweat rates for preadolescent children are lower than those of adolescent and adult athletes; however, when adjusted for size and body mass, losses are similar. The impacts of dehydration on performance are also similar between young and adult athletes: As little as a 1% loss of fluid can equate to a drop in physical performance. Young athletes should aim to consume 6 ml/lb (6 ml/0.45 kg) of body weight for each hour of exercise. For a 60 lb (27 kg) athlete, this would equate to 12 oz (0.35 L)/hour or 3 oz. (0.09 L) every 15 minutes; for the 100 lb (45 kg) athlete, the comparable amount would be 20 oz (0.59 L)/hour or 5oz. (0.15 L) every 15 minutes. Electrolytes are also important in assisting in fluid absorption. A combination of water and carbohydrate-electrolyte drinks should be used during exercise to help prevent dehydration. Water is sufficient when consumed in combination with food containing sodium and other electrolytes.

TABLE 4.4 Supplement Options for Youth Athletes

Supplement	Potential benefit	Recommended dose (4- to 8-year-olds)	Recommended dose (9- to 13-year-olds)	Recommended dose (14- to 18-year-olds)
Calorie-replacement shakes and bars	Assist in meeting energy needs and promote weight gain	Varied depending on diet and calorie needs	Varied depending on diet and calorie needs	Varied depending on diet and calorie needs
Protein supplements (whey, casein, egg)	Assist in meeting protein needs and with nutrient timing	Used as a source of protein at meals and snacks to assist in meeting daily protein needs 0.55-0.9 g/lb (1.2-2 g/kg) of body weight, 15-25 g consumed pre- and postworkout	Used as a source of protein at meals and snacks to assist in meeting daily protein needs 0.55-0.9 g/lb (1.2-2 g/kg) of body weight, 15-25 g consumed pre- and postworkout	Used as a source of protein at meals and snacks to assist in meeting daily protein needs 0.55-0.9 g/lb (1.2-2 g/kg) of body weight, 15-25 g consumed pre- and postworkout
Biotin	Enhances energy metabolism	12 mcg/day	20 mcg/day	25 mcg/day
Folate	Supports RBC formation, DNA synthesis, and protein metabolism	200 mcg/day	300 mcg/day	400 mcg/day
Niacin	Enhances energy metabolism; supports healthy skin, nervous system, and digestive tract	8 mg/day	12 mg/day	14-16 mg/day
Pantothenic acid	Enhances energy metabolism	2 mg/day	4 mg/day	5 mg/day
Riboflavin	Enhances energy metabolism	600 mcg/day	900 mcg/day	1,000-1,300 mcg/day
Thiamin	Enhances energy metabolism and supports nervous system function	600 mcg/day	900 mcg/day	1,000-1,200 mcg/day
Vitamin A	Protects vision, provides antioxidant and immune support, stabilizes cell membranes, and supports growth and repair of tissues	1,333 IU/day	2,000 IU/day	2,000 IU/day
Vitamin B12	Supports RBC formation, DNA synthesis, and neurological function	1.2 mcg/day	1.8 mcg/day	1.8 mcg/day
Vitamin C	Provides antioxidant and immune support, enhances collagen formation, and improves absorption of iron	25 mg/day	45 mg/day	45 mg/day

>continued

TABLE 4.4 *(continued)*

Supple-ment	Potential benefit	Recommended dose (4- to 8-year-olds)	Recommended dose (9- to 13-year-olds)	Recommended dose (14- to 18-year-olds)
Vitamin D	Assists in protein synthesis, provides immune support, and promotes bone health	600-1,000 IU	600-1,000 IU	1,000-2,000 IU
Vitamin E	Provides antioxidant support	10.5 IU/day (7 mg/day)	16.5 IU/day (11 mg/day)	22.4 IU/day (15 mg/day)
Calcium	Supports skeletal health and muscle contraction	1,000 mg/day	1,300 mg/day	1,300 mg/day
Chromium	Enhances insulin sensitivity	15 mcg/day	25 mcg/day	25 mcg/day
Copper	Supports health of bones, muscle, and blood vessels	440 mcg/day	700 mcg/day	900 mcg/day
Iodine	Supports thyroid function	90 mcg/day	120 mcg/day	150 mcg/day
Iron	Supports RBC function	10 mg/day	8 mg/day	11-15 mg/day
Magnesium	Assists in bone formation, nerve transmission, enzyme homeostasis, and muscle contraction	130 mg/day	240 mg/day	360 mg/day
Manganese	Assists in the forma-tion of connective tissue and bones and in fat and carbohy-drate metabolism	1.5 mg/day	1.9 mg/day	1.9 mg/day
Phosphorus	Supports develop-ment of the skeletal system	500 mg/day	1,250 mg/day	1,250 mg/day
Potassium	Controls electrolyte and fluid balance	3,800 mg/day	4,500 mg/day	4,500 mg/day
Selenium	Provides antioxidant and immune function support	30 mcg/day	40 mcg/day	55 mcg/day
Sodium	Controls electrolyte and fluid balance	1,200 mg/day	1,500 mg/day	1,500 mg/day
Zinc	Supports growth and provides immune system and antioxi-dant support	5 mg/day	8 mg/day	9-11 mg/day
Choline	Assists in neurotrans-mitter synthesis and cell signaling	250 mg/day	375 mg/day	400-550 mg/day
Omega-3 fatty acids	Supports brain and neuromuscular devel-opment and immune function	0.5-1 g/day of EPA and 0.5-1 g/day of DHA	1-3 g/day of EPA and 1-3 g/day of DHA	1-3 g/day of EPA and 1-3 g/day of DHA

5. **Eating consistently:** Developing a daily nutritional routine that consists of consuming 5-6 balanced meals or snacks throughout the day will help young athletes ensure they are getting adequate calories, protein, fat, carbohydrates, vitamins, and minerals.

If a young athlete wants to begin taking a dietary supplement, parents and coaches should be comfortable with vitamins, minerals, calorie replacements, protein powders, and fish oils. These are supplements that can assist athletes in meeting some of the nutritional guidelines mentioned above. However, if the athlete is looking at more advanced supplements containing creatine, beta-alanine, amino acids, herbs, caffeine, prohormones, or other ingredients, caution is warranted. The American College of Sports Medicine (ACSM) has recommended explicitly that anyone younger than 18 should not take creatine because possible side effects in the young are not known. Despite this recommendation, it's reported that 5%-8% of all 10-18 year olds report having used creatine (Nemet & Eliakim, 2009). Taking this into consideration, the following criteria might assist parents, coaches, and younger athletes in understanding when it would be appropriate to begin supplementing with some of these more advanced products. Before doing so, nutritional needs through foods must be met, and the athlete should be habitually practicing the five guidelines mentioned previously.

Child and Adolescent Athlete Criteria for Using Dietary Supplements

1. The athlete has a solid food foundation and is consistently practicing sport nutrition principles of adequate calorie intake, nutrient timing, consumption of a balanced and varied diet, adequate fluid and electrolyte intake, and consistent fueling.

2. The athlete has reached full maturity and is nearing the end of adolescence.

3. The athlete has consistently trained and used a resistance-training program or structured endurance-training program for 2 consecutive years.

The second criterion is that the athlete has reached full maturity and is nearing the end of adolescence. As mentioned previously, optimum levels of anabolic hormones such as testosterone are needed before an athlete can begin to realize his or her maximum performance potential. Most dietary supplements aim to assist athletes during training by enabling them to work at higher intensities, delay fatigue, or enhance recovery. As a result, most athletes will make substantial improvements once full maturity is reached, and their bodies can respond to a proper training program. Initially, the athlete should respond in such a positive way to the training program itself that a dietary supplement is not essential. If this is not the case, it may be advisable for parents and coaches to consult with a strength and conditioning specialist in the development of a proper training program rather than turn to dietary supplements. Most dietary supplements can provide only mild benefits ranging from 3% to 15% improvement; the majority result in only a 3%-5% improvement.

All athletes have a genetic ceiling above which further improvement cannot be achieved. This genetic ceiling takes years (10-15+) to achieve, and improvements in performance get smaller the more well-trained the athlete becomes. As a result, athletes might benefit most from using dietary supplements once they have seen the greatest improvements from training, and improvements in performance become smaller and more difficult to achieve.

These criteria can assist parents, coaches, and athletes in making decisions about when and which supplements to consider. The A-Z guide in chapter 3 can provide athletes with added information on effective and high-quality supplements to consider for various performance variables.

Female Athletes

Since the passage of Title IX—the law that expanded opportunities for females in sports over 40 years ago—the number of females participating in various sport activities has skyrocketed. For example, it is no longer unusual to see female finishers outnumber male finishers in major marathons. Such milestones are a cause for celebration. However, in order to truly embrace the obvious benefits of sport participation, it is essential that athletes and coaches alike understand the unique nutritional demands that face females during sport training and competition.

Performance Obstacles

Perhaps the most important nutritional consideration for women engaged in sport is an increased need for energy in the form of carbohydrate, fat, and protein to help fuel the working body. Inadequate caloric and macronutrient intake is a major problem among female athletes who tend to be much more concerned about their weight than male athletes, especially those engaged in sports where leanness is emphasized: gymnastics, dance, diving, and distance running, among others. The sad irony is that female athletes are far more likely to achieve an optimal performance physique by increasing their intake of appropriate nutrients than by enforcing unhealthy dietary restrictions. They will also perform much better in practice and competition and recover more efficiently due to reduced muscle breakdown and injury.

Nutrition Note

If an athlete's energy (calorie) intake falls below 13 kcal/lb (13 kcal/0.45 kg) of fat-free mass/day, hormonal balance and functionality of other metabolic systems may significantly deteriorate, hurting both health and performance.

A negative energy balance, whether it is a subconscious result of failing to consume enough calories to offset the deficit incurred during training or a conscious effort to achieve a perceived ideal body weight, not only can compromise performance but is also a known risk factor for lower estrogen levels and amenorrhea, or the cessation of menstrual flow. In turn, low estrogen levels can hurt bone mineral density and predispose the female athlete to stress fractures as well as an increased probability for developing osteopenia and osteoporosis, also known as brittle bones. Further medical problems arise when weight-control behaviors become recognized diagnoses of eating disorders, including anorexia nervosa (severe energy restriction) and bulimia nervosa (binge and purge disorder). The combination of disordered eating, which conscious restriction of calories falls under, menstrual irregularities, and diminished bone health has been labeled the female athlete triad and is becoming an increasingly prevalent problem in sport (Torstveit and Sundgot-Borgen, 2005; Hoch, Stravrakos, and Schimke, 2007; Nattiv et al., 2007; Quah et al., 2009; Doyle-Lucas, Akers, and Davy, 2010; Thein-Nissenbaum and Carr, 2011; Arieli and Constantini, 2012).

Trigger Factors for Disordered Eating

1. Prolonged periods of dieting or weight fluctuations
2. Traumatic events such as illness or injury, new coach, causal comments about weight, leaving home (college), failure at school or work, family problems, relationship issues, loss
3. Large increase in training volume and significant weight loss associated with increase in training volume
4. Belief that menarche (first period) has been reached too early
5. Early start of sport-specific training
6. Large discrepancy between self-denied ideal weight and ideal weight
7. Recommendation to lose weight without guidance
8. Social influences for thinness
9. Performance anxiety
10. Negative self-appraisal, generally as it relates to performance

Beyond a heightened risk for altered hormonal status and diminished bone health, female athletes, especially those following restrictive diets, are vulnerable to both macro- and micronutrient deficiencies that can result in fatigue, stunted growth (for adolescent athletes), poor immune function, loss of motivation, inability to concentrate, and significant declines in both strength and endurance. Several studies have found lower than recommended intakes for carbohydrate, which can significantly compromise glycogen stores and put an athlete at risk for the mental bonk and muscle-fatiguing wall, and for protein, which can inhibit strength gains as well as compromise muscle recovery and immune function (Rodriguez, Di Marco, Langley, 2009; Bilsborough and Crowe, 2003; Adam-Perrot et al., 2006). Iron is one of the most prevalent micronutrient deficiencies found in female athletes, partially due to restrictive energy intake that may include elimination of such iron-rich foods as red meat and dark meat (poultry). In addition, blood loss during menstruation along with a phenomenon known as exercise-induced hemolysis (red blood cells rupture when the foot strikes the ground) can cause hemoglobin (the protein that carries iron) levels to drop and can increase the risk for iron deficiency. Declines in both physical and cognitive performance have been demonstrated in female athletes with poor dietary intake of iron and especially iron deficiency anemia (blood deficiency) (Della Valle and Haas, 2011; McClung, 2012). Female athletes are also at increased risk for calcium, vitamin D, and zinc deficiencies; these nutrients play a role in building bone and muscle as well as supporting immune function (Gabel, 2006).

Another practice commonly employed by women trying to suppress hunger while dieting is to sip on calorie-free beverages such as water, tea, and diet soda—and consume large volumes of these beverages. Drinking excessive amounts of any type of fluid, especially water, outside of or during exercise, can cause blood sodium levels to drop, triggering a potentially fatal condition known as hyponatremia, or water intoxication, marked by one or several of the following symptoms: clear urine, muscle fatigue, pressure headache, dizziness, confusion, nausea, and vomiting. Coupled with sodium losses during exercise, female athletes, especially those new to endurance sports who may be on a race course for a longer duration, seem to be at greatest risk for hyponatremia and associated symptoms (Rosner and Kirven, 2007). Vulnerability may be further heightened during menstruation since both estrogen and progesterone hinder the function of the sodium-potassium pump, which helps maintain sodium levels and protect against hyponatremia.

Therefore, nutrition education for female athletes, especially during the formative preadolescent and adolescent years, becomes of paramount importance for prevention of health issues as well as success in sport.

Nutritional Recommendations

While the bulk of performance nutrition advice is not sex-specific, there are a few nutritional considerations that female athletes should pay particular attention to. For one, because women carry less metabolically active muscle tissue and, on average, 10% more body fat than their male counterparts, women's resting metabolic rates tend to fall about 5%-10% lower than men's. As a result, many health professionals believe energy and macronutrient calculations should focus on lean body mass (fat-free mass) versus total mass. Use of a body fat scale, even though error rate tends to be higher than other body fat–testing methods, can provide an estimate of fat-free mass for athletes and coaches to use to calculate needs.

Nonetheless, for both sexes, an energy intake that matches both resting and training metabolic needs, which will vary on a daily basis especially when comparing in- and off-season training protocols, and includes appropriate

TABLE 4.5 Calorie and Macronutrient Intake Recommendations for Athletes

Daily training	<1 hour	1-2 hours	2+ hours
Calories per lb (per 0.45 kg) fat-free mass	16-20	21-25	25-30
Carbohydrate g/lb (g/0.45 kg) fat-free mass	2.7-3.0	3.0-3.5	3.6-4.5
Protein g/lb (g/0.45 kg) fat-free mass	0.5-0.8	0.5-0.8	0.5-0.8

amounts of carbohydrate and protein (see table 4.5) is absolutely critical to performance success. Those athletes needing to drop body fat for health and performance reasons preferably will focus attention on this goal during the off-season. However, if an athlete wants to shed body fat during a competitive season, energy restriction should be limited to 500 calories/day, ideally outside of heavy training cycles. A registered dietitian, preferably a board-certified specialist in sport dietetics, can help determine a healthy body composition goal as well as develop a menu plan for successful achievement while maintaining peak performance during a competitive season.

As a general rule, female athletes should aim at consuming 4-6 closely calorie-matched meals throughout the day. The three staple meals (breakfast, lunch, and dinner) should include a balance that incorporates 25% protein (e.g., edamame, Greek yogurt, cottage cheese, eggs, lean beef, skinless poultry, fish), 25% starch (e.g., sweet potato, oats, quinoa, brown rice, corn, peas, legumes, 100% whole grain breads), and 50% color (fruits and vegetables) along with small doses of healthy fat (e.g., avocado, olives, nuts, seeds, fatty fish, vegetable oils). Avoidance of major food groups is highly discouraged as deficiency risks, including those common among female athletes (e.g., iron, calcium, vitamin D, zinc), tend to be heightened with food restriction. To improve iron intake, female athletes should include more animal protein such as beef in the diet. Plant sources of iron such as whole grains, fortified cereals, and legumes should be combined with foods rich in vitamin C (e.g., oranges) to aid iron absorption. To boost intake of bone-building nutrients, calcium and vitamin D, female athletes should aim to consume 3-4 servings of dairy or fortified dairy alternatives such as soy or almond milk (1 serving = 1 cup [0.24 L] milk, three-fourths cup [170 g] yogurt, 1 ounce [28 g] cheese, one-half cup [113 g] cottage cheese). To avoid a zinc deficiency and better support immune function and metabolism, inclusion of zinc-rich foods such as chicken breast, oysters, peanut butter, legumes, milk, yogurt, tofu (soy), and peanut butter is encouraged. It is also desirable to consume prepared foods with short, recognizable ingredient lists: Those failing to meet these criteria tend to be highly processed and generally score low on the nutrition grading scale—a system that grades foods on a scale of A to F based on overall nutrient density, with F being a failing score.

Additional calorie intake of about 100-250/hour is appropriate for most females and is warranted when training exceeds 90 minutes. Perhaps the most convenient method of replenishing lost fluids, electrolytes, and carbohydrate during prolonged sport activity is through a sport drink containing these nutrients. For aerobic activities lasting longer than 4 hours (e.g., long-distance cycling, walking a marathon), the addition of small amounts of protein (up to 5 g/hour) can help offset the hunger that creeps into the calorie-deprived body as well as possibly delay fatigue and speed recovery.

It is estimated that two out of every three female athletes walk around chronically dehydrated, which is a definite cause for concern since dehydration tends to be the primary dietary-contributing factor to poor performance. On the other hand, some female athletes drink excessive amounts of water throughout the day, which can promote hyponatremia. To maintain fluid balance, athletes should aim at drinking approximately half their body weight in fluid ounces each day, or so urine runs a pale or straw-like yellow (not clear) color. For example, a 150 pound (68 kg) woman would aim to consume 75 oz (2.2 L) of fluid (not just water)/day. An additional 4-8 oz (0.12-0.24 L) of fluid should be consumed every 15 minutes or so that body weight losses stay under 2% (e.g., 3 lb [1.4 kg] for a 150 lb athlete) during training. For training sessions lasting longer than an hour, a sport drink that contains carbohydrate, sodium, and other electrolytes to enhance fluid uptake is preferable to water.

Supplement Options

Because there is no research suggesting that supplementation with vitamins and minerals is beneficial to performance (except when an athlete has a deficiency of certain nutrients), the first line of defense for the female athlete—and any athlete for that matter—should always be via whole food intake. If a deficiency is detected by a doctor, therapeutic levels of specific vitamins and minerals in supplement form may help blood levels normalize and allow the athlete to regain optimal health and peak performance (see table 4.6). Female athletes without blood deficiencies yet who consistently fail to consume recommended daily intake amounts of key nutrients, especially iron, zinc, calcium, and vitamin D, through whole food intake may benefit from supplementation with a once-a-day multivitamin and multimineral supplement. Multivitamin and multimineral supplements generally provide lower doses (up to 100% of the current RDA) of nutrients and can serve as nutritional insurance for concerned athletes.

Injured Athletes

Sport-related injuries are common to athletes in all sports. Some injuries are much more serious than others; however, recovery from all types of injury can be improved with appropriate nutritional strategies. Athletes are constantly defying the norms in rehabilitation from injury. ACL reconstructive surgeries often required 12 months of rehabilitation 15-20 years ago; some athletes are now returning to play or compete in 6-7 months.

TABLE 4.6 Supplement Options for Female Athletes

Supplement	Potential benefit	Dose recommended
Beta-alanine	Helps protect against muscle acidosis and consequent fatigue during intense training	3.2-6.4 g/day
Calcium	Supports bone health; may help reduce cramping associated with PMS	Premenopausal: 1,000-1,200 mg/day Postmenopausal, adolescents: 1,500 mg/day
Carbohydrate	Enhances endurance	30-60 g/hour during prolonged training
Iron	Offsets losses seen with menstruation; facilitates oxygen delivery to working muscles and ATP energy production	Current RDA: 18 mg/day (Therapeutic doses for anemia generally range from 50 to 100 mg 3×/day for adult athletes.)
Magnesium	May help reduce cramping associated with PMS	100-350 mg/day
Tart cherry juice	Helps fight inflammation; aids recovery	12 oz (.35 L) taken 1-2×/day
Vitamin D	Supports bone health	600-800 IU/day
Whey or soy protein	Promotes nitrogen balance and recovery; protects against muscle breakdown when restricting calorie intake	0.5-0.8 g/lb (0.5-0.8 g/0.45 kg) fat-free mass
Zinc	Supports immune function and healthy metabolism	Current RDA: 8 mg/day (Therapeutic doses for deficiency generally range from 30 to 40 mg/day.)

Any type of tissue damage—muscle, tendon, ligament, cartilage, or bone—goes through distinct stages of repair. Immediately following injury, an important inflammatory response is initiated that can last from a few hours to several days (48-72 hours). This is a vital step toward optimal recovery and trying to prevent this response may be counterproductive. Following this phase is a period of repair and regeneration for the damaged tissue; it begins with the formation of scar tissue, which is later broken down and replaced by type II collagen. Over time, new tissue is formed, and repair is complete. Providing the body with essential nutrients to assist in these steps is essential.

Performance Obstacles

Some injuries require immobilization of muscles, joints, or bones for extended time to allow appropriate healing. This will result in significant losses in lean body mass in the muscles surrounding the immobilized joints. Other muscles not affected by injury will also be affected because the athlete's training program will be significantly altered as a result of injury. Preventing these losses in lean body mass is a key component to speeding recovery. In addition, athletes must provide the proper stimulation for muscle recovery. Tension and stress placed on the injured joint or muscle during rehabilitation will affect the formation and repair of new tissue. Initiating blood flow to the injured area will also assist in providing the adequate nutrients needed to speed healing.

Nutritional Recommendations

Injured athletes must first focus on calorie (energy) intake. A significant amount of protein synthesis and rebuilding of tissue takes place following injury, requiring additional calories. Many athletes significantly reduce caloric intake, believing their needs to be dramatically less as a result of decreased activity. While this is true, an injured athlete must be aware of his or her body's increased caloric need to facilitate regeneration. Depending on the severity of injury, caloric needs can increase by as much as 20% from injury alone. Inadequate caloric intake has been shown to reduce protein synthesis by as much as 19%; as a result, athletes not meeting calorie needs will have decreased ability to repair and regenerate muscle (Tipton, 2010). Athletes should also be aware that the calorie costs of using crutches are 2-3 times that of walking, further increasing needs. The Harris Benedict equation, presented earlier in the Master's-Level Athletes section, can be used to calculate resting metabolic rate based on height, weight, age, and sex. Injured athletes should calculate an adjusted RMR by multiplying RMR by an injury factor of 1.1-1.2. Once RMR-IFa (injury factor adjusted) is calculated, it can be multiplied by the activity factors in table 4.1 to calculate calorie needs.

Adequate protein intakes are also important. Proteins can assist in preventing the loss of muscle mass as well as initiate and provide the building blocks for repair and rebuilding of new tissue. While needs are elevated, an intake of 0.75-0.9 g/lb (per/kg) of body weight/day is sufficient. A balanced intake of macronutrients (fat, carbohydrate, protein) is important. As the intensity and duration of training activity significantly decrease, the need for carbohydrate is slightly reduced. Injured athletes should aim to consume 20%-25% of their calories from protein, 40%-45% from carbohydrates, and 30%-35% from healthy sources of fat. Healthy fats, including olive oil, mixed nuts (e.g., walnuts, almonds, pecans), avocados, coconut oil or milk, and flaxseeds or oil, can provide powerful fatty acids that limit inflammation and decrease pain in injured tissues. Injured athletes should also emphasize fruit and vegetable intake. Consuming a variety of colored fruits and vegetables will provide an array of nutrients with antioxidant and antiinflammatory benefits.

The benefits of nutrient timing experienced by noninjured athletes fueling before and after training also apply during injury and rehabilitative workouts. Rehabilitative exercise facilitates the use of injured muscles and joints, resulting in increased blood flow and delivery of nutrients. Providing important nutrients during these types of exercise will assist in delivering important nutrients to the injured site. Protein and carbohydrates should be consumed both before and after rehabilitative exercise. Due to the lowered intensity of this form of exercise, carbohydrate needs are decreased relative to those of noninjured athletes. A ratio of 3:1 or 4:1 carbohydrates to protein is often prescribed to noninjured athletes before and after exercise. This ratio can be reduced to 1:1 or 2:1 for injured athletes choosing lowered ratios of carbohydrates:protein depending upon the duration and intensity of rehabilitative exercise. It is important that injured athletes not eliminate carbohydrates from the diet, especially during these nutrient-timing windows. Carbohydrates both before and after exercise can limit stress and immune suppression during training and increase levels of the powerful anabolic hormone insulin.

Adequate intakes of vitamins and minerals are also needed. A clear relationship between zinc, vitamin C, vitamin A, and wound healing has been found (Tipton, 2010). In addition, intakes of calcium and vitamin D are also important. Injured athletes should focus on a balanced diet, emphasizing whole foods such as fresh fruits, vegetables, whole grains, dairy, lean proteins, and healthy sources of fat. These are the best sources of a wide array of nutrients needed for proper recovery. Athletes restricting certain food groups or consuming inadequate quantities of these food groups will not recover as optimally as those who eat a variety of whole foods.

Supplement Options

Dietary supplements can assist athletes in meeting additional nutritional needs during periods of injury. Following is a list of areas dietary supplements might target and benefit (see table 4.7 for specific guidelines).

- **Preservation of lean body mass:** Protein supplements, including calorie- or meal-replacement shakes and bars, can assist injured athletes in meeting elevated calorie and protein needs. Consuming them can also help ensure proper nutrient timing in relation to exercise. Branched-chain amino acids (BCAA), particularly leucine, the leucine metabolite HMB, vitamin D, and fish oils also have evidence to suggest benefits in preventing losses in muscle mass.

- **Joint support:** Glucosamine, chondroitin, MSM, avocado soybean unsaponifiables, and SAMe are all thought to provide benefits in the preservation of joints and prevention of pain. Mechanically, all promote the synthesis and limit the degradation of cartilage. There is little evidence to suggest these types of supplements would provide benefit to inflammation-related

TABLE 4.7 Supplement Options for Injured Athletes

Supplement	Potential benefit	Recommended dose
Protein supplements (whey, casein, egg)	Prevents muscle atrophy	Used as a source of protein at meals and snacks to assist in meeting daily protein needs 0.55-0.9 g/lb (1.2-2 g/kg) of body weight daily, 15-25 g consumed pre- and postworkout
Leucine	Prevents muscle atrophy	0.015-0.022 g/lb consumed pre- and postworkout
Branched-chain amino acids	Prevent muscle atrophy	6-14 g/day (ratio of leucine:valine:isoleucine = 3:1:1)
Arginine	Prevents muscle atrophy	2-14 g/day (7 g, 2× daily)
HMB	Prevents muscle atrophy	3 g/day (1.5 g, 2× daily)
Glutamine	Provides immune support and preserves muscle mass	5-15 g/day (7-8 g, 2× daily)
Omega-3 fatty acids	Preserves muscle mass and provides immune and joint support	1-3 g/day of EPA and DHA
Vitamin D	Preserves muscle mass and provides immune and joint support	2,000-5,000 IU/day
Calcium	Supports skeletal repair	1,200 mg/day
Copper	Supports repair and regeneration	100 mg/day
Vitamin C	Supports repair and regeneration	500-1000 mg/day
Zinc	Supports repair and regeneration	10-30 mg/day
Garlic	Antiinflammatory	2-4 g/day (600-1,200 mg of aged garlic extract)
Boswellia	Antiinflammatory	600-3,000 mg/day
Bromelain	Antiinflammatory	200-2,000 mg/day
Curcumin	Antiinflammatory	0.5-3 g/day
Ginger	Antiinflammatory	0.5-2 g/day
Tart cherry juice	Antiinflammatory and aids in recovery	12 oz. (350 mL) 1-2×/day
Quercetin	Antiinflammatory and aids in recovery	200-400 mg 2-3×/day
Glucosamine	Provides joint support	1,500 mg/day
Chondroitin	Provides joint support	800-1,200 mg/day
Avocado soybean unsaponifiables	Provides joint support	300 mg/day
Methylsulfonylmethane	Provides joint support	1,500-3,000 mg/day (500-1,000 mg 3× daily)
SAMe	Provides joint support	1,200 mg/day (400 mg 3× daily)

joint conditions such as tendonitis, with the exception of SAMe and avocado soybean unsaponifiables.

• **Anti-inflammatory:** While preventing inflammation within the first 48-72 hours appears counterproductive to injury repair, it is beneficial for speeding long-term recovery. Dietary supplements can often provide natural antiinflammatory protection.

Athletes With Diabetes

Diabetes is a metabolic disorder in which the body either fails to produce insulin (type 1) or is unable to use what is produced (type 2). Secreted by the pancreas, insulin influences the metabolism of all body fuels and regulates blood glucose (sugar), helping to facilitate muscle development, growth, and storage of fuel for energy use. Without insulin, sugar from food could not reach cells, causing muscle and fat stores to shrink, energy levels to plummet, and performance to suffer. People with type 1 diabetes are insulin dependent, meaning injection through a syringe or pump is necessary; those with type 2 diabetics, in many cases, can manage the disease with changes to diet and exercise. Due to the correlation between greater body fat and type 2 diabetes, athletes who have diabetes, especially those at the competitive or professional level where body fat levels tend to be low, are more apt to have type 1. The Centers for Disease Control and Prevention (2011) estimates that there are 18.8 million people in the United States who have been diagnosed with diabetes, with an alarming 23% and 21% rise in the incidence of type 1 and type 2 diabetes, respectively, in American youth from 2001 to 2009. By 2025, trends indicate that over 300 million people worldwide, athletes included, will have the disorder, making education regarding all treatment options, including potentially beneficial dietary supplements, essential.

> I'm not counting on a cure, but I'm not going to let this (type 1 diabetes) control me.
>
> Jay Cutler, NFL quarterback

Performance Obstacles

The primary goal of diabetes management is maintenance of optimal blood glucose levels, which is not always an easy feat for the athletes with diabetes due to the combined challenges of diminished or nonexistent insulin activity and the physical demands of training and competition. Both exercise-induced hypoglycemia (low blood sugar) and hyperglycemia (high blood sugar) are serious issues that athletes with diabetes face every time they compete. Athletes should monitor and log their blood glucose before, during, and after exercise to ensure levels remain in the normal range of 80-120 mg/dL, adjusting medications as necessary.

Drug Testing Warning

Insulin is on the current World Anti-Doping Association (WADA) List of Prohibited Substances and Methods. Therefore, in order to compete legally, athletes with diabetes who take insulin and are exposed to drug testing must complete a Therapeutic Use Exemption (TUE) form, found on the WADA website, before competition. See the WADA banned substances list from the References and Resources file at www. HumanKinetics.com/products/all-products/Athletes-Guide-to-Sports-Supplements-The.

The mere stress associated with sporting competition, including pre-event jitters and any trauma or injury during the event, can trigger a fight-or-flight hormonal response where blood glucose levels rise. For the athletes with diabetes, hyperglycemia can further ensue during exercise when glucose uptake by the muscles is decreased; this is due to inadequate insulin being available for transport coupled with increased glucose release from the liver. Outside of training, a high dietary intake of refined carbohydrates and sugar can also promote a negative blood sugar response. Left untreated, hyperglycemia can lead to a dangerous metabolic disturbance called ketoacidosis, where, in the absence of insulin, fatty acids are broken down to create ketones for energy production. This causes the pH of the blood to drop and the kidneys to work overtime trying to achieve homeostasis, which causes a plethora of problems detrimental to health and performance. Among these problems are dehydration, falling blood pressure often coupled with passing out, kidney failure, tachycardia (rapid heartbeat), blindness, poor wound healing, and damage to nerve endings. Thus, it is critical that athletes with diabetes make note of precompetition blood glucose levels to ensure personal safety. If blood glucose levels rise above 250 mg/dl, especially in the presence of ketosis, athletic participation is discouraged.

On the opposite end of the blood sugar spectrum, hypoglycemia ensues when uptake of blood glucose by the muscles during exercise exceeds that released by the liver or supplied from carbohydrate sources (e.g., sport drinks). Inadequate energy intake to support training demands, common among athletes following various dieting strategies to achieve a perceived ideal body weight for competition, may also trigger or exacerbate an episode. Furthermore, nearly all people with diabetes using insulin will experience a hypoglycemic episode at some point. Mild cases elicit hunger, fatigue, and dizziness, hardly a prescription for athletic success. In moderate or severe cases, these symptoms intensify and are often joined by poor concentration, shaking, cold skin, blurred vision, seizures, or loss of consciousness. Consequently, athletes with diabetes are encouraged to always carry emergency sources of sugar such as juice, glucose tablets, sport drinks, energy gels, energy chews, and raisins to combat hypoglycemia should such a situation arise during training or competition. An athlete with these symptoms should not return to competition until blood glucose rises to normal levels.

Nutritional Recommendations

Success in sport for any athlete, including those with diabetes, requires consuming adequate amounts of macronutrient energy (calories) to support daily training demands. A joint position statement issued by the ACSM, the American Dietetic Association, and the Dietitians of Canada (Rodriguez et al., 2009) offers general nutrient requirements for athletes, which include the following recommendations:

1. As a means to maintain optimal blood glucose levels and replenish depleted muscle glycogen stores during training, daily carbohydrate consumption should be 2.7-4.5 g/lb (2.7-4.5 g/0.45 kg) of body weight with the variations being dependent on the athlete's daily total energy expenditure, sport type, sex, and environmental circumstances. Low-glycemic and nutrient-dense carbohydrate sources such as whole grains, legumes, and whole fruits and vegetables are recommended for optimal blood sugar control (see table 4.8).

2. To promote nitrogen balance, daily protein consumption for endurance-trained athletes should fall between 0.5 and 0.6 g/lb (0.5-0.6 g/0.45 kg) of body weight. To allow for accretion and maintenance of muscle mass, strength-trained athletes should aim for a daily protein intake of 0.7-0.8 g/lb (0.7-0.8 g/0.45 kg) of body weight. High-quality protein sources include soy beans, eggs, fish, poultry, dairy foods, and meat. Protein supplements are rarely needed provided energy intake is adequate to maintain body weight and are highly discouraged for athletes with diabetes who have diminished kidney function.

3. Fat intake should round out an athlete's caloric demands; the majority should be derived from unsaturated sources such as fish oils, vegetable oils, nuts, seeds, and avocado.

4. While daily energy requirements are highly variable based on daily training as well as activity levels outside of training, recommendations range from 16 to 18 calories/lb (16-18 calories/.045 kg) of body weight for endurance athletes and 20-22+ calories/lb (20-22+ calories/0.45 kg) body weight for strength-trained athletes.

5. In addition to consuming the right quantity and balance of macronutrient energy, a key component of sport success for athletes with diabetes is proper supplementation with carbohydrate energy (calories) before, during, and after competition to help protect against exercise-induced hypoglycemia,

TABLE 4.8 Carbohydrate Intake Recommendations for Sport Activity

Type of activity	Blood glucose level	Carbohydrate intake recommendations	Example of snack
Short duration at low- to-moderate-intensity exercise (e.g., walk .5 mi [800 m], leisurely bike ride <30 minutes)	<80 mg/dL	30 g	Medium banana
	>80 mg/dL	10-15 g	One-half cup (.12 L) juice
Moderate intensity exercise (e.g., swim, jog, cycle for 1 hour)	<80 mg/dL	30 g + small amount of protein	One-half peanut butter sandwich
	80-180 mg/dL	10-15 g	1-2 figs
	180-300 mg/dL	No extra food	n/a
	300+ mg/dL	Exercise not recommended	n/a
High-intensity, strenuous exercise (e.g., racing, interval workout, scrimmaging)	<80 mg/dL	~50 g + some protein	Blend three-fourths cup (.18 L) nonfat milk with 2 tbsp nonfat Greek yogurt, 1 banana, one-half cup 113 g) mango.
	80-180 mg/dL	~30 g + some protein	1 banana sliced into one-half cup (113 g) nonfat Greek yogurt
	180-300 mg/dL	10-15 g + some protein	One-third energy bar (e.g., PowerBar)
	300+ mg/dL	Exercise not recommended	n/a

sustain peak levels of performance, and promote recovery. Because blood sugars can be affected by such factors as exercise intensity, exercise duration, time of day, environmental conditions, emotional stress or excitement, and absorption of insulin and dietary supplements, there is not a standard recommendation for athletes with diabetes. Therefore, frequent self-monitoring of blood glucose levels and maintenance of a journal that logs such data are important for determining an optimal dietary management plan for safe participation in the sport. Until a dietary management plan is created, general guidelines can be followed.

Preworkout Fueling

For exercise lasting less than hour, additional carbohydrates are generally not needed unless blood sugars are less than 100 mg/dL, in which case a small snack consisting of approximately 15-30 g of low-glycemic carbohydrates can be consumed to help prevent a hypoglycemic event. In preparation for aerobic exercise lasting longer than 1 hour, a more substantial meal is recommended unless blood sugars are over 200 mg/dL. For every hour before the start of exercise, athletes with diabetes should consume a well-balanced meal that includes approximately 30-50 g of carbohydrate. Adequate time should be allowed for digestion. As a general rule of thumb, 1 hour digestion time should be allotted for every 200-300 calories consumed preworkout. In addition, consuming approximately 16 oz (0.47 L) of fluids—water or a sport drink with less than 10% carbohydrate—within the hour leading up to exercise is also recommended.

Fueling During Competition

While supplementation with carbohydrate exerts the greatest benefit during prolonged exercise sessions (>60 minutes), athletes with diabetes whose blood sugars run low preworkout or whose insulin levels are too high may need to eat small amounts of carbohydrate during competition to avoid a hypoglycemic episode. Recommendations for carbohydrate fueling during exercise include consuming 30-60 g of carbohydrate each hour of exercise; carbohydrate needs for lower-intensity sports (e.g., golf) are approximately 50% lower (see table 4.9). Athletes with diabetes competing in endurance sports such as an Ironman triathlon may benefit from using multiple carbohydrate sources at intake levels up to 90 g/hour. The addition of small amounts of protein (up to 5 grams/hour) may enhance blood sugar control as well as stave off hunger during the later stages of aerobic competition. There is some evidence that treatment of corn starch with a heat-moisture process to create what is known as a SuperStarch, which is currently used in a sport nutrition product called UCAN, helps to optimize blood sugar control during exercise (Roberts et al., 2011). It's lower-glycemic response than other commonly used carbohydrate sources in sport foods makes it of potential benefit to athletes with diabetes.

Postcompetition Fueling

Consuming carbohydrate with small amounts of protein immediately postcompetition has been shown to significantly increase glucose uptake by the muscles as well as reduce postworkout muscle damage, thereby enhancing recovery. Athletes with diabetes may further benefit from prevention of late-onset hypoglycemia, which can occur up to 24 hours after exercise. In general, athletes should aim at consuming about 0.5 g of carbohydrate and 1/8 gram of protein/lb (0.5 g carbohydrate/0.45 kg and 1/8 g protein/0.45 kg) of body weight within 30 minutes after finishing an event. A simple, inexpensive option that fits these recommendations and is proven to aid recovery is low-fat milk. Those with diabetes may have to adjust their insulin accordingly depending on blood glucose level. Because glycogen repletion occurs at a rate of only 5%-7% per hour, those with diabetes should

TABLE 4.9 Carbohydrate Content of Select Sport Nutrition Products

Product	Carbohydrate content	Other ingredients
Sport drinks	**Per 8 oz (.24 L)**	
Accelerade www.pacifichealthlabs.com	14 g	Whey protein, electrolytes
Carbo-Pro Hydra C-5 www.sportquestdirect.com	18 g	D-ribose, electrolytes, beta-alanine, betaine
Clif Electrolyte www.clifbar.com	19 g	Electrolytes
Cytomax www.cytomax.com	15 g	Electrolytes
EFS Drink www.firstendurance.com	16 g	Electrolytes, amino acids, vitamin C, malic acid
Gatorade www.gatorade.com	14 g	Electrolytes
Hammer Heed www.hammernutrition.com	13 g	Electrolytes, L-carnosine, glycine, tyrosine
Hammer Perpeteum www.hammernutrition.com	18 g	Soy protein, electrolytes, L-carnosine, caffeinated flavors
Infinit Nutrition Run www.infinitnutrition.com	22 g	Electrolytes
Infinit Nutrition Ride www.infinitnutrition.com	26 g	Whey protein, amino acids, electrolytes
PowerBar Perform www.powerbar.com	17 g	Electrolytes
UCAN www.generationucan.com	15 g	SuperStarch, electrolytes, vitamin C
Energy gels	**Per gel packet**	
Accel Gel www.pacifichealthlabs.com	20 g	Whey protein, vitamin C, vitamin E, caffeinated varieties
Clif Shot www.clifbar.com	22 g	Electrolytes, vitamin A, vitamin C, caffeinated varieties
Gu Energy www.guenergy.com	25 g	Electrolytes, amino acids, caffeinated varieties
Hammer Gel www.hammernutrition.com	21 g	Electrolytes, amino acids, caffeinated varieties
Honey Stinger Gel www.honeystinger.com	29 g	Electrolytes, B vitamins, ginseng varieties
Infinit Napalm www.infinitnutrition.com	25 g	Electrolytes, caffeine
PowerBar Gel www.powerbar.com	27 g	Electrolytes, green tea extract, caffeinated varieties
Vega Sport Endurance Gel	22 g	Electrolytes
Energy chews	**Per 3 pieces**	
Clif Shot Blocks www.clifbar.com	24 g	Electrolytes, caffeinated varieties
Gu Chomps www.guenergy.com	22 g	Electrolytes, amino acids, antioxidants, caffeinated varieties
Honey Stinger www.honeystinger.com	12 g	Electrolytes
PowerBar Gel Blasts www.powerbar.com	15 g	Sodium citrate, caffeinated varieties

continue to consume additional carbohydrate-focused meals throughout the day until energy stores are replenished.

Supplement Options

The power that blood sugar control can have on the performance and health of athletes with diabetes cannot be emphasized enough. Premature fatigue and sluggishness brought on by a downward or upward swing in blood sugars are proven detriments to several aspects of performance, including recovery, as well as to the overall health of athletes with diabetes. Chronically elevated blood sugars can also cause permanent damage to nerves, triggering a burning sensation, numbness, tingling, and pain, most commonly in the legs and feet. Several dietary supplements are purported to help protect against such blood sugar swings and the consequent detriments associated with the stress of poor glycemic control.

Supplements That May Increase Blood Sugar	Supplements That May Decrease Blood Sugar
Caffeine	Alpha-lipoic acid
DHEA	Biotin
Fish oil (high doses)	Chromium
Ginkgo biloba	Fenugreek
Glucosamine sulfate	Fiber
Melatonin	Ginseng, American
Niacin	*Gymnema sylvestre*
Vitamin C (high doses)	Magnesium
	Thiamin
	Vanadyl sulfate
	Zinc

A key area of research is the impact of antioxidant supplementation on ameliorating damage from unstable oxygen molecules called free radicals that can increase in numbers to levels beyond the body's own defense capabilities during times of extreme stress, as often seen with strenuous exercise, especially in the presence of uncontrolled blood sugars. According to health scientists from Duke University Medical Center, poor control of blood glucose in itself can deplete the body's stores of antioxidant nutrients (Opara et al., 1999; Opara, 2004). Add the stress of intense training and competition, and athletes with diabetes may find themselves recovering poorly, getting sick, and experiencing some of the serious complications of diabetes such as nerve damage. Supplementation with antioxidants—vitamins C and E, coenzyme Q10, pycnogenol, resveratrol, quercetin, and alpha-lipoic acid—may help protect against these complications as well as aid recovery and performance, particularly during intense training cycles (Ansar et al., 2011; Brasnyo et al., 2011; Chao et al., 2009; Dakhale et al., 2011; Halmai et al., 2011; Gupta et al., 2011; Kobori et al., 2009; Koh et al., 2011; Porasuphatana et al., 2012; Sing and Jialal, 2008). Megadoses, especially with vitamin C, are contraindicated because they can actually elevate blood sugars as well as be of detriment to both performance and health.

B vitamins, which include thiamin, riboflavin, niacin, pantothenic acid, vitamin B6, biotin, folic acid, and vitamin B12, play in important role in production of enzymes that aid the conversion of glucose into energy. Furthermore, though not consistently supported in research, B vitamins may help protect an athlete against nerve ending damage associated with poor blood sugar control. Some research has shown the blood levels of certain B vitamins to be significantly lower in those with diabetes than in those without, making supplementation of possible benefit (Davis, Calder, and Curnow, 1976; Satyanarayana et al., 2011). For instance, blood levels of thiamin (B1) have been shown to be 75% significantly lower in those with diabetes due to increased clearance through the kidneys (Luong and Nguyen, 2012). Vascular health, regardless of glucose homeostasis, is ultimately hurt because of increased inflammation (Page, Laight, and Cummings, 2011. People with diabetes also seem to be at greater risk for deficiencies in pantothenic acid (B5) (Tahiliani and Beinlich, 1991). Biotin (B7) plays an especially important role in helping the body use glucose, its basic fuel. Administration of supplemental biotin has been shown to prevent the development of insulin resistance in skeletal muscles, thereby aiding the transport of glucose energy to muscle and fat cells (Sasaki et al., 2012). Of important note, high doses of niacin (B3) may increase blood sugars, possibly making adjustment of insulin dosing necessary with supplementation.

Perhaps the most studied mineral as it relates to the treatment and maintenance of diabetes, especially type 2, is chromium, which facilitates the transportation of glucose into cells by enhancing the action of insulin. A chromium deficiency, thought to be more prevalent among people with diabetes, impairs the body's ability to use glucose, compromising energy levels and increasing the need for insulin. Therefore, supplementation is purported to help, particularly in diabetics who are chromium deficient (Singer and Geohas, 2006). Magnesium and zinc are two additional minerals of pronounced importance to diabetics. Levels of magnesium, one of the most abundant minerals in the body, are known to be depleted with insulin use (Rosner and Goefien, 1968). Lowered magnesium levels can negatively affect glucose homeostasis as well as increase risk for muscle cramping, making supplementation of potential merit for athletes with diabetes. Deficiencies in zinc, which plays an integral role in the regulation of insulin production and consequent glucose use by muscle and fat cells, are also more common among those with diabetes, likely due to a reduced rate of intestinal absorption (Chooi, Todd, and Boyd, 1976; Huber and Gershoff, 1973). For this reason, zinc supplementation may be of potential benefit.

Finally, though evidence from well-controlled studies has not been conclusive, vanadium or vanadyl sulfate carries insulin-like properties that appear to help enhance the delivery of glucose energy to the muscles, making it another mineral of potential merit for athletes with diabetes (Crans, 2000; Willsky et al., 2011).

Several additional ingredients, including dietary fiber, American ginseng, cinnamon, flaxseed, fenugreek, taurine, garlic, and *Gymnema sylvestre,* have shown promise in promoting glucose homeostasis through improvements in insulin sensitivity and consequent decreases in blood sugars (Bartlett and Eperjesi, 2008; Benzie and Wachtel-Galor, 2011; Fabian et al., 2011; Lee and Dugoua, 2011; Moloney et al., 2010; Yeh et al., 2003). Because supplements are poorly regulated, and taking several may affect optimal glycemic control as well as interfere with kidney function, it is important that athletes with diabetes consult with physicians or registered dietitians (www.eatright. org) before implementing a supplementation protocol (see table 4.10). With an appropriate dietary management action plan, safe participation as well as achievement of personal performance goals are possibilities for athletes with diabetes.

Athletes With Food Allergies or Intolerances

The prevalence of food allergies has seemingly grown in the past several decades, with as many as 25% of adults believing that they or their children suffer from food allergies. Nevertheless, according to results from the National Health and Nutrition Examination Survey 2005-2006 (Liu et al., 2010), clinically proven diagnoses for true allergic reactions by an appropriate professional (board-certified allergist or immunologist who is a medical doctor) remain low, with only an estimated 2.5% of the US population affected. Slightly higher incidence numbers were reported for black subjects, male subjects, and children. Food intolerance, on the other hand, is much more common. Its associated gastrointestinal symptoms, including bloating, gas, diarrhea, and stomach cramping, present debilitating problems for many athletes. Thus, exploration of treatment options, including adjustments to whole food intake and possible introduction of dietary supplements, is important.

Performance Obstacles

When an allergy to a food or specific ingredient within a food product exists, an abnormal immune response occurs (see table 4.11). Initially, the food allergen triggers the production of substances called immunoglobulin E (IgE) antibodies, which cause particles found within large cells to release chemicals such as histamine that are responsible for the onset of inflammatory-oriented symptoms. These symptoms range in severity and generally

TABLE 4.10 Supplement Options for Diabetic Athletes

Dietary supplement	How it can help	Dose recommended
Alpha-lipoic acid	Lowers blood sugars; decreases nerve pain	150-200 mg 2-4×/day
B-complex with extra biotin	Improves metabolism of glucose	50 mg 3×/day
Carbohydrate	Prevents exercise-induced hypoglycemia (adjustment to insulin levels may be needed)	15-90 g/hour of exercise
Chromium picolinate	Lowers blood sugars; increases insulin sensitivity	150-200 mcg/day 3×/day with meals
Cinnamon	Lowers blood sugars	3-6 g/day
Coenzyme Q10	Lowers blood sugars; reduces oxidative stress associated with elevated blood sugars	60-80 mg/day
Fenugreek	Lowers blood sugars	5-30 g/meal
Fiber	Lowers blood sugars	Up to 50 g/day
Flaxseed	Lowers blood sugars	600 mg 3×/day of a flaxseed lignin extract
Garlic	Lowers blood sugars	300 mg (*Allium sativum*) 2× daily
Ginseng, American	Lowers blood sugars	1-3 g/day in capsule form or 3-5 ml 3×/day
Gymnema sylvestre	Lowers blood sugars; increases insulin sensitivity	200-250 mg 2×/day
Magnesium	Lowers blood sugars	250-500 mg 1-2×/day
Pycnogenol	Reduces oxidative stress associated with elevated blood sugars	50-200 mg/day
Quercetin	Lowers blood sugars	100 mg 3×/day
Resveratrol	Increased insulin sensitivity; reduces oxidative stress associated with elevated blood sugars	10 mg/day
Taurine	Facilitates the release of insulin	500 mg 2×/day on an empty stomach
Vanadium (vanadyl sulfate)	Lowers blood sugars; increases insulin sensitivity	No more than 1.8 mg/day
Vitamin C	Reduces oxidative stress associated with elevated blood sugars	1,000 mg/day
Vitamin E	Reduces oxidative stress associated with elevated blood sugars	200 mg/day
Zinc	Increases insulin sensitivity	30 mg/day

TABLE 4.11 Most Common Food Allergies

Child athlete		Adult athlete
Cow's milk	Shellfish	Fish
Eggs	Soy	Peanuts
Fish	Tree nuts	Shellfish
Peanuts	Wheat	Tree nuts

arise within a couple minutes although they can sometimes appear a few hours after consuming the allergen; the symptoms are thought to intensify postexercise. On the mild-to-moderate end of the symptom spectrum are hives (red, itchy skin), stuffy or itchy nose, sneezing, itchy or teary eyes, vomiting, stomach cramps, shortness of breath and asthma, diarrhea, and swelling of the tissue beneath the skin. On the severe end of the symptom spectrum, and indicative of a reaction known as anaphylaxis, are a tingling sensation in the mouth, swelling of the tongue and throat, wheezing, chest tightness, difficulty breathing, hoarseness, intense stomach cramping, vomiting, pale or red color to face and body, and loss of consciousness. If not treated immediately with an injection of adrenalin from an EpiPen, anaphylaxis can be fatal.

Unlike food allergy that is immunity based and can be life threatening, food intolerance relates to the inability of the digestive system to properly process a food ingredient, generally as a result of deficiencies in digestive enzymes such as lactose in milk, an imbalance of bacteria and yeast in the intestines, sensitivities to food additives and dyes, or reactions to naturally occurring chemicals in foods (see table 4.12). This can cause partially or undigested food to enter the bloodstream, which triggers the production of substances called immunoglobulin G antibodies (IgG) and onset of uncomfortable, yet not life-threatening, gastro-intestinal focused symptoms such as nausea, bloating, gas, stomach cramping, and diarrhea that can linger

TABLE 4.12 Common Food Intolerances

Ingredient	Food sources
Lactose	Dairy foods
Gluten	Wheat, barley, rye
Monosodium glutamate (MSG)	Meat, fish, poultry, many vegetables, sauces, soups, marinades
Sulfites	Red wine
Nitrites	Processed meats
Salicylate	Several fruits and vegetables, some cheeses, tomato paste, soy sauce, vinegar, some nuts, coffee, wine, beer, rum, jams, jellies, mint
Amines	Fish, cheese, some meats, bananas, avocados, mushrooms, chocolate, sauerkraut, soy sauce

as long as the food ingredient remains in the diet and certainly hinder an athlete's ability to perform at peak.

Athletes experiencing symptoms, especially those gastrointestinal driven, may be at greater risk for energy imbalances and consequent nutrient deficiencies that can cause performance to plummet. If diarrhea ensues, dehydration and electrolyte imbalances also can present serious risks to the athlete's performance, recovery, and overall health. Those with multiple food allergies and intolerances are generally instructed to avoid all food triggers and may, therefore, struggle to put together a menu plan that includes enough calories and nutrition to support training demands.

Nutritional Recommendations

Treatment of a food allergy or intolerance is as simple as limiting intake or eliminating the culprit food. The first step in discovering a food allergy or intolerance is to develop a list of suspect foods over a period of a month that, in one way or another, seem to trigger the onset of one or more unpleasant symptoms. Once this list is compiled, the suspect foods can be eliminated from the diet over the next month to see if the recorded symptoms disappear. After a month's period, one suspect food can be reintroduced into the diet to determine if symptoms reappear. A positive reaction will almost always manifest itself with one or more symptoms in coordination with a spike in heart rate. A board-certified immunologist, commonly referred to as an allergist, is the health professional most qualified to diagnose a food allergy and can confirm a food allergy by running a series of tests that generally includes a skin test. Upon confirmation from a doctor, the athlete is encouraged to consult with a registered dietitian, preferably one board-certified in sport dietetics, to help create a custom training menu that is allergy friendly and incorporates the right balance of nutrition to support peak performance.

Supplement Options

The National Center for Complementary and Alternative Medicine (NCCAM), an outreach of the National Institutes of Health, is responsible for investigating the effectiveness of alternative forms of allergy treatment, including dietary supplements. While avoidance of the culprit food is currently the only proven effective nutritional treatment for food allergies, preliminary evidence suggests that certain dietary supplements may help alleviate specific allergy-driven symptoms, such as gastrointestinal distress, inflammation, and asthma, making them of potential benefit for the affected athlete (see table 4.13).

Probiotics are one increasingly popular ingredient under investigation for the treatment of food-related allergies. Probiotics, also known as friendly bacteria or microorganisms within the gut, are found in such foods as yogurt and kefir as well as in dietary supplement form; they seem to help enhance the immune response by introducing beneficial bacteria into the gut. While research is still in an infancy state, a probiotic supplement containing at least 10 billion CFU of bifidobacteria species and lactobacillus species may be helpful for athletes with food allergies (Isolauri, Rautava, and Salminen, 2012; Fiocchi et al., 2012; Isolauri and Salminen, 2008).

Spices such as tumeric and ginger, easily added into the diet through their use in cooking, have demonstrated potent antiinflammatory properties that may help mute the inflammatory responses, including asthma, associated with allergic reaction (Maeda-Yamamoto, Ema, and Shibuichi, 2007; Zhou, Beevers, and Huang, 2011; Ghayur, Gilani, and Janssen, 2008). It has also been postulated that the apparent rise in food allergy and intolerance is associated with the modern diet that emphasizes omega-6 fatty acids versus omega-3 fatty acids, which is a recipe for inflammation. Research has found increased intake of omega-3 fatty acids from such sources as fish oil, flaxseed, and chia seed reduces symptoms associated with food allergies (de Matos et al., 2012).

Deficiencies in vitamin D, the sunshine vitamin, have recently been correlated with increased incidence of allergic diseases, including food allergy, asthma, and allergic rhinitis, with one study demonstrating a significantly higher prevalence of severe vitamin D deficiency in patients with allergic rhinitis than the normal population (30% versus 5.1%) (Arshi et al., 2012).

TABLE 4.13 Supplement Options for Athletes With Food Allergies and Corresponding Symptoms

Supplement	How it may help	Dose recommended
Boswellia serrata	Reduces inflammation; alleviates asthma symptoms	600-3,000 mg/day
Bromelain	Reduces inflammation; enhances action of quercetin	500 mg split into 3-4 doses and taken with meals
Folic acid	Lowers IgE antibodies; alleviates asthma symptoms	400 mcg/day
Ginger	Reduces inflammation	0.5-2 g/day
Omega-3 fatty acids (fish oil, chia seeds, flaxseed oil)	Reduce inflammation	EPA and DHA: 1-3 g/day (3:2 ratio) ALA: 3-5 g/day
Probiotics	Enhance immune function	Should contain >10 billion CFU of bifidobacteria and lactobacillus species
Quercetin	Reduces inflammation; alleviates asthma symptoms	200-400 mg 2-3 ×/day before meals
Tumeric	Reduces inflammation	500 mg-3 g/day
Vitamin D	Reduce inflammations; alleviates allergy symptoms	1,000-2,000 IU/day

Additional research is needed, however, to determine if supplementation is effective in alleviating symptoms. Folic acid, or vitamin B9, is another vitamin that may help suppress allergic reactions and lessen the severity of allergy and asthma symptoms, according to researchers from John Hopkins. Specifically, the study investigators found that people with higher levels of folate (the naturally occurring form of folic acid) had fewer IgE antibodies, fewer reported allergies, less wheezing, and lower likelihood of asthma. People with the lowest folate levels (<8 ng/ml) had a 40% greater risk of wheezing than people with the highest folate levels (>18 ng/ml) (Matsui and Matsui, 2009).

Quercetin, a dietary flavonoid found naturally within apple skin, has been shown to ameliorate allergy-driven inflammation, especially that associated with asthma, by lowering levels of IgE antibodies (Lee, Ji, and Sung, 2010; Chirumbolo, 2011). Bromelain, an enzyme found naturally in pineapple, enhances the action of quercetin and thus is commonly paired with quercetin in dietary supplements. *Boswellia serrata* is another ingredient that presents strong -antiinflammatory properties of particular promise for athletes with allergy-driven asthma (Ammon, 2006; Houssen et al., 2010).

While preliminary evidence demonstrates potentially beneficial applications of supplement ingredients for alleviating food allergies and corresponding symptoms, continued research is needed to confirm their effectiveness as well as determine optimal dosing for therapeutic use.

Vegetarian Athletes

There are a variety of well-balanced plant-based diets, which vary from exclusion of all animal products and byproducts (vegan) to exclusion of select animal products (semivegetarian, lacto-vegetarian, lacto-ovo-vegetarian). The health and performance benefits of plant-based diets are profound due to a generally higher intake of such cardioprotective nutrients as dietary fiber, folic acid, potassium, magnesium, and antiinflammatory phytonutrients as well as a lower intake of proinflammatory saturated fat. Indeed, for well over 100 years, there has been documentation of plant-eating athletes from all types of sporting competitions outperforming their meat-eating counterparts. Scott Jurek, for example, is an ultramarathoner and self-proclaimed vegan athlete who has racked up wins in many of the sport's most prestigious races, including Badwater (2005, 2006) and the Western States 100 Mile Endurance Run (1999-2005); in 2010 he set a new U.S. record for distance run in 24 hours with 165.7 miles (266.7 km) at the 24-Hour World Championships in Brive-la-Gaillarde, France. The plant-focused eating habits of successful athletes like Jurek, who chronicles his journey as a vegan athlete in his book *Eat & Run,* has garnered the attention of other athletes, leading to an increased number taking on a vegetarian approach to fueling performance.

Vegetarian Eating Explained

Semivegetarian: Includes some but not all animal-derived products, including meat, poultry, fish, seafood, eggs, and dairy foods.

Lacto-vegetarian: Includes dairy foods but excludes eggs, fish, seafood, and meat.

Lacto-ovo-vegetarian: Includes only dairy foods and eggs.

Ovo-vegetarian: Includes only eggs.

Vegan: Excludes all animal products, including eggs, dairy, and foods that include animal byproducts.

Performance Obstacles

A well-balanced diet containing adequate amounts of calories, protein, vitamins, and minerals is a proven component of an athlete's health and success in sport. Even so, many athletes struggle to strike the right nutritional balance to adequately meet the metabolic demands of training. This holds true especially for those following specialized dietary plans such as vegetarianism, where restriction of various foods can make nutritional planning more challenging and increase the risk for nutritional deficiencies. Numerous studies have demonstrated vegetarian diets to be deficient in several nutrients, including protein, iron, zinc, calcium, and vitamin B12 (Craig, 2009; Craig, 2010). The greatest risk for deficiency is with those athletes who restrict intake of animal foods as a way to control weight, a common practice among female athletes and athletes involved in sports such as running, where achievement of a perceived ideal body weight is thought to influence performance, as well as those athletes who simply lack the knowledge to be able to create a menu plan suitable to meet the demands of training and competition. The impact that a poorly implemented vegetarian menu plan can have on athletic performance cannot be overstated. Beyond nutrient deficiency, risks include unfavorable changes in metabolic efficiency, altered hormonal status, and diminished bone health, all of which can significantly compromise the health and performance of an athlete.

Unfavorable Changes in Metabolic Efficiency

Athletes can expend extraordinary amounts of energy during training and competition. In fact, it has been estimated that athletes require anywhere from 16-30 calories/lb (16-30 calories/0.45 kg) of lean body weight to meet the high demands of competitive sport. Energy needs in vegetarian athletes may be even higher since resting energy expenditure has been shown to be approximately 11% higher in vegetarians compared to nonvegetarians (Toth and Poehlman, 1994). Because vegetarians eat lots of high-fiber, low-fat foods (e.g., whole grains, fruits, vegetables), it is not uncommon to discover inadequate energy intakes in vegetarian endurance athletes, especially those expending greater than 1,000 calories/day. When energy expenditure exceeds intake by over 1,000 calories, there is significant catabolism of lean body mass, leading to a drop in metabolic efficiency and athletic performance. For those vegetarian athletes who have trouble keeping weight on, it is recommended to eat 6 or more medium-sized meals and snacks containing such energy-dense plant foods as nuts, avocado, dried fruit, and dairy products.

Altered Hormonal Status

There has been some concern that vegetarian athletes are at increased risk for altered hormonal status, especially for the sex hormones estrogen and testosterone. In a study of 8 male athletes, engagement in a lacto-ovo-vegetarian diet over a period of 6 weeks caused a slight decrease in total testosterone levels, although performance detriments were negligible (Raben et al., 1992). Similarly, female vegetarian athletes have reported lower circulating estrogen levels as compared to their meat-eating counterparts (Goldin et al., 1982). It is thought that the cessation of hormonal function is merely an energy-conserving adaptation to an energy-deficit profile, which can be caused by reduced energy intake or by a high energy expenditure from chronic, intense exercise, or by a combination of the two. In addition, some studies have found that those eating plant-based diets, with their high-fiber content, report greater loss of sex hormones in feces compared to nonvegetarian diets (Gorbach and Goldin, 1987). Furthermore, vegetarians tend to have lower intakes of protein, fat, and zinc compared to omnivores (Craig and Mangels, 2009). However, it is unclear whether hormonal function diminishes as a result of the food composition in a vegetarian diet or simply because of a reduction in total energy intake. Regardless of the cause, altered hormonal status can lead to serious health and fitness implications. Symptoms of altered hormonal status include fatigue, weight loss, frequent infections, decreased physical performance, diminished bone health, and increased injury. In order to maintain normal hormonal status, vegetarians should follow a well-balanced diet that meets individual energy needs.

Nutrient Deficiency

Beyond energy intake, adequate intakes of both macro- and micronutrients are critical to the health and performance of a vegetarian athlete. Protein is perhaps the most recognized nutrient of concern for vegetarians due to the incomplete nature and reduced digestibility of most plant sources of protein. With the exception of soybeans, milk, and egg whites, other vegetarian food choices lack some of the essential amino acids necessary for maximal tissue growth and repair. Most vegetarian foods need to be combined to attain all the essential amino acids; for example, tortillas and beans, rice and lentils, peanuts and wheat bread. Endurance-trained athletes require 0.5-0.6 g of protein/lb (0.5-0.6 g of protein/0.45 kg) of body weight; strength-trained athletes require 0.7 to 0.8 g of protein/lb (0.7 to 0.8 g of protein/0.45 kg) of body weight, which is approximately 150%-200% the U.S. RDA for protein intake. Additional amounts of protein are needed to replace the loss of amino acids during exercise and to help repair exercise-induced muscle damage that occurs during weight-bearing activities such as running. The World Health Organization (WHO) suggests that vegetarian endurance athletes consume 110% of their calculated protein requirement because of the reduced protein digestibility of plant foods, attributable to the high-fiber content of such foods. Vegetarian diets providing adequate energy and a variety of protein-containing plant foods will supply all the essential amino acids needed for efficient protein metabolism, thereby enhancing recovery from exercise and helping to prevent muscle injury.

Micronutrients of particular concern to vegetarian athletes include calcium, vitamin D, vitamin B12, iron, and zinc. Calcium and vitamin D become especially vulnerable nutrients for vegetarians who do not consume dairy products. A chronically low calcium intake, especially when combined with an inadequate energy intake, is associated with decreased bone mineral density, leading to elevated risk for bone fracture (Talbott et al., 1998; Zanker and Swaine, 1998; Myburgh et al., 1990). Because vitamin D enhances the intestinal absorption of calcium, low serum levels (<40 ng/ml) can also increase risk for fracture (McCabe, Smyth, and Richardson, 2012). In addition, a calcium deficiency may play a part in muscle cramping and weakness during exercise since calcium plays a critical role in normal muscle function (Yu-Yahiro, 1994). Recommended intake of calcium ranges from 1,000 mg to 1,500 mg and 600 to 800 IU for vitamin D depending on the individual. Good nondairy sources of calcium include calcium-fortified foods, calcium-processed tofu (4 oz [113 g] = 145 mg), almonds (1 oz [28 g] = 332 mg), legumes (1 cup [227 g] = 90 mg), and collard greens (0.5 cup [113 g] = 179 mg). Vitamin D is found in fortified dairy foods as well as fatty fish.

Vitamin B12, which is present naturally only in animal products, is essential for maintaining healthy red blood cells and nerve fibers. Vegetarians who restrict calorie intake may be at elevated risk for a deficiency, leading to premature fatigue during exercise and potential nerve damage. Furthermore, a relationship between poor vitamin B12 status in vegetarians and increased bone turnover and risk for fracture has been demonstrated (Hermann et al., 2009). Fortunately, the U.S. RDA (2.4 mcg) for vitamin B12 is very small and quite easy to attain through such fortified plant sources as soy milk, nutritional yeast, and breakfast cereals.

Iron, a trace mineral, is a major component of the body's red blood cells, or hemoglobin, whose role is to carry oxygen to various body tissues, including muscle, for use during aerobic activity. A blood deficiency in iron may lead to premature fatigue during exercise due to lack of oxygen transport to working muscles. While iron is found extensively in several plant foods, the absorption is reduced by 20% compared to the iron found in animal products (Hurrell, 1997). Therefore, the risk for iron deficiency is increased in vegetarian athletes even if total iron intake meets the U.S. RDA of 10-15 mg. For added absorption of vegetarian iron sources, consume those with foods rich in vitamin C, such as orange juice.

Along with iron, zinc deficiency tops the list of the most common dietary deficiencies among vegetarian athletes. This is likely due in part to urinary and sweat losses during heavy training and the fact that plant sources of zinc (e.g., legumes, whole grains, wheat germ, fortified cereals, nuts, tofu, miso) are not absorbed as efficiently as animal sources of zinc (LuKaski, 1995). A study of female distance runners discovered that 50% fell below the recommended daily intake for zinc (12 mg/day), which may lead to an altered zinc status (Duester et al., 1989). An altered zinc status will compromise immune function as well as basal metabolic rate and thyroid hormone levels, which can have a major impact on performance and health (Wada and King, 1986). Fortunately, data from the U.S. Department of Agriculture suggests that zinc status can be maintained within normal limits with a vegetarian (lacto-ovo) diet that includes such zinc-rich foods as beans, milk, yogurt, tofu, and peanut butter (Hunt, Matthys, and Hohnson, 1998).

Diminished Bone Health

Although the prevalence of osteoporosis, or brittle bones, has not established in the athletic population, scientists believe that vegetarian athletes may be at elevated risk due to energy imbalances, low calcium intake, and hormonal aberrations. In fact, over a period of just 1 year, an athlete with a restrictive eating pattern (often the case with vegetarians) may develop osteopenia, increasing the risk for stress fractures 8-fold (Pettersson et al., 1999; Bennel et al., 1995). Generally consistent with a low energy intake is low dietary calcium intake, especially in athletes who do not consume dairy. Dietary restriction of calcium over a mere 9-week period has been shown to elevate the rate of bone turnover and consequent loss of bone mass, also leading to increased risk for stress fractures (Talbott, Rothkopf, Shapses, 1998). Related to energy imbalances are hormonal imbalances, which also elevate the risk for stress fractures in athletes. In order to prevent loss of bone mass and consequent stress fracture, vegetarian athletes are encouraged to consume an energy-sufficient diet that includes a variety of calcium-rich foods.

Nutritional Recommendations

As the popularity of plant-based diets increases among athletes, the risk for poorly planned diets and consequent nutritional deficiencies also increases. A negative energy imbalance not only compromises metabolic efficiency but also seems to negatively affect hormonal status, bone health, and nutritional intake of protein, calcium, vitamin B12, iron, and zinc. Subsufficient intakes of these nutrients will have a profound negative effect on health and endurance performance. However, an athlete can reap many benefits, both performance based and health based, from a balanced vegetarian diet. The following tips offer a framework for achieving a healthy vegetarian lifestyle:

• **Achieve energy balance by consuming enough calories to meet training demands.** The average athlete requires anywhere from 16 to 30 calories/lb (16-30 calories/0.45 kg) of body weight to meet the high demands of endurance training; vegetarian endurance athletes may need about 10% more. To meet the demands of endurance training, vegetarian athletes are encouraged to eat 6 or more medium-sized meals or snacks containing such energy-dense plant foods as nuts, avocado, dried fruit, and dairy products.

• **Keep in touch with your hormones.** Despite popular belief, absence of hormones, specifically loss of a menstrual cycle for female athletes, does not mean that training is going well. For male athletes, low testosterone levels also can be problematic for bone density and performance. Listen to your body. If you are feeling tired, training is not going well, and illness becomes common, your hormones may be out of whack. Try reducing your training load or adding more energy-dense foods to your daily meal plan to see if normal hormone function returns.

• **Include a variety of protein-containing plant foods throughout the day.** The average athlete requires 0.5-0.8 g of protein/lb (0.5-0.8 g of protein/0.45 kg) of body weight daily to allow for efficient tissue growth and repair. Vegetarian athletes benefit from an estimated 10% greater amount due to the reduced digestibility of plant proteins.

• **Don't skimp on bone-building nutrients.** Vegetarians should include 3-4 servings of dairy (e.g., 1 cup [.24 L] skim milk, soy milk, almond milk, three-fourths cup [170 g] Greek yogurt, one-half cup [113 g] nonfat cottage cheese) to fulfill daily calcium needs.

• **Pump up the iron.** Recommended daily allowances of iron can be fulfilled on one day by consuming one-half cup (113 g) firm tofu and one-half cup (113 g) lentils, for example. Plant sources of iron are absorbed better when taken with vitamin C.

• **Enhance dietary intake of vitamin B12.** While additional amounts of B12 will not enhance oxygenation of blood, B12 is essential for maximal energy and normal nervous system function. Good vegetarian sources include fortified soy milks, meat analogs, and breakfast cereals.

• **Zinc up.** Help keep the bugs away: Consume a well-balanced vegetarian diet that includes lentils, beans, whole grains, nuts, and soy.

Supplement Options

While dietary supplements should never serve as a crutch to a poorly planned diet, there are several nutrients found primarily in animal-based foods that are often lacking in the diets of plant-eating athletes; as a result, supplementation may be warranted to avoid deficiency and consequent declines in performance. As discussed earlier, protein, zinc, iron, calcium, vitamin D, and vitamin B12 are among these nutrients (see table 4.14).

Additional supplements of potential merit for the vegetarian athlete include beta-alanine and creatine monohydrate. Studies have shown the plasma concentration of creatine to be lower among vegetarian athletes (Lukaszuk et al., 2005); supplementation with oral creatine monohydrate provides a boost to muscle stores and consequent abilities to resynthesize ATP energy needed to propel performance, especially that of explosive nature. Similarly, muscle carnosine levels have been shown to be 2+ times greater in meat eaters as compared to vegetarians, making supplementation with beta-alanine, a key limiting factor in the storage of carnosine, of potential benefit to the vegetarian athlete. Athletes with higher levels of muscle carnosine have an enhanced ability to buffer hydrogen ions that can trigger a state of acidosis and consequent muscle fatigue during intense training and competition (Harris et al., 2012).

TABLE 4.14 Supplement Options for Vegetarian Athletes

Supplement	How it may help	Dose recommended
Beta-alanine	Provides a boost to muscle carnosine levels, which helps reduce muscle fatigue associated with acidosis	3.2-6.4 g/day for 12-weeks
Calcium	Supports bone health	1,000-1,500 mg/day
Creatine monohydrate	Promotes the resynthesis of ATP energy for use during explosive periods of activity, helping enhance speed and overall strength gains	5 g/day or utilize a loading phase consuming 0.3 g/kg for 3-5 days following a maintenance dose of 3-5 g/day
Iron	Increases oxygen delivery to muscles; increases ATP energy production	20-30 mg/day (Higher doses may be warranted for deficiency.)
Protein powder Soy (vegan) Whey Casein Egg	Promotes nitrogen balance, supports maintenance and growth of muscle, and aids recovery	Up to 25 g per serving to help an athlete achieve daily goal of 0.5-0.8 g/lb (0.5-0.8 g/0.45 kg) body weight
Vitamin B12	Enhances energy and endurance	25-100 mcg/day
Vitamin D	Supports bone health	600-800 IU/day (Higher levels may be warranted for deficiency.)
Zinc	Enhances recovery; improves immune function	25-30 mg/day

Before using any dietary supplements, however, athletes who have concerns regarding nutritional status and supplemental ingredients of potential benefit to health and performance are encouraged to consult with a doctor as well as a registered dietitian, preferably one who is a board-certified specialist in sport dietetics.

Athletes Competing in Heat or Cold

Most athletes, whether in training or competition, have been forced to perform in either hot and humid or cold conditions. American football players typically begin training camps and two-a-day practices during some of the hottest and most humid times of the year. Many athletes can lose over a gallon (3.8 L) of fluid during one practice. Besides the obvious impact on sweat rates, fluid, and electrolyte losses, the heat can produce other physiological effects that influence performance. The 1996 decision to hold the Olympic Games in Atlanta created a lot of interest in the impact of heat and humidity on performance. Many scientific experts believed it would be impossible for some athletes to reach performance norms under those conditions. Cold temperatures, however, do not affect performance unless combined with wind chills or rain, which could result in hypothermia. Scientists have determined that for the endurance athlete, a temperature of 10°C-12°C (50°F-54°F) is optimal. Less scientific data is available for strength and power sports, but it's reasonable to assume these same optimal temperatures would apply.

Performance Obstacles

Core temperature and fluid balance present the greatest concerns for athletes in the heat. Exertion during training and competition expend energy, which is dissipated in the form of heat. Dissipating heat from the body can take many forms including convection (using a fan to blow heat away from the body), conduction (using cold water towels on the back of the neck or sitting on a cool bench), and evaporation (sweating). Some of these forms of heat dissipation can be limited by equipment or gear worn by athletes (e.g., helmets, shoulder pads, pants). These types of equipment trap heat close to the body. As a result, many athletes rely heavily on sweating for thermoregulation. The loss of fluids results in drops in blood plasma and a subsequent drop in stroke volume, cardiac output, and maximal aerobic capacity. In addition, blood flow to working muscles declines. A secondary concern is that warm environments increase an athlete's reliance on carbohydrates for fuel. Interestingly, while reliance on carbohydrates increases, it has not been shown to affect muscle glycogen levels at the point of fatigue, leaving scientists to conclude that decreased performance is not a result of fuel availability but thermoregulation.

Hot conditions can also affect the brain. Recently, a theory has been developed related to the brain's role as the central governor of the body.

Elevation of core and brain temperature could be responsible for preventing the body from working harder or longer in hot conditions. Other mechanisms could be related to neurotransmitters, such as serotonin, which act on sites in the brain and affect fatigue. Scientists have shown that the administration of buproprion results in enhanced performance in the heat. Buproprion promotes the activity of dopamine, a powerful neurotransmitter, which positively influences motivation and perceptions of fatigue. As a result athletes tend to perform at higher intensities for longer in hot and humid conditions when taking buproprion. However, buproprion does not have beneficial effects in more temperate conditions. More research will further increase scientists' understanding of the brain's role in these conditions.

Nutritional Recommendations

Athletes should focus on fueling strategies to improve thermoregulation and potentially affect mechanisms in the brain related to fatigue. Maintaining fluid balance and plasma volume during exercise are most vital for athletes. This is accomplished through proper fluid and electrolyte intake. American football players restricted in thermoregulation because of the equipment (helmets, shoulder pads, etc.) they wear have been found to lose over 2 L (2 qt) of fluids/hour during practices in hot environments; this is compared to average losses by runners of 1.75 L/hour (1.8 qt/hr) in hot temperatures, 1.6 L/hour (1.7 qt/hr) by basketball players training indoors, and 1.25 L/hour (1.3 qt/hr) by soccer players (Godek, Bartolozzi, and Godek, 2005). When fluids are consumed, not 100% of intake is absorbed; therefore, it is recommended that athletes consume roughly 125% of losses. Both carbohydrates and electrolytes affect the absorption of fluid. Both assist in optimal absorption, and both can be obtained from food sources or from the beverage itself.

Losses of electrolytes, specifically sodium, are highly variable and can range between 200-1,700 mg/L of sweat lost. This is typically greater than the amount commonly found in sport drinks. In addition, athletes prone to muscle cramps typically lose 2 times (or more) the amount of sodium as athletes less prone to cramping. Other electrolytes lost in sweat include potassium, calcium, and magnesium; the amounts of these nutrients lost in sweat are significantly less than those of sodium and chloride. Unless a dietary deficiency exists as a result of a poor diet, added supplementation of these electrolytes does not appear to be beneficial. While electrolytes are important, athletes should guard against overconsuming sodium in one dose. High intakes of electrolytes should be accompanied by large intakes of fluid. An intake of 500-700 mg of sodium/L (500-700 mg of sodium/1.1 qt) of fluid consumed is advised by the American College of Sports Medicine, much higher than that found in sport drinks. Athletes should guard against consuming small volumes of fluid containing large amounts of sodium or exceeding the amount of sodium per liter recommended by the ACSM as this can have a negative effect on restoring fluid balance.

Athletes should consider the following guidelines for fueling before, during, and after exercise to limit the impact of the heat on fluid balance and thermoregulation.

- Before exercise, consume 16-20 oz (0.47-0.59 L) of fluid in combination with carbohydrates or electrolytes in the form of food or sport drinks 30-45 minutes before exercise.
- During exercise, consume 4-8 oz (0.12-0.24 L) of fluid every 15 minutes of activity. Fluid intake should come from a combination of water and carbohydrate–electrolyte beverages.
- Carbohydrate intake during longer periods of exercise (>1 hour) is needed to optimize performance in the heat. A recommended intake is 22-60 g/hour of activity.
- Additional sodium should be provided for athletes prone to cramping or in extremely hot and humid conditions at a rate of 500-700 mg/L (500-700 mg of sodium/1.1 qt) of fluid consumed, or roughly 500-700 mg/hour of activity. Extreme cases do exist where higher amounts of sodium are recommended.

Supplement Options

In addition to protecting against issues of thermoregulation, certain dietary supplements or nutrition ingredients can affect serotonin and dopamine receptors regulating the brain's involvement in the onset of fatigue especially in hot conditions. Table 4.15 includes a list of potential dietary supplements to consider.

TABLE 4.15 Supplement Options for Athletes Training in the Heat

Supplement	Potential benefit	Recommendations
Fluids	Balances fluids	16-20 oz (0.47-0.59 L) prior to exercise; 16-32 oz (0.47-0.95 L)/hour of training; 20 oz/lb (0.59 L/0.45 kg) lost following exercise
Carbohydrate and electrolyte replacements (gels, fluids)	Prevents central nervous system (CNS) fatigue, fuel depletion; balances fluids	22-45 g carbohydrate/hour; 0.5-1 L (17-34 oz)/hour of activity
Sodium (Na)	Balances fluids	500-700 mg/hour of activity in hot environments
Tyrosine	Prevents central nervous system (CNS) fatigue	75 mg/lb (75 mg/0.45 kg) of body weight 1 hour prior to exercise

Athletes Competing at Altitude

Altitude training was brought to the forefront of sports in 1968 when Mexico City, at an elevation of 2,240 m (7,300 ft) was chosen to host the Olympic Games. Many athletes believed that living and training at altitude was superior to training at sea level, and that altitude training would enhance performance at sea level. Colorado Springs was chosen as the site of the U.S. Olympic Training Center in 1978 because of its high altitude. Since that time, debate has focused on the theory and benefits. Currently, most scientists suggest that living at a higher altitude and training at low altitudes is best for enhancing performance (Millet et al., 2010). Whether living, competing, or training at altitude, special nutritional considerations should be taken to ensure optimal performance. Altitude is typically defined as being at an elevation above 2,600 meters (8,600 feet). Higher elevations reduce the amount of oxygen available in the air and create a state of hypoxia, in which the rate of oxygen supply cannot meet demands of the muscles. This forces the muscles to rely heavily on pathways of anaerobic metabolism such as the creatine-phosphate energy system and anaerobic lactate energy system.

Performance Obstacles

Training at elevation can decrease exercise capacity by 3% for every 300 m (982 ft) above 1,500 m (4,921 ft). Weight loss is common among athletes training at altitude. Appetite is suppressed at altitude, decreasing calorie intake and resulting in weight loss. Athletes training or competing at altitude must ensure optimal calorie intake to maintain performance and prevent losses in lean body mass.

Higher-altitude environments increase the amount of fluids lost through the urine and ventilation. These environments cause the kidneys to increase urine production, which speeds the loss of fluids, and puts athletes at a much higher risk of dehydration. Dehydration can have multiple detrimental effects on the athlete including decreases in physical and cognitive performance and increased risk of injury. As little as 1%-2% losses in body water can equate to 5%-15% drops in performance. A combination of adequate fluid and electrolyte intake will ensure athletes are staying well hydrated.

As the body is forced to rely more heavily on anaerobic metabolism, optimal carbohydrate intake is of even greater importance. Athletes will need to rely heavily on carbohydrate and muscle glycogen stores at altitude and will deplete stores much more quickly during training and competition. Low glycogen stores have been shown to decrease high-intensity work capacity by as much as 33% in strength and power sports (Balsom, 1999). Altitude will also increase the total stress of training or competition since athletes will produce greater amounts of stress hormones and free radicals than normal due to the hypoxic conditions. Training or competing at high altitude can also result in poor sleep and slow recovery. Athletes should put extra thought into training volumes and intensities to account for these changes.

Nutritional Recommendations

Nutritionally, athletes must focus on calorie and carbohydrate intake as well as fluids, electrolytes, and possibly higher intakes of antioxidants such as vitamins E and C. Weight loss is common but can be prevented if calorie needs are met. Calorie recommendations are similar at altitude verses at sea at sea level, and scientists believe reduced appetite and calorie intake are responsible for the weight loss commonly experienced by athletes. Caloric intake should emphasize carbohydrates. Roughly 65% of caloric intake should come from high-carbohydrate foods since athletes will rely heavily on anaerobic pathways of metabolism and use carbohydrates and glycogen stores extensively. Recommendations for carbohydrate intake during exercise at altitude are speculative. It is obvious that needs significantly increase from the recommended 22-45 g of carbohydrates/ hour of activity recommended for athletes at sea level. Remaining on the higher end of these recommendations and consuming slightly more—45-75 g/hour of activity—is advised. Consuming 3-5 L/day (3.2-5.2 qt/day) of fluid is recommended. Keeping fluid volumes high, especially with meals when adequate amounts of electrolytes such as sodium and potassium are provided in foods will assist with absorption. Athletes should also aim to consume an electrolyte beverage when drinking fluids alone without food. No altitude-specific recommendations are available for fluid intake during exercise; general guides for athletes at sea level should be applied.

Adding support by using antioxidant supplements lacks a significant amount of scientific data to make definitive recommendations; however, some evidence exists to suggest benefits from supplementation with antioxidant vitamins and minerals, including vitamin A, vitamin E, vitamin C, selenium, and zinc. Subudhi and colleagues (2006) at the University of Colorado found that supplementation of these vitamins and minerals was capable of improving ventilator threshold at high altitude (4,300 m; 14,107 ft) but was ineffective in altering markers of oxidative stress. Hagobian and colleagues (2006) examined the effects of 10,000 IU beta-carotene, 200 IU vitamin E, 250 mg vitamin C, 50 mcg of selenium, and 15 mg of zinc on markers of inflammation at moderate altitude (4,300 m; 14,107 ft) and found no effects. In contrast, a review of antioxidant needs concluded that providing antioxidants via the diet or supplements does reduce oxidative stress at altitude (Askew, 2002). Current research is inconclusive. It is clear that altitude increases markers of stress, free radical production, and inflammation. Antioxidant vitamins and minerals might assist athletes in combating these increases.

Supplement Options

Table 4.16 provides information about a variety of sports supplements that provide support for these added nutritional needs:

- Increased caloric intake and carbohydrates
- Fluids and electrolytes
- Antioxidants

TABLE 4.16 Options for Athletes Training at Altitude

Supplement	Potential benefit	Recommendations
Calorie replacement shakes and bars	Assists in meeting energy needs and promotes weight gain	Varies depending on diet and calorie needs
Electrolyte drinks	Balances fluids	Varies depending on diet and fluid intake
Electrolytes (sodium, potassium)	Balances fluids	Sodium: 1,000-2,000 mg/day; 500-700 mg/L of sweat lost Potassium: 300-600 mg/day
Vitamin A	Provides antioxidant support	10,000 IU/day
Vitamin C	Provides antioxidant support	250 mg/day
Vitamin E	Provides antioxidant support	200 IU/day
Zinc	Provides antioxidant support	15 mg/day
Selenium	Provides antioxidant support	50 mcg/day

Summary

While general nutritional recommendations can serve as solid framework for a successful sporting season, the power of customized nutrition, including the addition of specific dietary supplements, can be profound and often helps take an athlete to a more competitive level. There are a multitude of conditions, with just a sprinkling explained in this chapter, which may warrant further customization. Athletes with specialized concerns are encouraged to work closely with a registered sport dietitian as well as a doctor in developing both a nutritional and supplementation plan best suited to their needs.

ABOUT THE AUTHORS

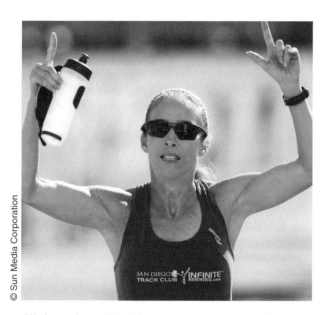

© Sun Media Corporation

Kimberly Mueller, MS, RD, CSSD is a registered dietitian and board-certified specialist in sport dietetics with immense experience working with athletes competing within the endurance and team-sport arena. She grew up competing in club-level soccer before focusing her attention on the sport of running as a Division I collegiate cross-country and track-and-field athlete. She has also earned accolades as an All-American Triathlete, as well as an elite runner chasing after the Olympic trials standard for the marathon. Kim enjoys using her own practical sport experiences and knowledge of nutrition science to help fellow athletes achieve optimal health and peak fitness performance via creation of custom menu plans and personalized nutrition coaching with her company, Fuel Factor (www.Fuel-Factor.com). Kim's passion for customized nutrition also led her to help develop and launch Infinit Nutrition (www.infinitnutrition.com), a company that custom-blends functional ingredients to address the performance and health goals of recreational and professional athletes, including those competing in such prestigious events as Tour de France and Formula 500. She is well known for her nutrition clinics and as a contributor to books such as *The Performance Zone, The Woman Triathlete, Triathlon Revolution, Racing Weight, The New Rules of Marathon, and Half Marathon Nutrition.* As a nutrition coach for Infinite Running (www.infiniterunning.org), Kim helps elite runners develop daily and race-day nutrition strategies that enhance endurance, facilitate optimal recovery, and protect against performance staleness. Kim lives in San Diego, where she is actively involved with several athletic groups, including the San Diego Track Club and Triathlon Club of San Diego. In 2013, she began a new journey as mom to her beautiful baby girl, Kaia Lyn.

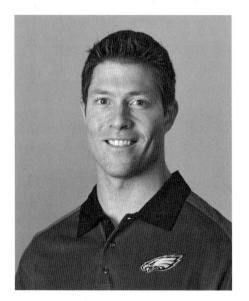

Josh Hingst, MS, RD, CSCS, head strength coach with the Philadelphia Eagles, is a specialist in the fields of nutrition and strength and conditioning, giving him unique expertise in understanding how nutrition and supplementation can complement strength training. He has worked extensively with strength and power athletes in sports such as Olympic weightlifting, powerlifting, bodybuilding, football, basketball, and baseball. His professional licenses and certifications include registered dietitian and certified strength and conditioning specialist.

Prior to his work with the Philadelphia Eagles, Hingst was assistant strength and conditioning coach of the Jacksonville Jaguars. He also spent three years as the director of sport nutrition at the University of Nebraska. In that role he directed programs in body composition analysis, nutrition education, performance fueling strategies, eating disorder prevention and counseling, and sports supplements and hydration. Before joining the Nebraska Cornhuskers, Hingst served as team nutritionist for the Atlanta Falcons during their 2008 season, after spending five years in strength and conditioning and sport nutrition capacities at Florida State. During his time at FSU, Hingst earned his master's degree in clinical nutrition with an emphasis in sport nutrition. He received bachelor's degrees in nutrition sciences and dietetics and exercise science from Nebraska in 2001.